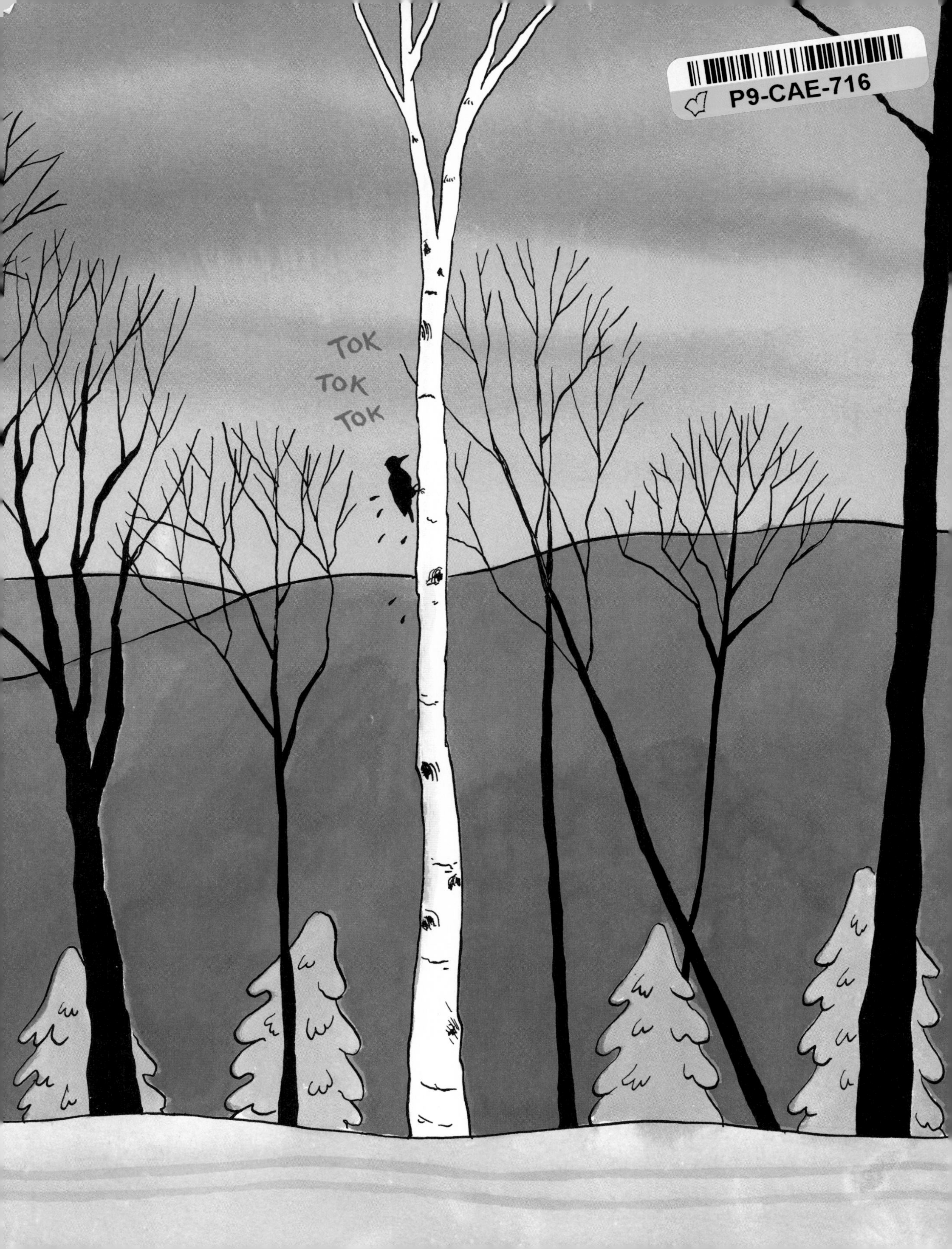
TOK
TOK
TOK

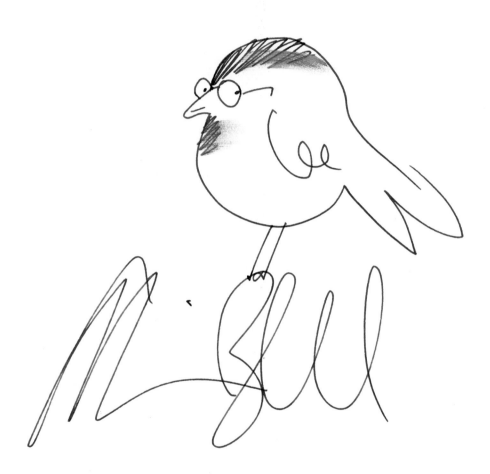

THE
SECRET TO
SUPERHUMAN
STRENGTH

ALSO BY ALISON BECHDEL

FUN HOME: A FAMILY TRAGICOMIC

THE ESSENTIAL DYKES TO WATCH OUT FOR

ARE YOU MY MOTHER?: A COMIC DRAMA

THE SECRET TO SUPERHUMAN STRENGTH

ALISON BECHDEL

WITH THE EXTREMELY EXTENSIVE COLORING COLLABORATION OF
HOLLY RAE TAYLOR

HOUGHTON MIFFLIN HARCOURT
BOSTON | NEW YORK
2021

For Hol

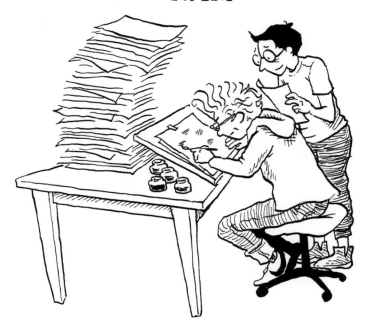

COPYRIGHT © 2021 BY ALISON BECHDEL

ALL RIGHTS RESERVED

FOR INFORMATION ABOUT PERMISSION TO REPRODUCE SELECTIONS FROM THIS BOOK,
WRITE TO TRADE.PERMISSIONS@HMHCO.COM OR TO PERMISSIONS, HOUGHTON MIFFLIN HARCOURT
PUBLISHING COMPANY, 3 PARK AVENUE, 19TH FLOOR, NEW YORK, NEW YORK 10016.

HMHBOOKS.COM

LIBRARY OF CONGRESS CATALOGING-IN-PUBLICATION DATA IS AVAILABLE.
ISBN 978-0-544-38765-2
ISBN 978-0-358-55484-4 (SIGNED EDITION)

LINES FROM "TRANSCENDENTAL ETUDE" BY ADRIENNE RICH FROM *THE DREAM OF A COMMON
LANGUAGE: POEMS 1974–1977.* COPYRIGHT © 1978 BY W. W. NORTON & COMPANY, INC.
USED BY PERMISSION OF W. W. NORTON & COMPANY, INC.

BOOK DESIGN BY ALISON BECHDEL

PRINTED IN CHINA

SCP 10 9 8 7 6 5 4 3 2 1

First there is a mountain, then there is no mountain, then there is.

—Donovan

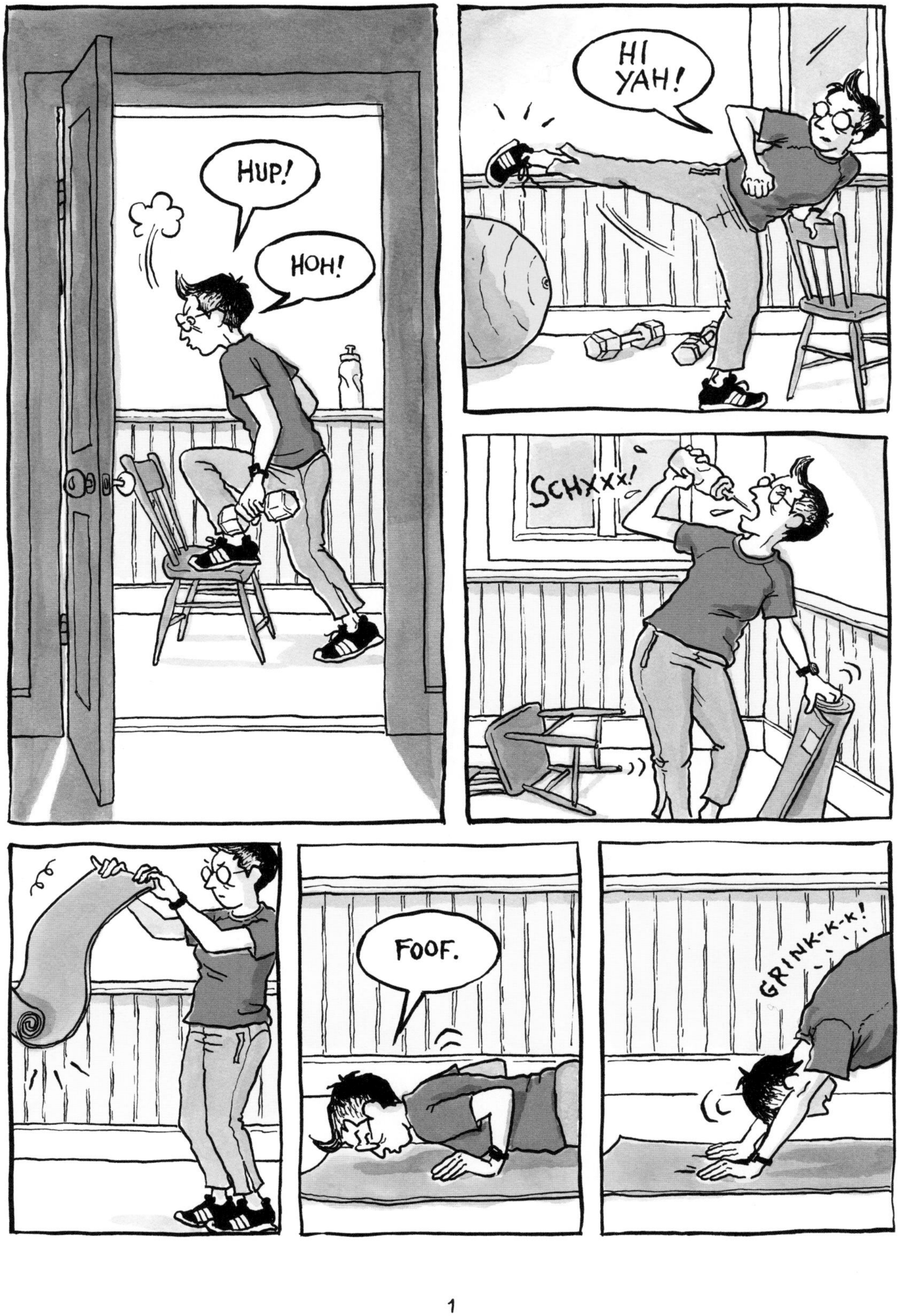
HUP!
HOH!
HI YAH!
SCHXXX!
FOOF.
GRINK-K-K!

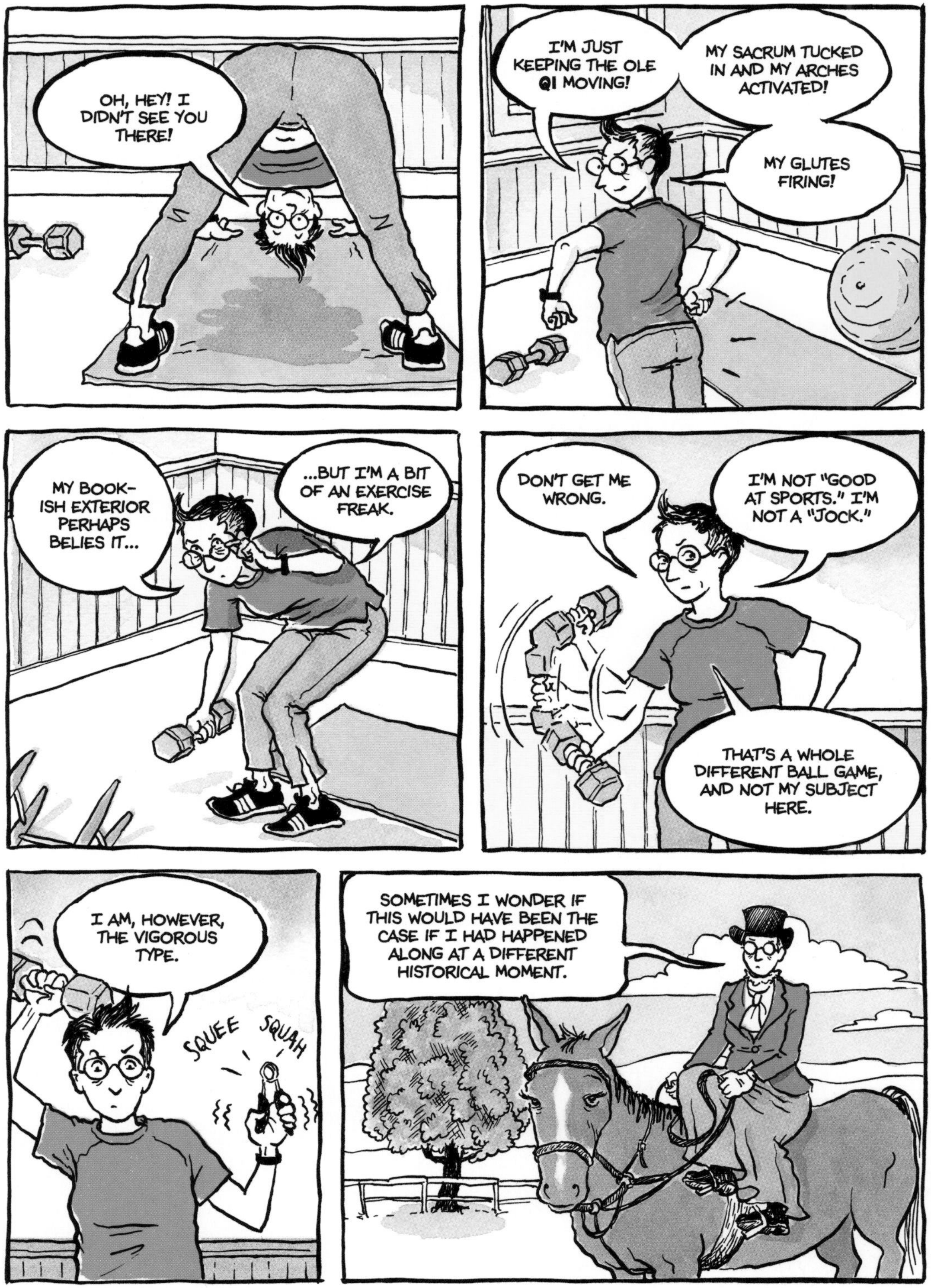
OH, HEY! I DIDN'T SEE YOU THERE!
I'M JUST KEEPING THE OLE QI MOVING!
MY SACRUM TUCKED IN AND MY ARCHES ACTIVATED!
MY GLUTES FIRING!
MY BOOK-ISH EXTERIOR PERHAPS BELIES IT...
...BUT I'M A BIT OF AN EXERCISE FREAK.
DON'T GET ME WRONG.
I'M NOT "GOOD AT SPORTS." I'M NOT A "JOCK."
THAT'S A WHOLE DIFFERENT BALL GAME, AND NOT MY SUBJECT HERE.
I AM, HOWEVER, THE VIGOROUS TYPE.
SQUEE
SQUAH
SOMETIMES I WONDER IF THIS WOULD HAVE BEEN THE CASE IF I HAD HAPPENED ALONG AT A DIFFERENT HISTORICAL MOMENT.

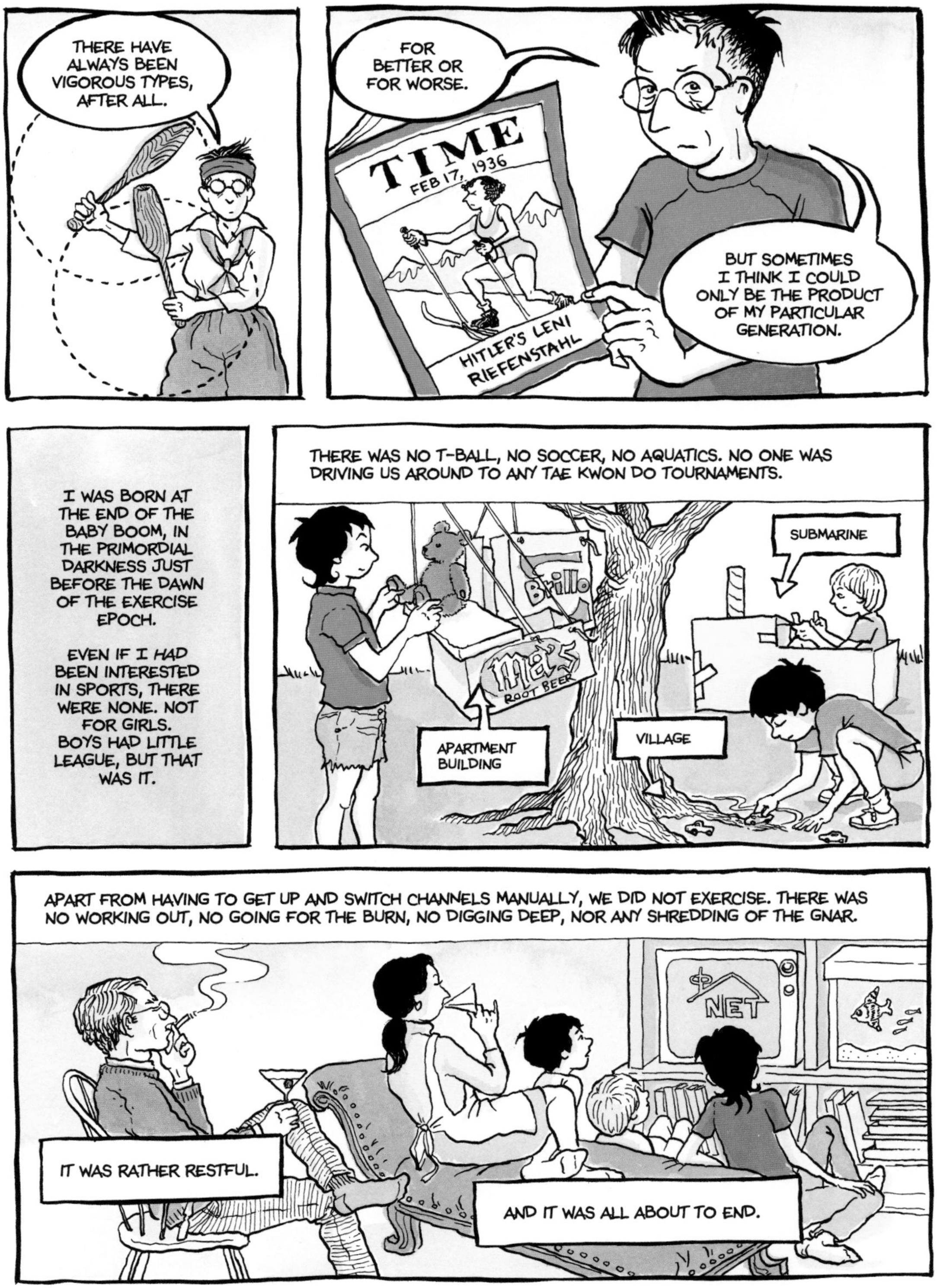
THERE HAVE ALWAYS BEEN VIGOROUS TYPES, AFTER ALL.
FOR BETTER OR FOR WORSE.
TIME
FEB 17, 1936
HITLER'S LENI RIEFENSTAHL
BUT SOMETIMES I THINK I COULD ONLY BE THE PRODUCT OF MY PARTICULAR GENERATION.
I WAS BORN AT THE END OF THE BABY BOOM, IN THE PRIMORDIAL DARKNESS JUST BEFORE THE DAWN OF THE EXERCISE EPOCH.
EVEN IF I *HAD* BEEN INTERESTED IN SPORTS, THERE WERE NONE. NOT FOR GIRLS. BOYS HAD LITTLE LEAGUE, BUT THAT WAS IT.
THERE WAS NO T-BALL, NO SOCCER, NO AQUATICS. NO ONE WAS DRIVING US AROUND TO ANY TAE KWON DO TOURNAMENTS.
Brillo
ma's
ROOT BEER
SUBMARINE
APARTMENT BUILDING
VILLAGE
APART FROM HAVING TO GET UP AND SWITCH CHANNELS MANUALLY, WE DID NOT EXERCISE. THERE WAS NO WORKING OUT, NO GOING FOR THE BURN, NO DIGGING DEEP, NOR ANY SHREDDING OF THE GNAR.
NET
IT WAS RATHER RESTFUL.
AND IT WAS ALL ABOUT TO END.

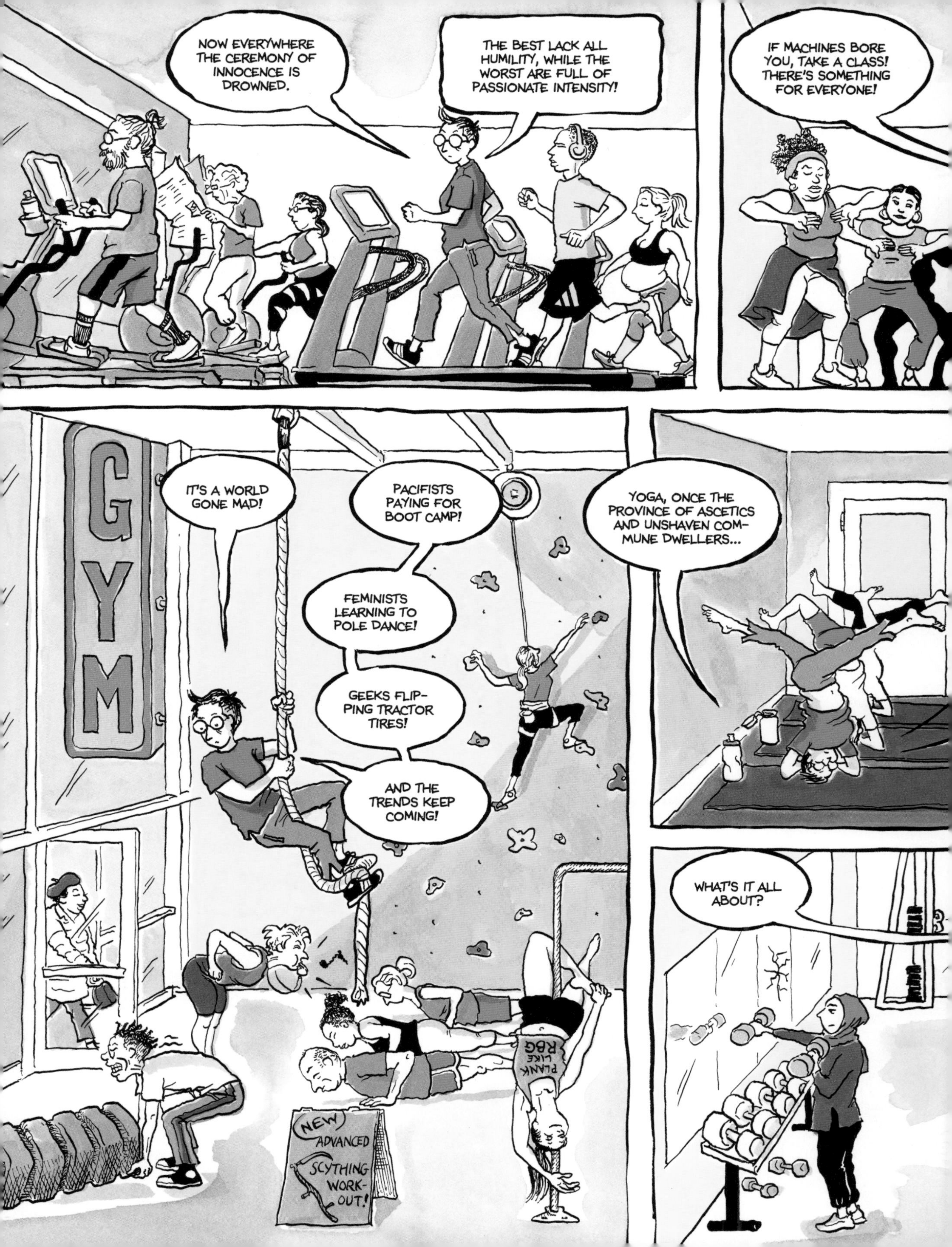
NOW EVERYWHERE THE CEREMONY OF INNOCENCE IS DROWNED.
THE BEST LACK ALL HUMILITY, WHILE THE WORST ARE FULL OF PASSIONATE INTENSITY!
IF MACHINES BORE YOU, TAKE A CLASS! THERE'S SOMETHING FOR EVERYONE!
GYM
IT'S A WORLD GONE MAD!
PACIFISTS PAYING FOR BOOT CAMP!
FEMINISTS LEARNING TO POLE DANCE!
GEEKS FLIP-PING TRACTOR TIRES!
AND THE TRENDS KEEP COMING!
PLANK LIKE RBG
NEW ADVANCED SCYTHING WORK-OUT!
YOGA, ONCE THE PROVINCE OF ASCETICS AND UNSHAVEN COM-MUNE DWELLERS...
WHAT'S IT ALL ABOUT?

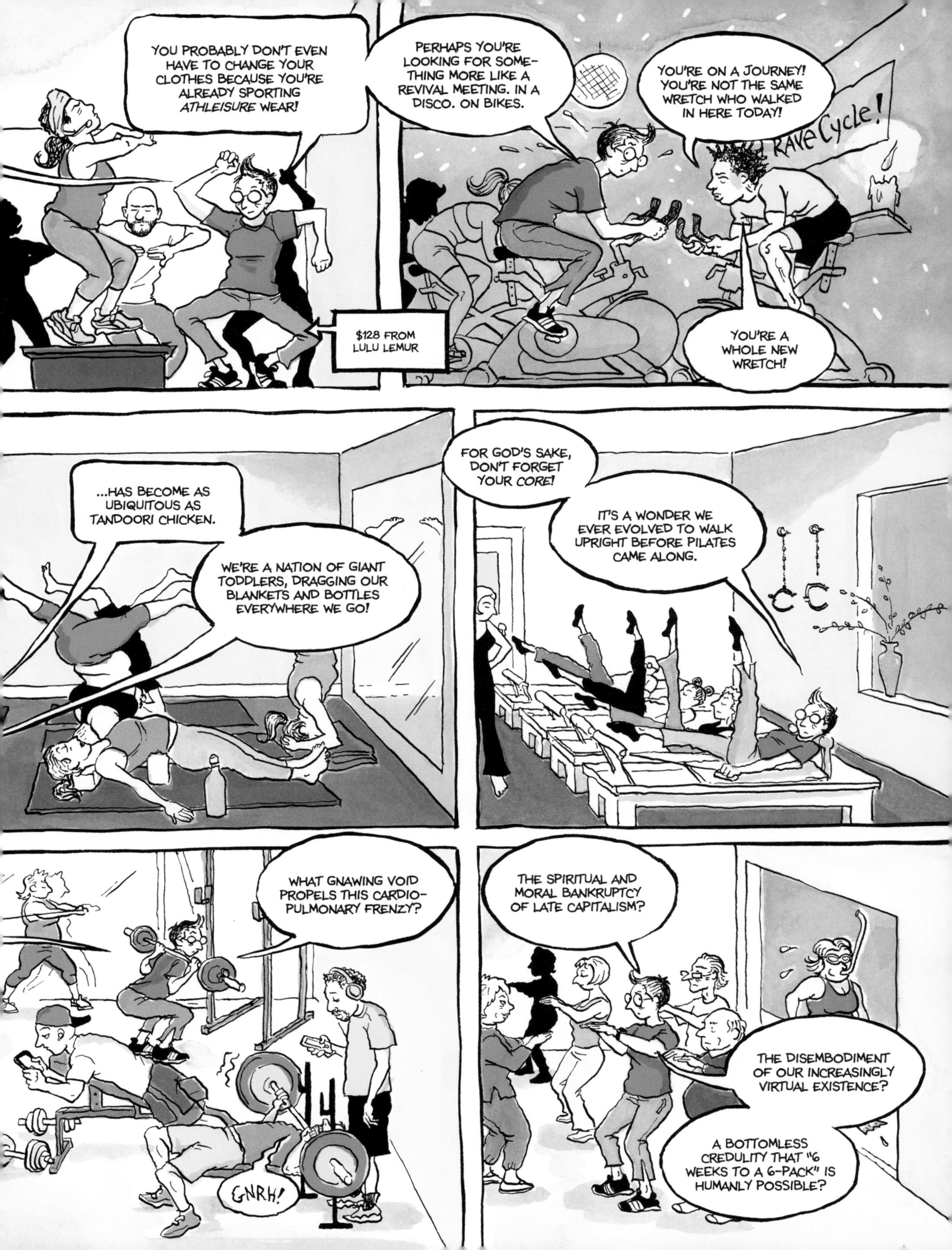

YOU PROBABLY DON'T EVEN HAVE TO CHANGE YOUR CLOTHES BECAUSE YOU'RE ALREADY SPORTING *ATHLEISURE* WEAR!
$128 FROM LULU LEMUR
PERHAPS YOU'RE LOOKING FOR SOME-THING MORE LIKE A REVIVAL MEETING. IN A DISCO. ON BIKES.
YOU'RE ON A JOURNEY! YOU'RE NOT THE SAME WRETCH WHO WALKED IN HERE TODAY!
RaveCycle!
YOU'RE A WHOLE NEW WRETCH!
...HAS BECOME AS UBIQUITOUS AS TANDOORI CHICKEN.
WE'RE A NATION OF GIANT TODDLERS, DRAGGING OUR BLANKETS AND BOTTLES EVERYWHERE WE GO!
FOR GOD'S SAKE, DON'T FORGET YOUR *CORE*!
IT'S A WONDER WE EVER EVOLVED TO WALK UPRIGHT BEFORE PILATES CAME ALONG.
WHAT GNAWING VOID PROPELS THIS CARDIO-PULMONARY FRENZY?
GNRH!
THE SPIRITUAL AND MORAL BANKRUPTCY OF LATE CAPITALISM?
THE DISEMBODIMENT OF OUR INCREASINGLY VIRTUAL EXISTENCE?
A BOTTOMLESS CREDULITY THAT "6 WEEKS TO A 6-PACK" IS HUMANLY POSSIBLE?

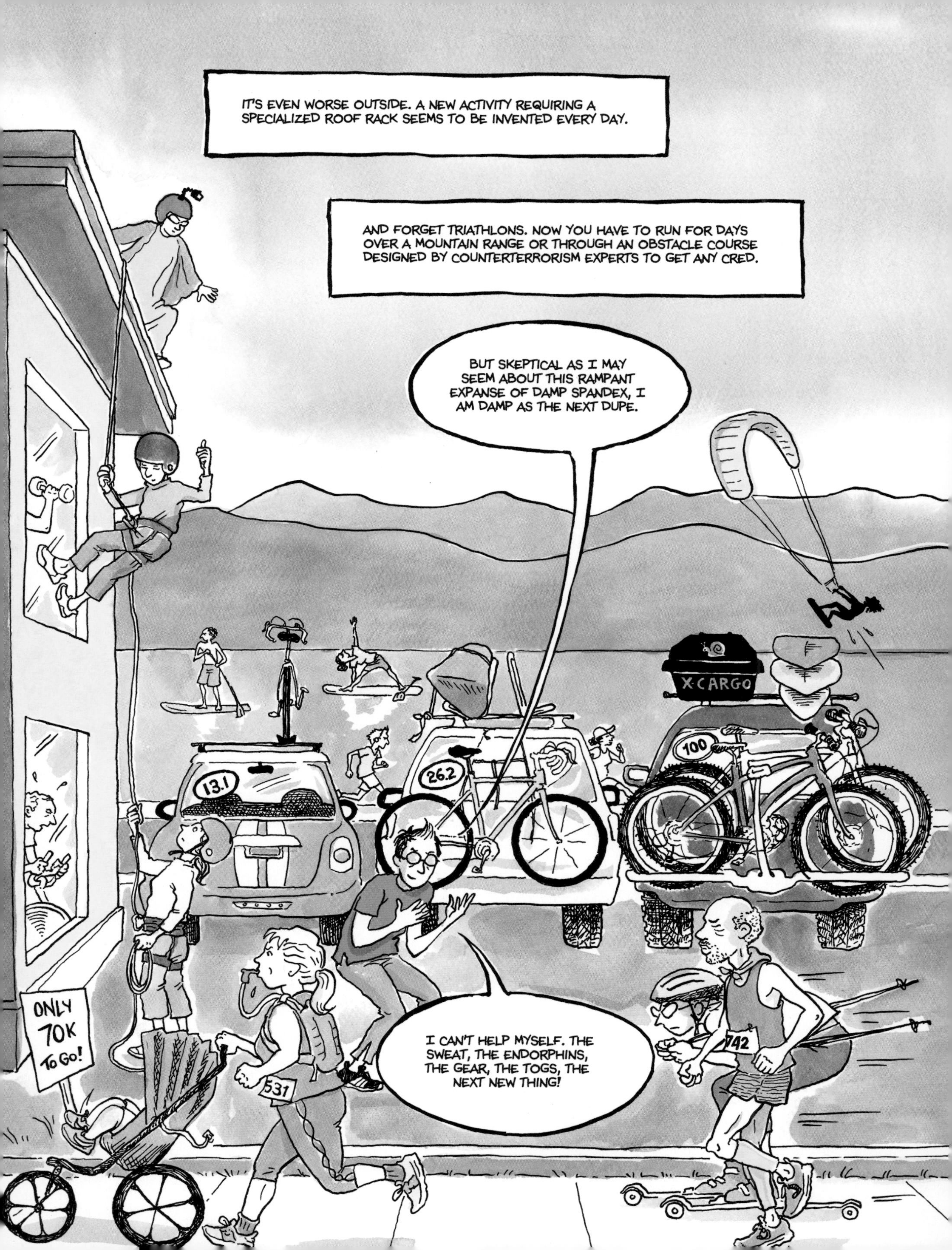
IT'S EVEN WORSE OUTSIDE. A NEW ACTIVITY REQUIRING A SPECIALIZED ROOF RACK SEEMS TO BE INVENTED EVERY DAY.
AND FORGET TRIATHLONS. NOW YOU HAVE TO RUN FOR DAYS OVER A MOUNTAIN RANGE OR THROUGH AN OBSTACLE COURSE DESIGNED BY COUNTERTERRORISM EXPERTS TO GET ANY CRED.
BUT SKEPTICAL AS I MAY SEEM ABOUT THIS RAMPANT EXPANSE OF DAMP SPANDEX, I AM DAMP AS THE NEXT DUPE.
X-CARGO
13.1
26.2
100
ONLY 70K TO GO!
531
742
I CAN'T HELP MYSELF. THE SWEAT, THE ENDORPHINS, THE GEAR, THE TOGS, THE NEXT NEW THING!

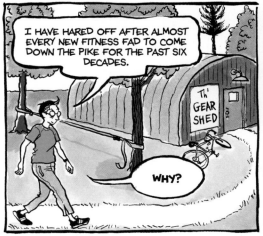

I HAVE HARED OFF AFTER ALMOST EVERY NEW FITNESS FAD TO COME DOWN THE PIKE FOR THE PAST SIX DECADES.

Th' GEAR SHED

WHY?

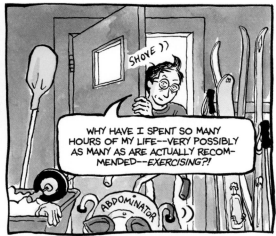

SHOVE))

WHY HAVE I SPENT SO MANY HOURS OF MY LIFE--VERY POSSIBLY AS MANY AS ARE ACTUALLY RECOMMENDED--*EXERCISING?!*

ABDOMINATOR

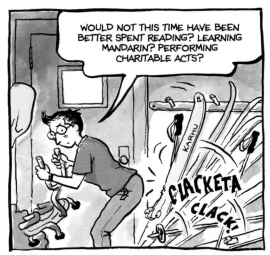

WOULD NOT THIS TIME HAVE BEEN BETTER SPENT READING? LEARNING MANDARIN? PERFORMING CHARITABLE ACTS?

KARHU

CLACKETA CLACK!

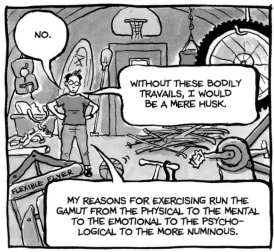

NO.

WITHOUT THESE BODILY TRAVAILS, I WOULD BE A MERE HUSK.

FLEXIBLE FLYER

MY REASONS FOR EXERCISING RUN THE GAMUT FROM THE PHYSICAL TO THE MENTAL TO THE EMOTIONAL TO THE PSYCHOLOGICAL TO THE MORE NUMINOUS.

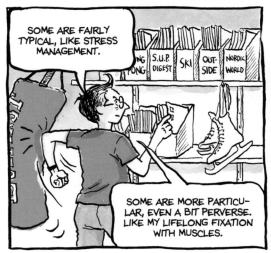

SOME ARE FAIRLY TYPICAL, LIKE STRESS MANAGEMENT.

NG PONG | S.U.P. DIGEST | SKI | OUT-SIDE | NORDIC WORLD

SOME ARE MORE PARTICULAR, EVEN A BIT PERVERSE. LIKE MY LIFELONG FIXATION WITH MUSCLES.

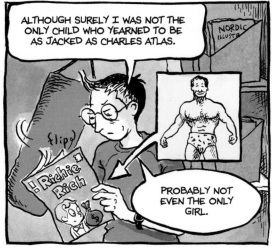

ALTHOUGH SURELY I WAS NOT THE ONLY CHILD WHO YEARNED TO BE AS JACKED AS CHARLES ATLAS.

NORDIC ILLUSTR.

flip

Richie Rich

PROBABLY NOT EVEN THE ONLY GIRL.

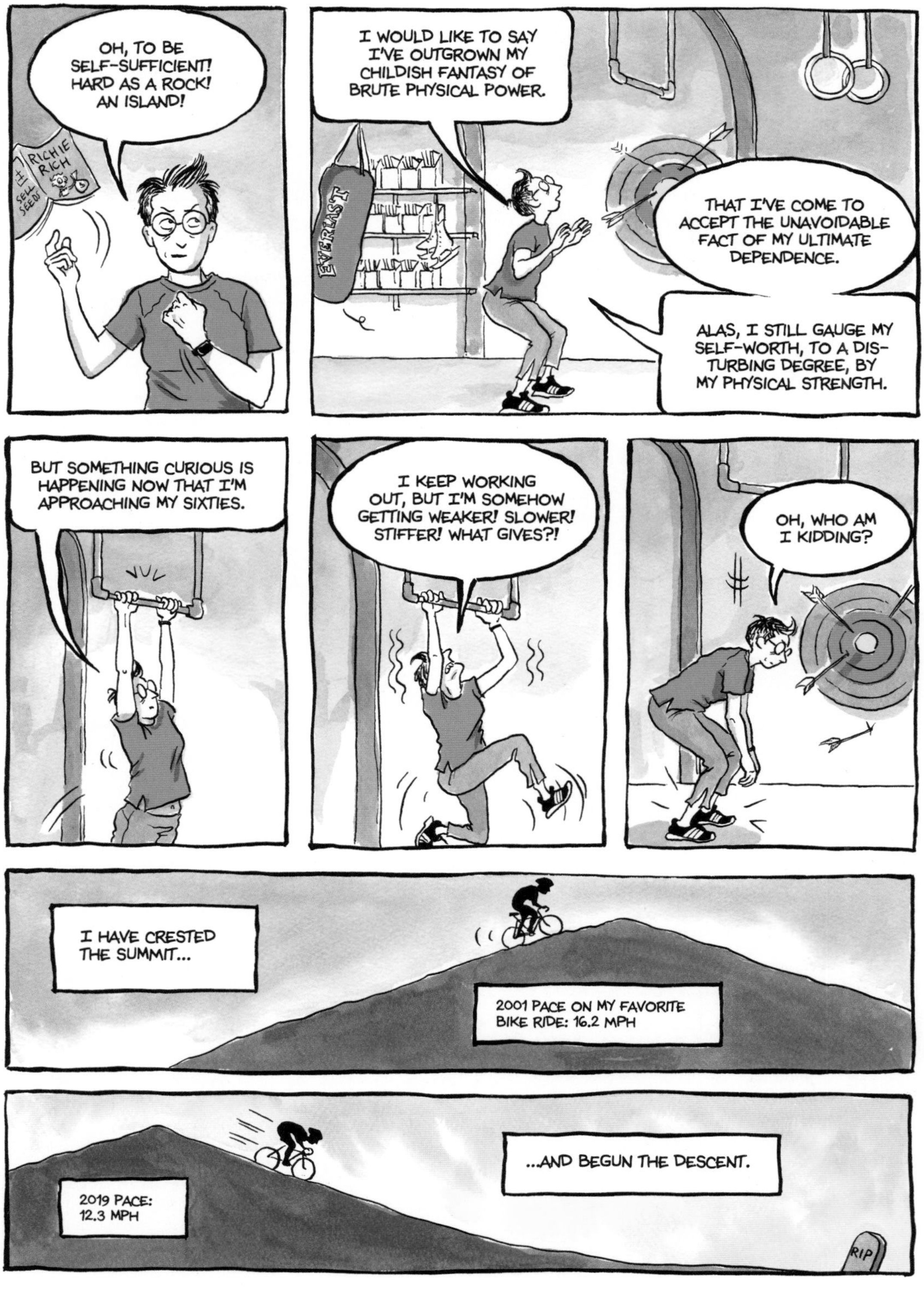
OH, TO BE SELF-SUFFICIENT! HARD AS A ROCK! AN ISLAND!
RICHIE RICH
SELL SEEDS
I WOULD LIKE TO SAY I'VE OUTGROWN MY CHILDISH FANTASY OF BRUTE PHYSICAL POWER.
EVERLAST
THAT I'VE COME TO ACCEPT THE UNAVOIDABLE FACT OF MY ULTIMATE DEPENDENCE.
ALAS, I STILL GAUGE MY SELF-WORTH, TO A DISTURBING DEGREE, BY MY PHYSICAL STRENGTH.
BUT SOMETHING CURIOUS IS HAPPENING NOW THAT I'M APPROACHING MY SIXTIES.
I KEEP WORKING OUT, BUT I'M SOMEHOW GETTING WEAKER! SLOWER! STIFFER! WHAT GIVES?!
OH, WHO AM I KIDDING?
I HAVE CRESTED THE SUMMIT...
2001 PACE ON MY FAVORITE BIKE RIDE: 16.2 MPH
...AND BEGUN THE DESCENT.
2019 PACE: 12.3 MPH
RIP

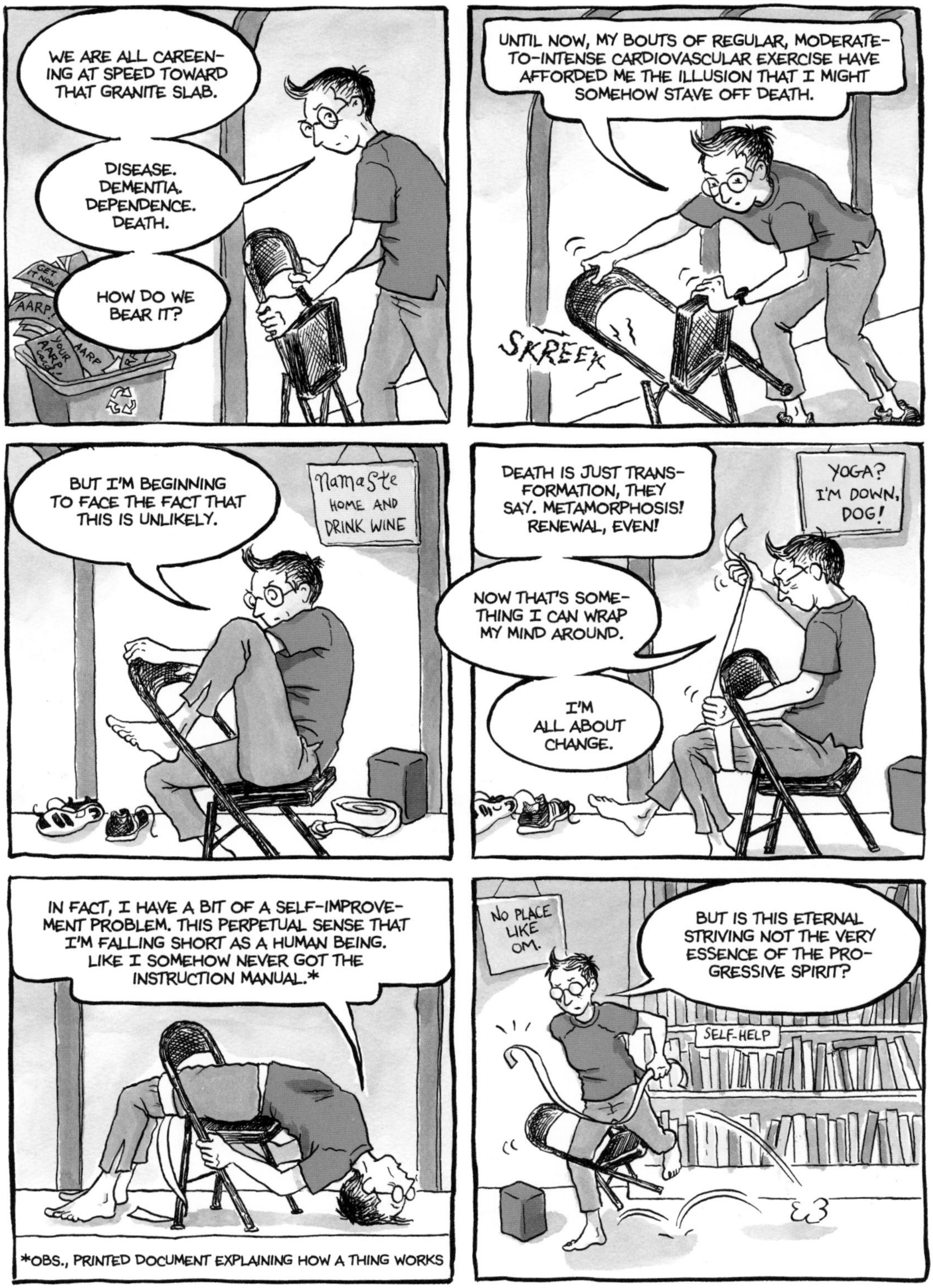
WE ARE ALL CAREENING AT SPEED TOWARD THAT GRANITE SLAB.
DISEASE. DEMENTIA. DEPENDENCE. DEATH.
HOW DO WE BEAR IT?
AARP!
AARP
UNTIL NOW, MY BOUTS OF REGULAR, MODERATE-TO-INTENSE CARDIOVASCULAR EXERCISE HAVE AFFORDED ME THE ILLUSION THAT I MIGHT SOMEHOW STAVE OFF DEATH.
SKREEK
BUT I'M BEGINNING TO FACE THE FACT THAT THIS IS UNLIKELY.
Namaste HOME AND DRINK WINE
DEATH IS JUST TRANSFORMATION, THEY SAY. METAMORPHOSIS! RENEWAL, EVEN!
YOGA? I'M DOWN, DOG!
NOW THAT'S SOMETHING I CAN WRAP MY MIND AROUND.
I'M ALL ABOUT CHANGE.
IN FACT, I HAVE A BIT OF A SELF-IMPROVEMENT PROBLEM. THIS PERPETUAL SENSE THAT I'M FALLING SHORT AS A HUMAN BEING. LIKE I SOMEHOW NEVER GOT THE INSTRUCTION MANUAL.*
*OBS., PRINTED DOCUMENT EXPLAINING HOW A THING WORKS
NO PLACE LIKE OM.
BUT IS THIS ETERNAL STRIVING NOT THE VERY ESSENCE OF THE PROGRESSIVE SPIRIT?
SELF-HELP

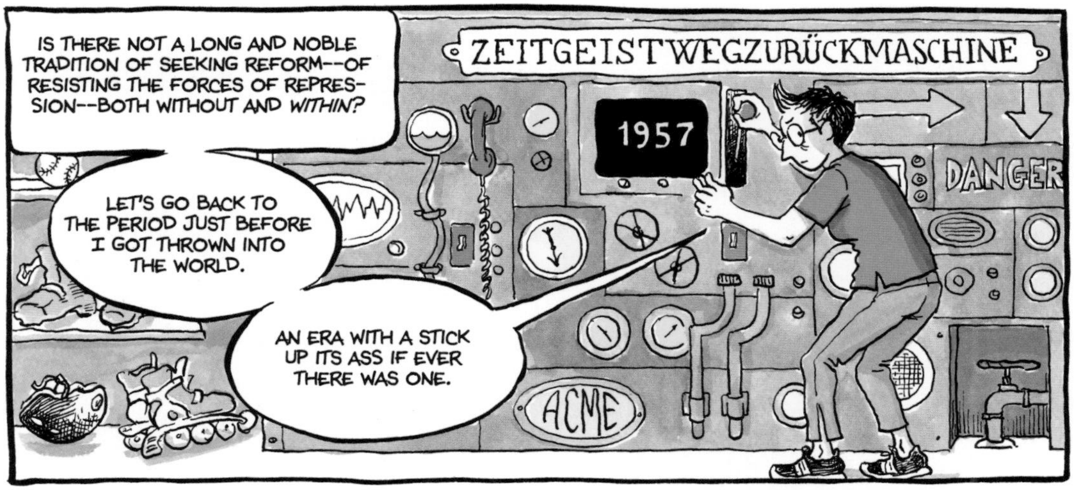
IS THERE NOT A LONG AND NOBLE TRADITION OF SEEKING REFORM--OF RESISTING THE FORCES OF REPRESSION--BOTH WITHOUT AND *WITHIN?*
ZEITGEISTWEGZURÜCKMASCHINE
1957
DANGER
LET'S GO BACK TO THE PERIOD JUST BEFORE I GOT THROWN INTO THE WORLD.
AN ERA WITH A STICK UP ITS ASS IF EVER THERE WAS ONE.
ACME

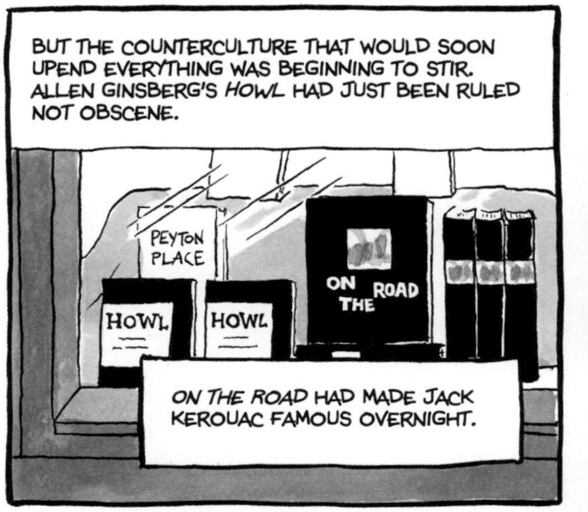
BUT THE COUNTERCULTURE THAT WOULD SOON UPEND EVERYTHING WAS BEGINNING TO STIR. ALLEN GINSBERG'S *HOWL* HAD JUST BEEN RULED NOT OBSCENE.
PEYTON PLACE
HOWL
HOWL
ON THE ROAD
ON THE ROAD HAD MADE JACK KEROUAC FAMOUS OVERNIGHT.

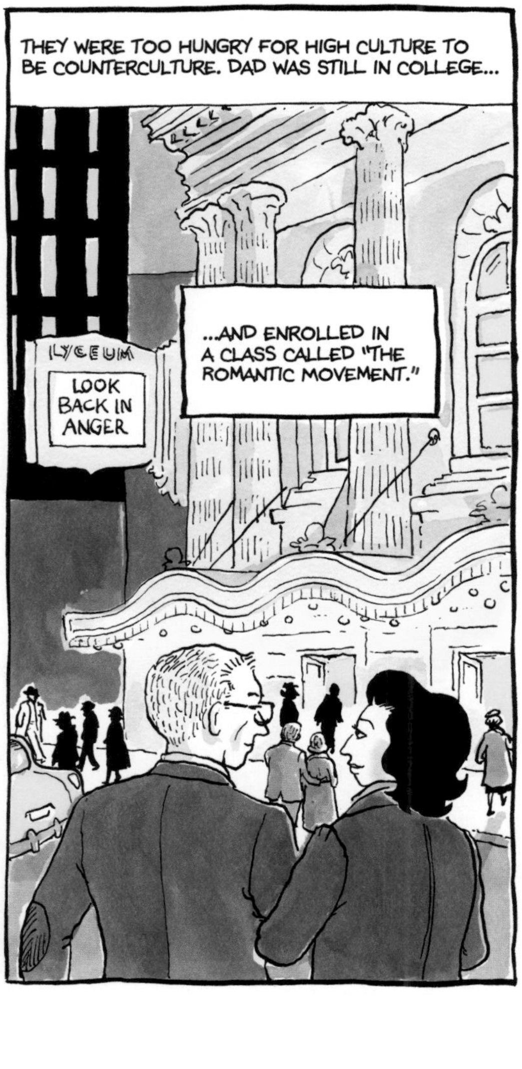
THEY WERE TOO HUNGRY FOR HIGH CULTURE TO BE COUNTERCULTURE. DAD WAS STILL IN COLLEGE...
LYCEUM
LOOK BACK IN ANGER
...AND ENROLLED IN A CLASS CALLED "THE ROMANTIC MOVEMENT."

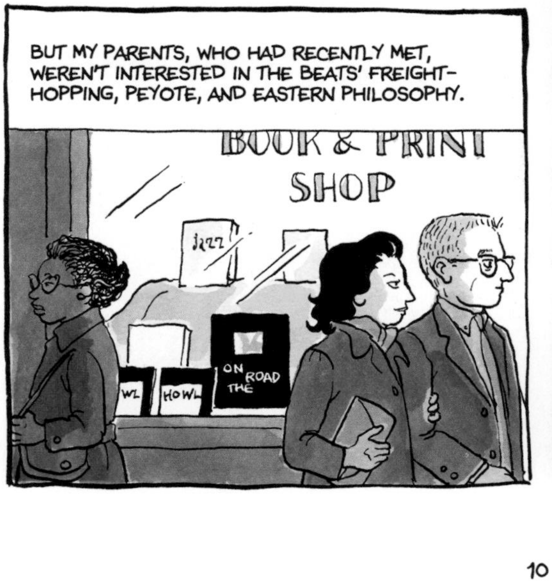
BUT MY PARENTS, WHO HAD RECENTLY MET, WEREN'T INTERESTED IN THE BEATS' FREIGHT-HOPPING, PEYOTE, AND EASTERN PHILOSOPHY.
BOOK & PRINT SHOP
JAZZ
HOWL
ON THE ROAD

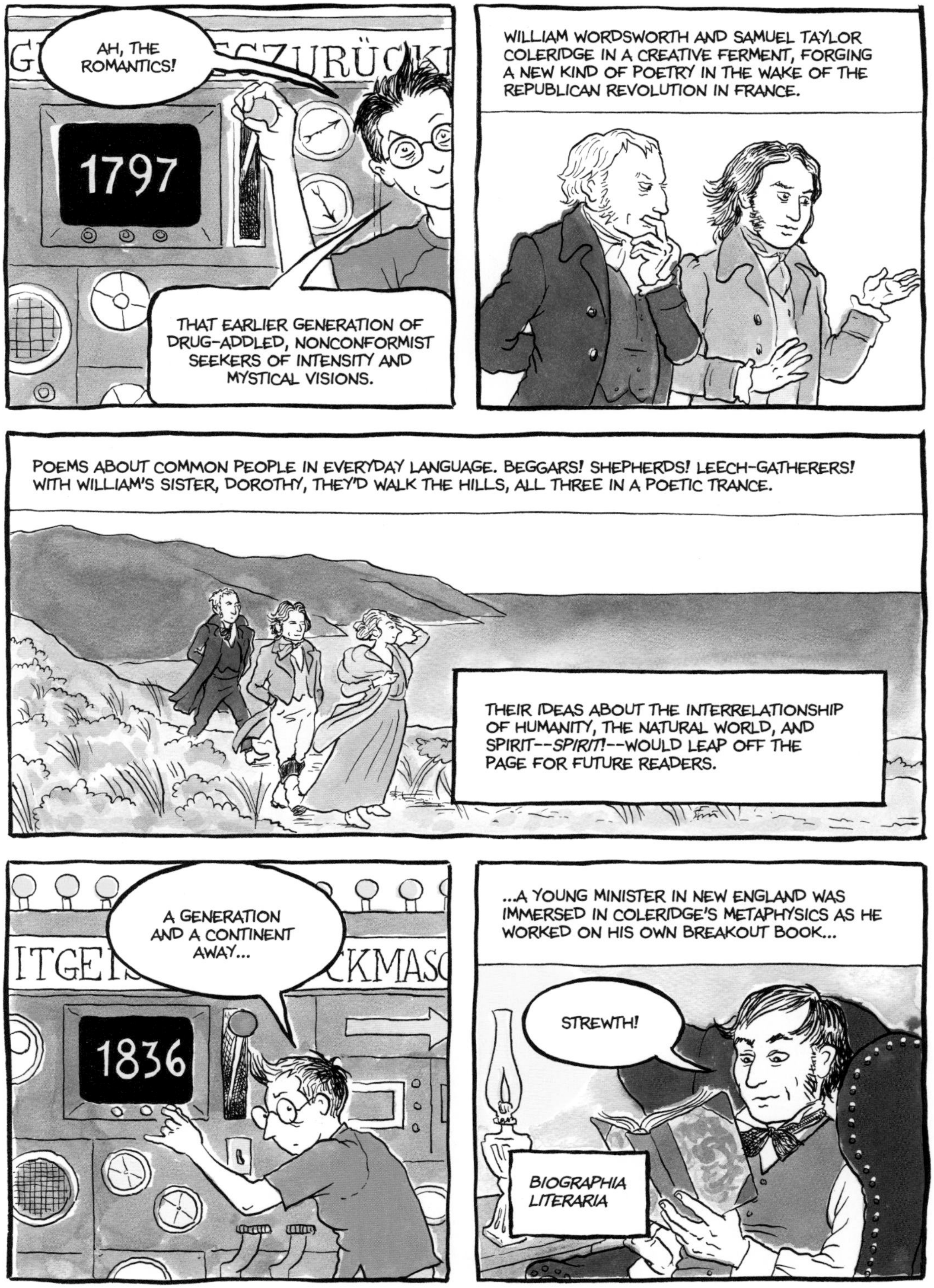

AH, THE ROMANTICS!
1797
THAT EARLIER GENERATION OF DRUG-ADDLED, NONCONFORMIST SEEKERS OF INTENSITY AND MYSTICAL VISIONS.
WILLIAM WORDSWORTH AND SAMUEL TAYLOR COLERIDGE IN A CREATIVE FERMENT, FORGING A NEW KIND OF POETRY IN THE WAKE OF THE REPUBLICAN REVOLUTION IN FRANCE.
POEMS ABOUT COMMON PEOPLE IN EVERYDAY LANGUAGE. BEGGARS! SHEPHERDS! LEECH-GATHERERS! WITH WILLIAM'S SISTER, DOROTHY, THEY'D WALK THE HILLS, ALL THREE IN A POETIC TRANCE.
THEIR IDEAS ABOUT THE INTERRELATIONSHIP OF HUMANITY, THE NATURAL WORLD, AND SPIRIT--*SPIRIT!*--WOULD LEAP OFF THE PAGE FOR FUTURE READERS.
A GENERATION AND A CONTINENT AWAY...
1836
...A YOUNG MINISTER IN NEW ENGLAND WAS IMMERSED IN COLERIDGE'S METAPHYSICS AS HE WORKED ON HIS OWN BREAKOUT BOOK...
STREWTH!
BIOGRAPHIA LITERARIA

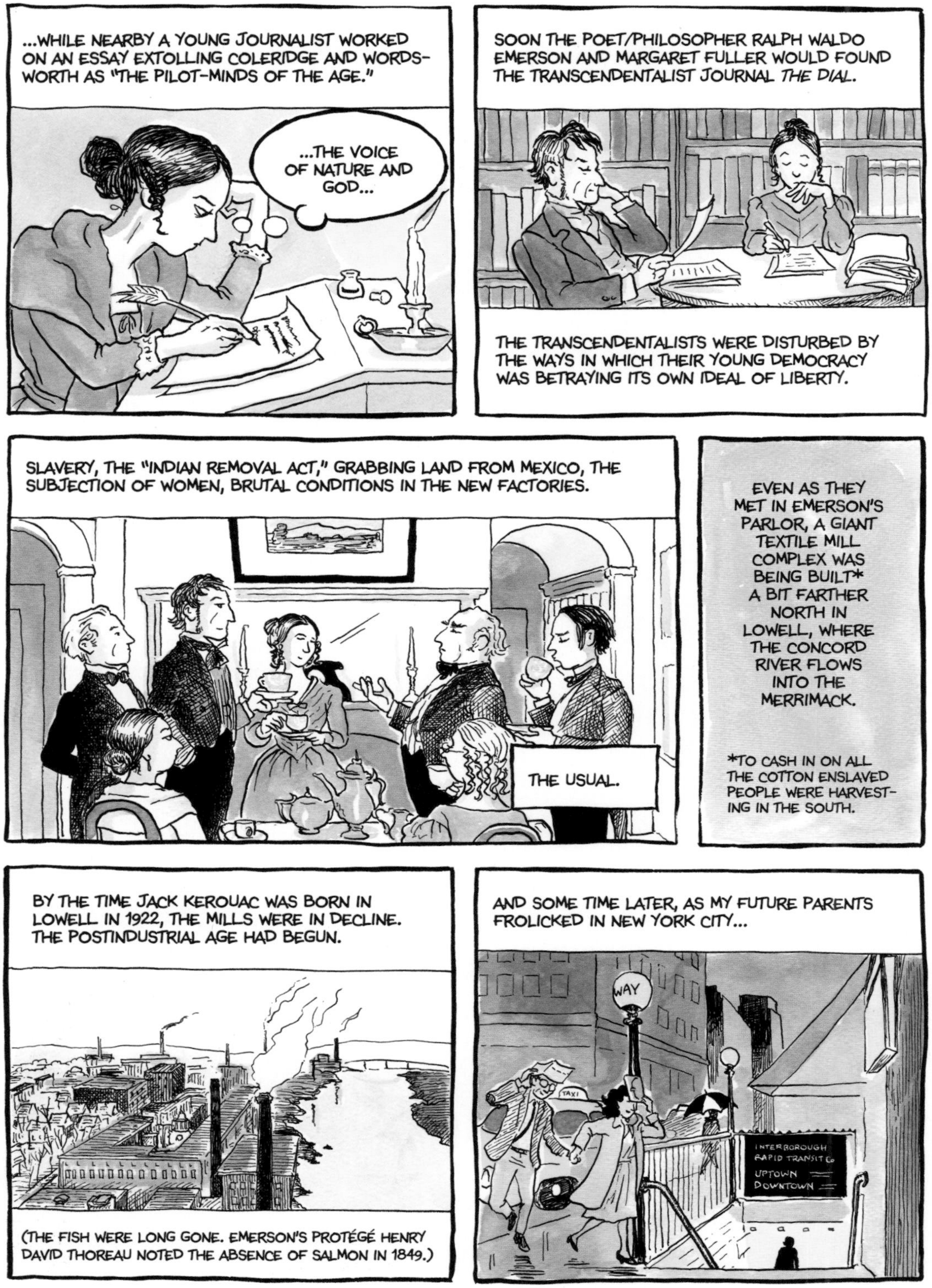
...WHILE NEARBY A YOUNG JOURNALIST WORKED ON AN ESSAY EXTOLLING COLERIDGE AND WORDS-WORTH AS "THE PILOT-MINDS OF THE AGE."
...THE VOICE OF NATURE AND GOD...
SOON THE POET/PHILOSOPHER RALPH WALDO EMERSON AND MARGARET FULLER WOULD FOUND THE TRANSCENDENTALIST JOURNAL *THE DIAL*.
THE TRANSCENDENTALISTS WERE DISTURBED BY THE WAYS IN WHICH THEIR YOUNG DEMOCRACY WAS BETRAYING ITS OWN IDEAL OF LIBERTY.
SLAVERY, THE "INDIAN REMOVAL ACT," GRABBING LAND FROM MEXICO, THE SUBJECTION OF WOMEN, BRUTAL CONDITIONS IN THE NEW FACTORIES.
THE USUAL.
EVEN AS THEY MET IN EMERSON'S PARLOR, A GIANT TEXTILE MILL COMPLEX WAS BEING BUILT* A BIT FARTHER NORTH IN LOWELL, WHERE THE CONCORD RIVER FLOWS INTO THE MERRIMACK.
*TO CASH IN ON ALL THE COTTON ENSLAVED PEOPLE WERE HARVESTING IN THE SOUTH.
BY THE TIME JACK KEROUAC WAS BORN IN LOWELL IN 1922, THE MILLS WERE IN DECLINE. THE POSTINDUSTRIAL AGE HAD BEGUN.
(THE FISH WERE LONG GONE. EMERSON'S PROTÉGÉ HENRY DAVID THOREAU NOTED THE ABSENCE OF SALMON IN 1849.)
AND SOME TIME LATER, AS MY FUTURE PARENTS FROLICKED IN NEW YORK CITY...
WAY
TAXI
INTERBOROUGH RAPID TRANSIT Co
UPTOWN
DOWNTOWN

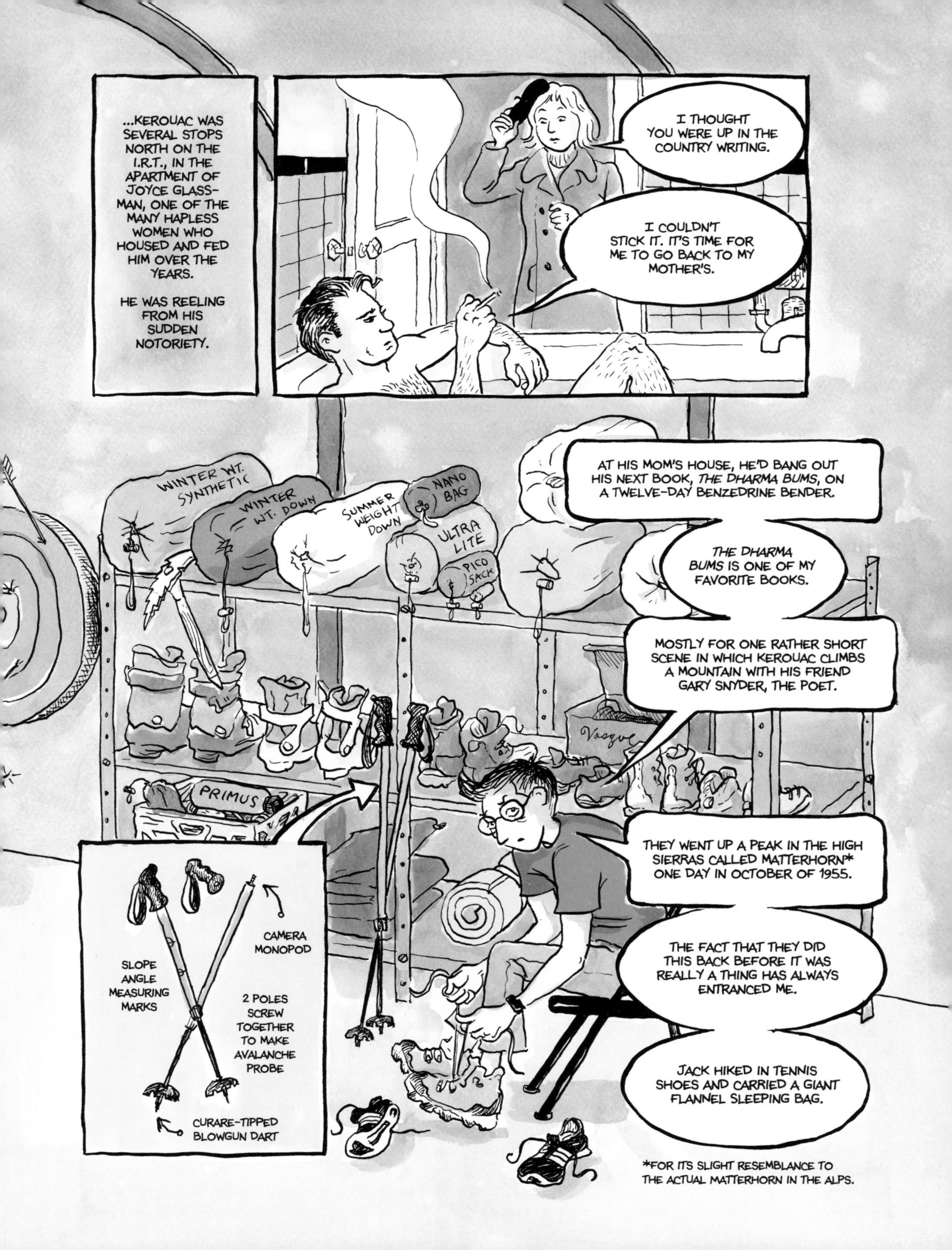

...KEROUAC WAS SEVERAL STOPS NORTH ON THE I.R.T., IN THE APARTMENT OF JOYCE GLASSMAN, ONE OF THE MANY HAPLESS WOMEN WHO HOUSED AND FED HIM OVER THE YEARS.
HE WAS REELING FROM HIS SUDDEN NOTORIETY.
I THOUGHT YOU WERE UP IN THE COUNTRY WRITING.
I COULDN'T STICK IT. IT'S TIME FOR ME TO GO BACK TO MY MOTHER'S.
AT HIS MOM'S HOUSE, HE'D BANG OUT HIS NEXT BOOK, *THE DHARMA BUMS*, ON A TWELVE-DAY BENZEDRINE BENDER.
THE DHARMA BUMS IS ONE OF MY FAVORITE BOOKS.
MOSTLY FOR ONE RATHER SHORT SCENE IN WHICH KEROUAC CLIMBS A MOUNTAIN WITH HIS FRIEND GARY SNYDER, THE POET.
WINTER WT. SYNTHETIC
WINTER WT. DOWN
SUMMER WEIGHT DOWN
NANO BAG
ULTRA LITE
PICO SACK
PRIMUS
Vasque
THEY WENT UP A PEAK IN THE HIGH SIERRAS CALLED MATTERHORN* ONE DAY IN OCTOBER OF 1955.
THE FACT THAT THEY DID THIS BACK BEFORE IT WAS REALLY A THING HAS ALWAYS ENTRANCED ME.
JACK HIKED IN TENNIS SHOES AND CARRIED A GIANT FLANNEL SLEEPING BAG.
CAMERA MONOPOD
SLOPE ANGLE MEASURING MARKS
2 POLES SCREW TOGETHER TO MAKE AVALANCHE PROBE
CURARE-TIPPED BLOWGUN DART
*FOR ITS SLIGHT RESEMBLANCE TO THE ACTUAL MATTERHORN IN THE ALPS.

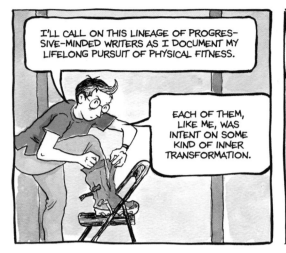

I'LL CALL ON THIS LINEAGE OF PROGRESSIVE-MINDED WRITERS AS I DOCUMENT MY LIFELONG PURSUIT OF PHYSICAL FITNESS.

EACH OF THEM, LIKE ME, WAS INTENT ON SOME KIND OF INNER TRANSFORMATION.

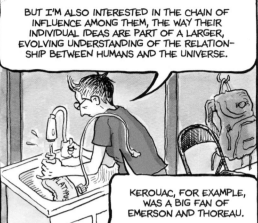

BUT I'M ALSO INTERESTED IN THE CHAIN OF INFLUENCE AMONG THEM, THE WAY THEIR INDIVIDUAL IDEAS ARE PART OF A LARGER, EVOLVING UNDERSTANDING OF THE RELATIONSHIP BETWEEN HUMANS AND THE UNIVERSE.

KEROUAC, FOR EXAMPLE, WAS A BIG FAN OF EMERSON AND THOREAU.

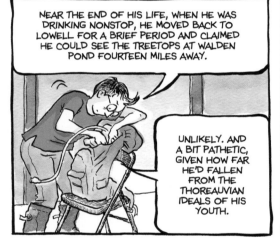

NEAR THE END OF HIS LIFE, WHEN HE WAS DRINKING NONSTOP, HE MOVED BACK TO LOWELL FOR A BRIEF PERIOD AND CLAIMED HE COULD SEE THE TREETOPS AT WALDEN POND FOURTEEN MILES AWAY.

UNLIKELY. AND A BIT PATHETIC, GIVEN HOW FAR HE'D FALLEN FROM THE THOREAUVIAN IDEALS OF HIS YOUTH.

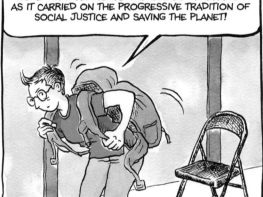

BUT JACK'S TRANSCENDENTALIST-INSPIRED WORK WOULD IN TURN INSPIRE THE SIXTIES GENERATION AS IT CARRIED ON THE PROGRESSIVE TRADITION OF SOCIAL JUSTICE AND SAVING THE PLANET!

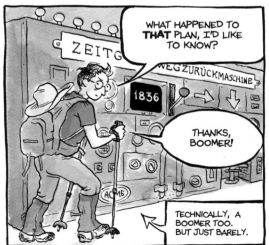

WHAT HAPPENED TO **THAT** PLAN, I'D LIKE TO KNOW?

THANKS, BOOMER!

TECHNICALLY, A BOOMER TOO. BUT JUST BARELY.

ZEITG

WEGZURÜCKMASCHINE

1836

ACME

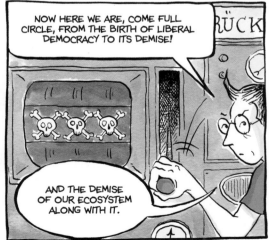

NOW HERE WE ARE, COME FULL CIRCLE, FROM THE BIRTH OF LIBERAL DEMOCRACY TO ITS DEMISE!

AND THE DEMISE OF OUR ECOSYSTEM ALONG WITH IT.

RÜCK

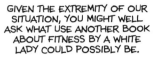

GIVEN THE EXTREMITY OF OUR SITUATION, YOU MIGHT WELL ASK WHAT USE ANOTHER BOOK ABOUT FITNESS BY A WHITE LADY COULD POSSIBLY BE.

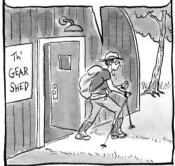

Th' GEAR SHED

...

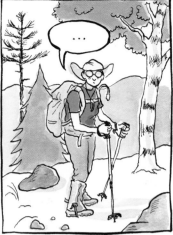

WELL, I'M NOT JUST WRITING ABOUT FITNESS.

I'M WRITING ABOUT HOW THE PURSUIT OF FITNESS HAS BEEN A VEHICLE FOR ME TO SOMETHING ELSE.

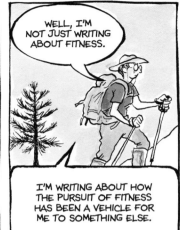

THE FEELING OF MY MIND AND BODY BECOMING ONE.

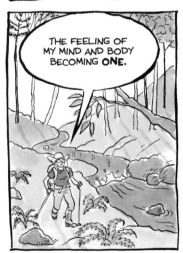

BUT WHAT IS THE MIND?

WHAT IS THE BODY?

WHAT IS THIS SELF THAT THEY SOMEHOW CONSTITUTE?!

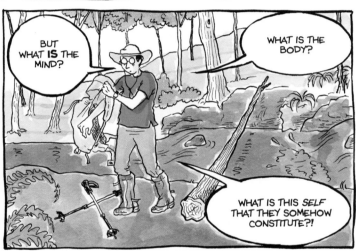

THESE QUESTIONS DEMAND RIGOROUS PHENOMENOLOGICAL, NEUROSCIENTIFIC, AND QUANTUM-MECHANICAL INVESTIGATION.

AND I MAJORED IN ART.

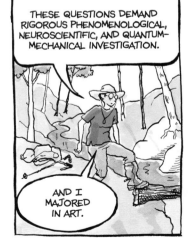

ALL I CAN DO IS OFFER UP MY OWN ANECDOTAL EVIDENCE.

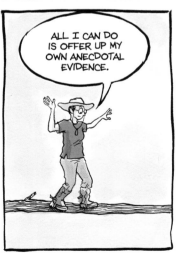

WHEN MY MIND SHUTS UP AND MY BODY TAKES OVER, I'M OUTSIDE THE DUALISTIC FRAMEWORK OF LANGUAGE.

OF SUBJECT AND OBJECT.

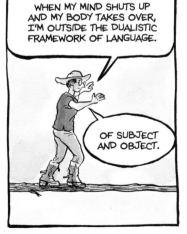

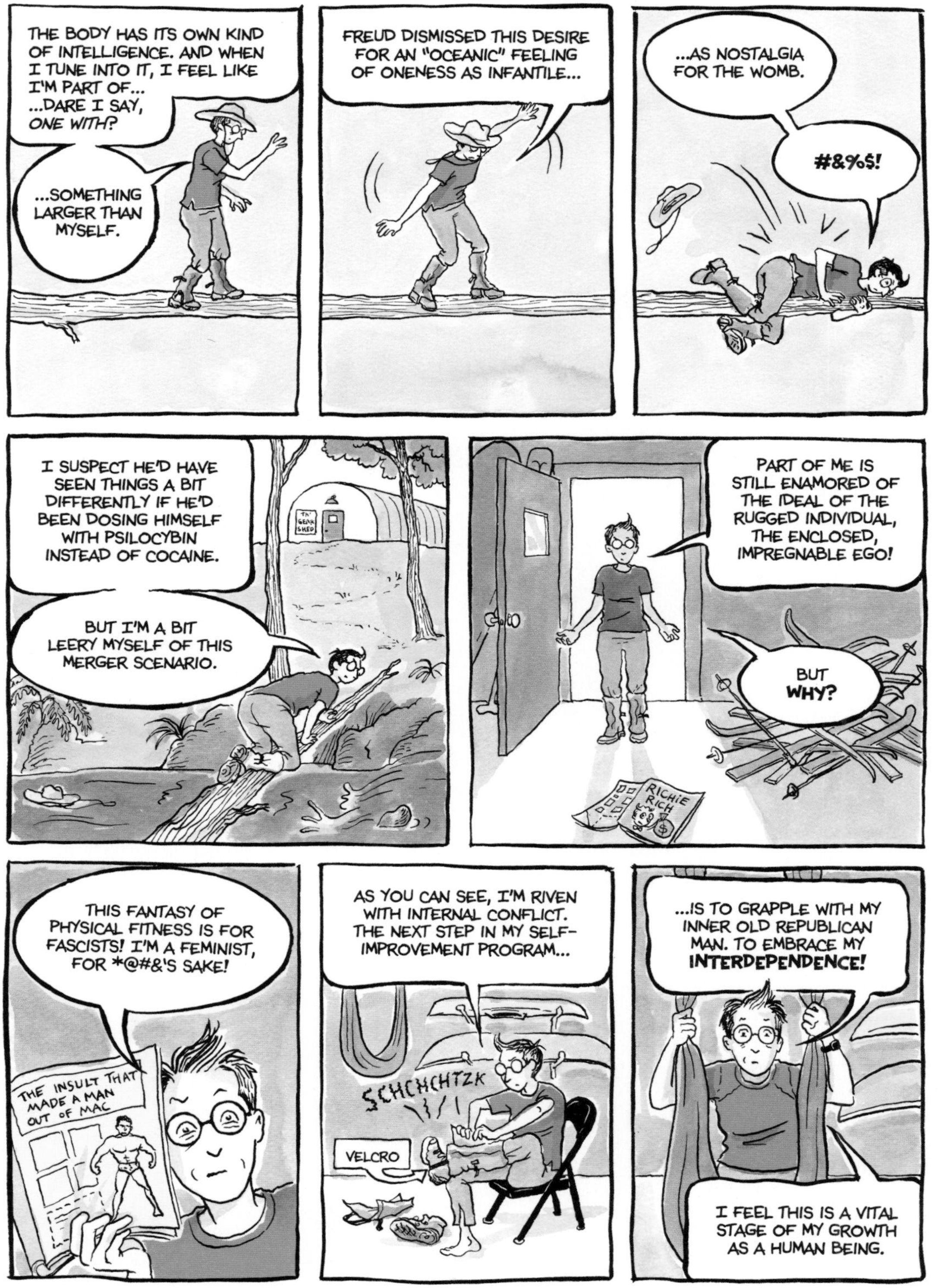
THE BODY HAS ITS OWN KIND OF INTELLIGENCE. AND WHEN I TUNE INTO IT, I FEEL LIKE I'M PART OF... ...DARE I SAY, *ONE WITH?*
...SOMETHING LARGER THAN MYSELF.
FREUD DISMISSED THIS DESIRE FOR AN "OCEANIC" FEELING OF ONENESS AS INFANTILE...
...AS NOSTALGIA FOR THE WOMB.
#&%$!
I SUSPECT HE'D HAVE SEEN THINGS A BIT DIFFERENTLY IF HE'D BEEN DOSING HIMSELF WITH PSILOCYBIN INSTEAD OF COCAINE.
BUT I'M A BIT LEERY MYSELF OF THIS MERGER SCENARIO.
PART OF ME IS STILL ENAMORED OF THE IDEAL OF THE RUGGED INDIVIDUAL, THE ENCLOSED, IMPREGNABLE EGO!
BUT **WHY?**
RICHIE RICH
THIS FANTASY OF PHYSICAL FITNESS IS FOR FASCISTS! I'M A FEMINIST, FOR *@#&'S SAKE!
THE INSULT THAT MADE A MAN OUT OF MAC
AS YOU CAN SEE, I'M RIVEN WITH INTERNAL CONFLICT. THE NEXT STEP IN MY SELF-IMPROVEMENT PROGRAM...
SCHCHCHTZK
VELCRO
...IS TO GRAPPLE WITH MY INNER OLD REPUBLICAN MAN. TO EMBRACE MY **INTERDEPENDENCE!**
I FEEL THIS IS A VITAL STAGE OF MY GROWTH AS A HUMAN BEING.

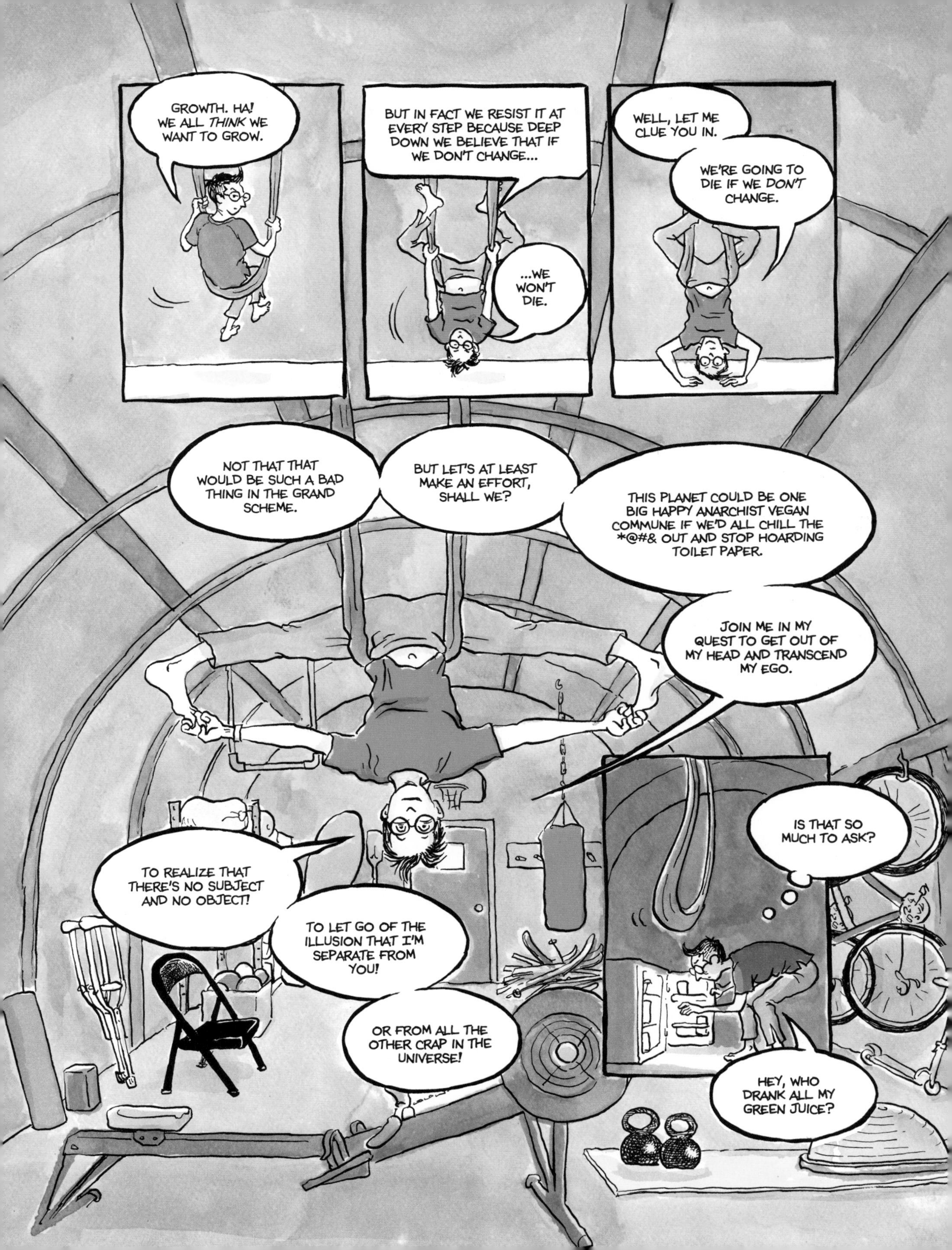
GROWTH. HA! WE ALL *THINK* WE WANT TO GROW.
BUT IN FACT WE RESIST IT AT EVERY STEP BECAUSE DEEP DOWN WE BELIEVE THAT IF WE DON'T CHANGE...
...WE WON'T DIE.
WELL, LET ME CLUE YOU IN.
WE'RE GOING TO DIE IF WE *DON'T* CHANGE.
NOT THAT THAT WOULD BE SUCH A BAD THING IN THE GRAND SCHEME.
BUT LET'S AT LEAST MAKE AN EFFORT, SHALL WE?
THIS PLANET COULD BE ONE BIG HAPPY ANARCHIST VEGAN COMMUNE IF WE'D ALL CHILL THE *@#& OUT AND STOP HOARDING TOILET PAPER.
JOIN ME IN MY QUEST TO GET OUT OF MY HEAD AND TRANSCEND MY EGO.
TO REALIZE THAT THERE'S NO SUBJECT AND NO OBJECT!
TO LET GO OF THE ILLUSION THAT I'M SEPARATE FROM YOU!
OR FROM ALL THE OTHER CRAP IN THE UNIVERSE!
IS THAT SO MUCH TO ASK?
HEY, WHO DRANK ALL MY GREEN JUICE?

1960s

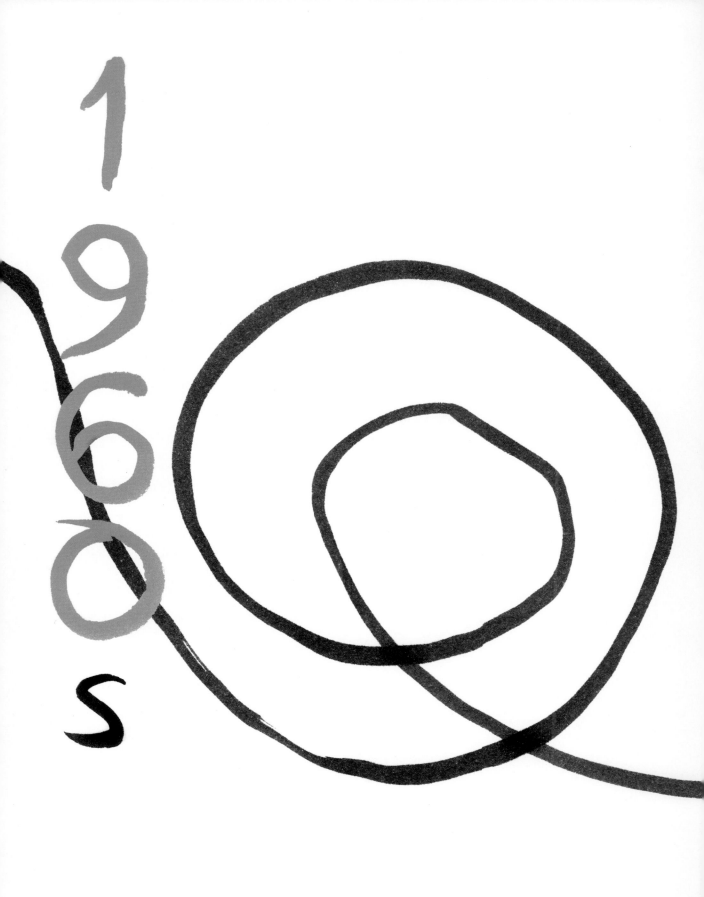

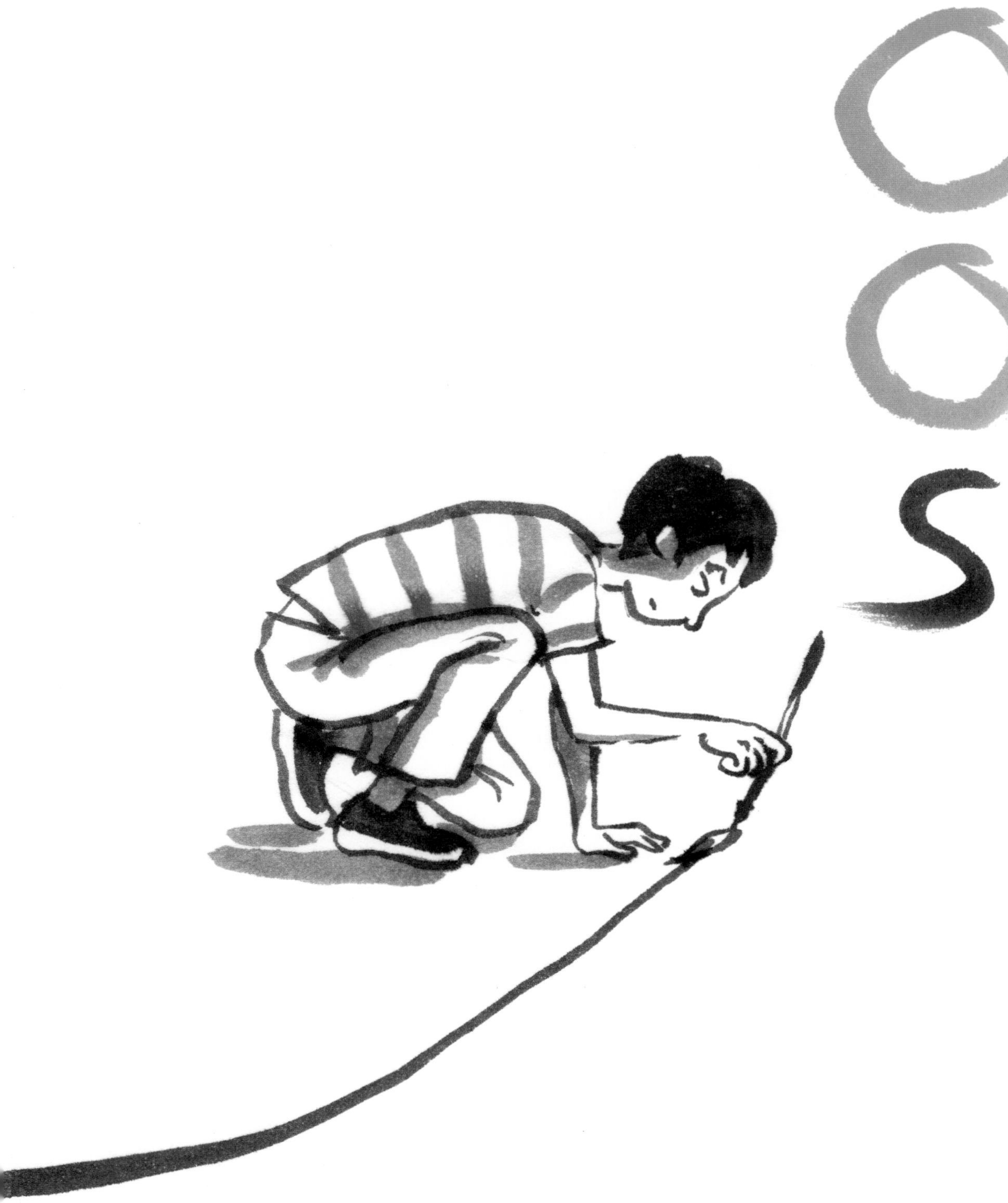

I ENTERED THE WORLD IN THE USUAL MIDCENTURY FASHION. NO RELAXATION TECHNIQUES, NO DIM LIGHTS. NO BIRTHING TUB. NO FAMILY MEMBERS. MY FATHER WASN'T EVEN OUT IN THE WAITING ROOM.

QUIT YELLING! IT'S NOT GONNA DO YOU ANY GOOD.

HE WAS OFF FETCHING A BODY FOR HIS OWN FATHER'S FUNERAL HOME.

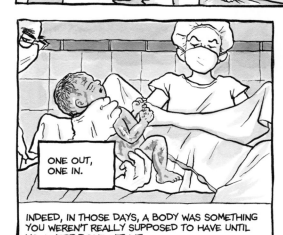

ONE OUT, ONE IN.

INDEED, IN THOSE DAYS, A BODY WAS SOMETHING YOU WEREN'T REALLY SUPPOSED TO HAVE UNTIL YOU WERE DONE WITH IT.

I WAS NOT LAID AGAINST MY MOTHER'S SKIN, BUT TOWELED OFF AND WHISKED AWAY TO THE NURSERY. I PROBABLY SPENT SEVERAL DAYS THERE. MATERNITY STAYS WERE LONGER THEN.

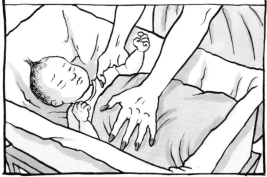

I WOULD BE BROUGHT BACK TO MOM FOR SHORT, RIGIDLY SCHEDULED VISITS.

TIME'S UP.

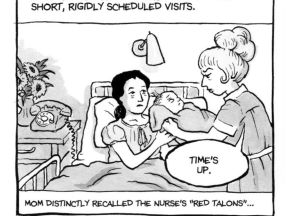

MOM DISTINCTLY RECALLED THE NURSE'S "RED TALONS"...

NO, AT MOST THE BODY WAS A WAY OF TRANS-PORTING YOUR HEAD AROUND. BUT SOON, THIS CARTESIAN STATE OF AFFAIRS WOULD BEGIN TO CHANGE.

TONK!

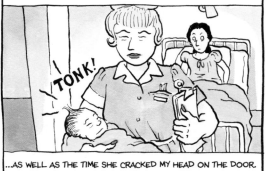

...AS WELL AS THE TIME SHE CRACKED MY HEAD ON THE DOOR.

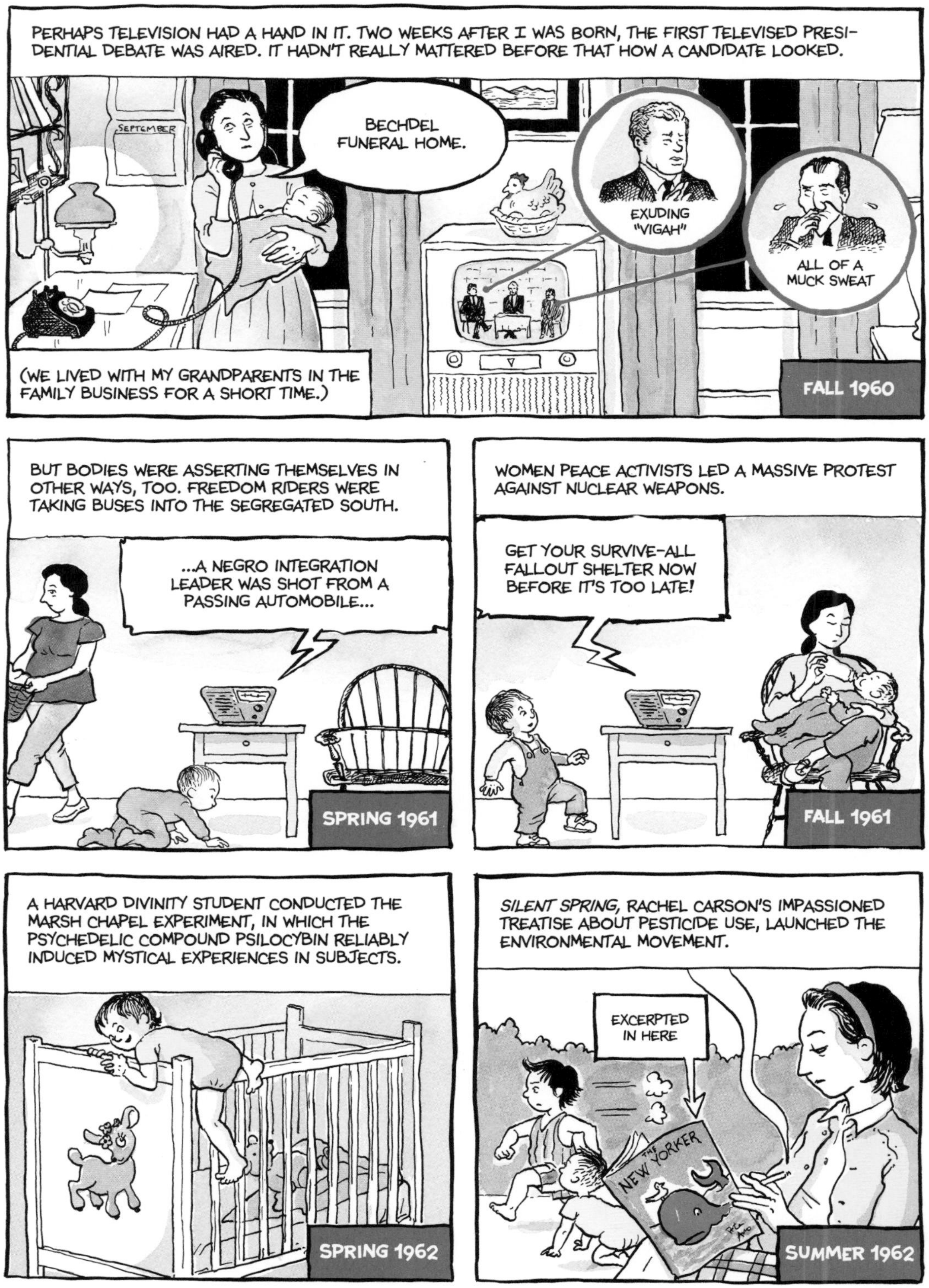
PERHAPS TELEVISION HAD A HAND IN IT. TWO WEEKS AFTER I WAS BORN, THE FIRST TELEVISED PRESIDENTIAL DEBATE WAS AIRED. IT HADN'T REALLY MATTERED BEFORE THAT HOW A CANDIDATE LOOKED.
SEPTEMBER
BECHDEL FUNERAL HOME.
EXUDING "VIGAH"
ALL OF A MUCK SWEAT
(WE LIVED WITH MY GRANDPARENTS IN THE FAMILY BUSINESS FOR A SHORT TIME.)
FALL 1960
BUT BODIES WERE ASSERTING THEMSELVES IN OTHER WAYS, TOO. FREEDOM RIDERS WERE TAKING BUSES INTO THE SEGREGATED SOUTH.
...A NEGRO INTEGRATION LEADER WAS SHOT FROM A PASSING AUTOMOBILE...
SPRING 1961
WOMEN PEACE ACTIVISTS LED A MASSIVE PROTEST AGAINST NUCLEAR WEAPONS.
GET YOUR SURVIVE-ALL FALLOUT SHELTER NOW BEFORE IT'S TOO LATE!
FALL 1961
A HARVARD DIVINITY STUDENT CONDUCTED THE MARSH CHAPEL EXPERIMENT, IN WHICH THE PSYCHEDELIC COMPOUND PSILOCYBIN RELIABLY INDUCED MYSTICAL EXPERIENCES IN SUBJECTS.
SPRING 1962
SILENT SPRING, RACHEL CARSON'S IMPASSIONED TREATISE ABOUT PESTICIDE USE, LAUNCHED THE ENVIRONMENTAL MOVEMENT.
EXCERPTED IN HERE
THE NEW YORKER
SUMMER 1962

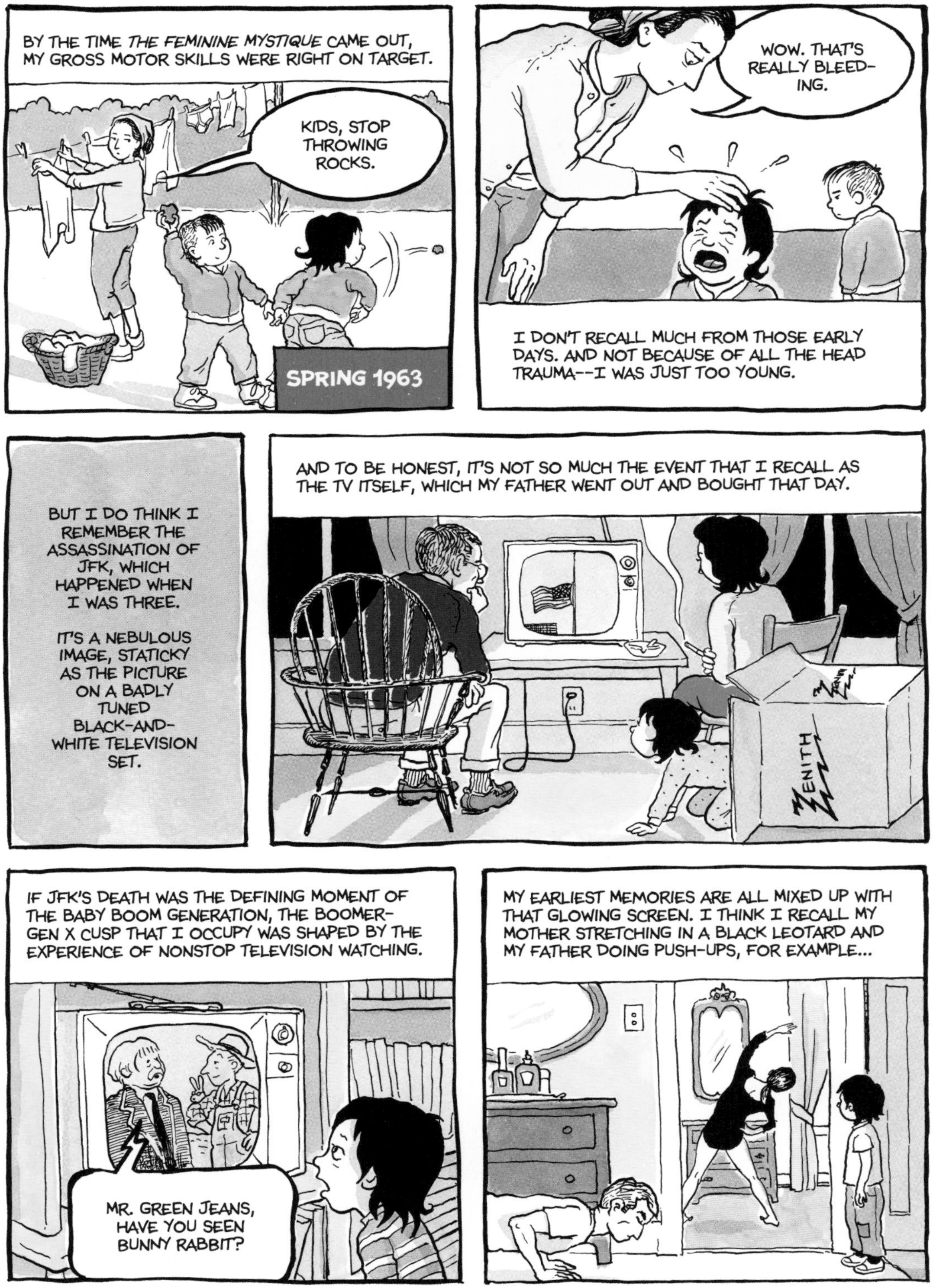
BY THE TIME THE FEMININE MYSTIQUE CAME OUT, MY GROSS MOTOR SKILLS WERE RIGHT ON TARGET.
KIDS, STOP THROWING ROCKS.
SPRING 1963
WOW. THAT'S REALLY BLEED-ING.
I DON'T RECALL MUCH FROM THOSE EARLY DAYS. AND NOT BECAUSE OF ALL THE HEAD TRAUMA--I WAS JUST TOO YOUNG.
BUT I DO THINK I REMEMBER THE ASSASSINATION OF JFK, WHICH HAPPENED WHEN I WAS THREE.
IT'S A NEBULOUS IMAGE, STATICKY AS THE PICTURE ON A BADLY TUNED BLACK-AND-WHITE TELEVISION SET.
AND TO BE HONEST, IT'S NOT SO MUCH THE EVENT THAT I RECALL AS THE TV ITSELF, WHICH MY FATHER WENT OUT AND BOUGHT THAT DAY.
ZENITH
IF JFK'S DEATH WAS THE DEFINING MOMENT OF THE BABY BOOM GENERATION, THE BOOMER-GEN X CUSP THAT I OCCUPY WAS SHAPED BY THE EXPERIENCE OF NONSTOP TELEVISION WATCHING.
MR. GREEN JEANS, HAVE YOU SEEN BUNNY RABBIT?
MY EARLIEST MEMORIES ARE ALL MIXED UP WITH THAT GLOWING SCREEN. I THINK I RECALL MY MOTHER STRETCHING IN A BLACK LEOTARD AND MY FATHER DOING PUSH-UPS, FOR EXAMPLE...

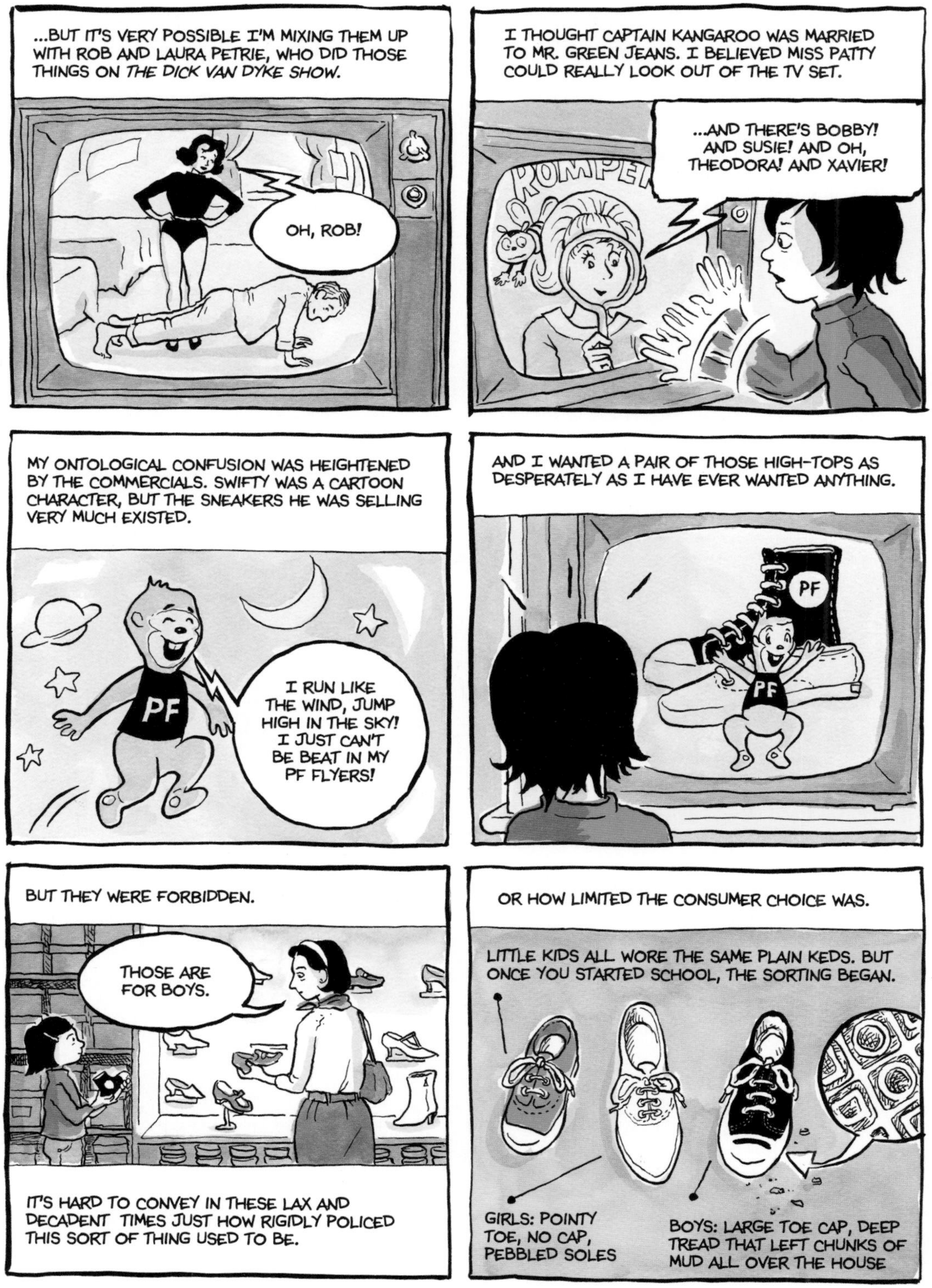
...BUT IT'S VERY POSSIBLE I'M MIXING THEM UP WITH ROB AND LAURA PETRIE, WHO DID THOSE THINGS ON *THE DICK VAN DYKE SHOW*.
OH, ROB!
I THOUGHT CAPTAIN KANGAROO WAS MARRIED TO MR. GREEN JEANS. I BELIEVED MISS PATTY COULD REALLY LOOK OUT OF THE TV SET.
...AND THERE'S BOBBY! AND SUSIE! AND OH, THEODORA! AND XAVIER!
MY ONTOLOGICAL CONFUSION WAS HEIGHTENED BY THE COMMERCIALS. SWIFTY WAS A CARTOON CHARACTER, BUT THE SNEAKERS HE WAS SELLING VERY MUCH EXISTED.
PF
I RUN LIKE THE WIND, JUMP HIGH IN THE SKY! I JUST CAN'T BE BEAT IN MY PF FLYERS!
AND I WANTED A PAIR OF THOSE HIGH-TOPS AS DESPERATELY AS I HAVE EVER WANTED ANYTHING.
PF
PF
BUT THEY WERE FORBIDDEN.
THOSE ARE FOR BOYS.
IT'S HARD TO CONVEY IN THESE LAX AND DECADENT TIMES JUST HOW RIGIDLY POLICED THIS SORT OF THING USED TO BE.
OR HOW LIMITED THE CONSUMER CHOICE WAS.
LITTLE KIDS ALL WORE THE SAME PLAIN KEDS. BUT ONCE YOU STARTED SCHOOL, THE SORTING BEGAN.
GIRLS: POINTY TOE, NO CAP, PEBBLED SOLES
BOYS: LARGE TOE CAP, DEEP TREAD THAT LEFT CHUNKS OF MUD ALL OVER THE HOUSE

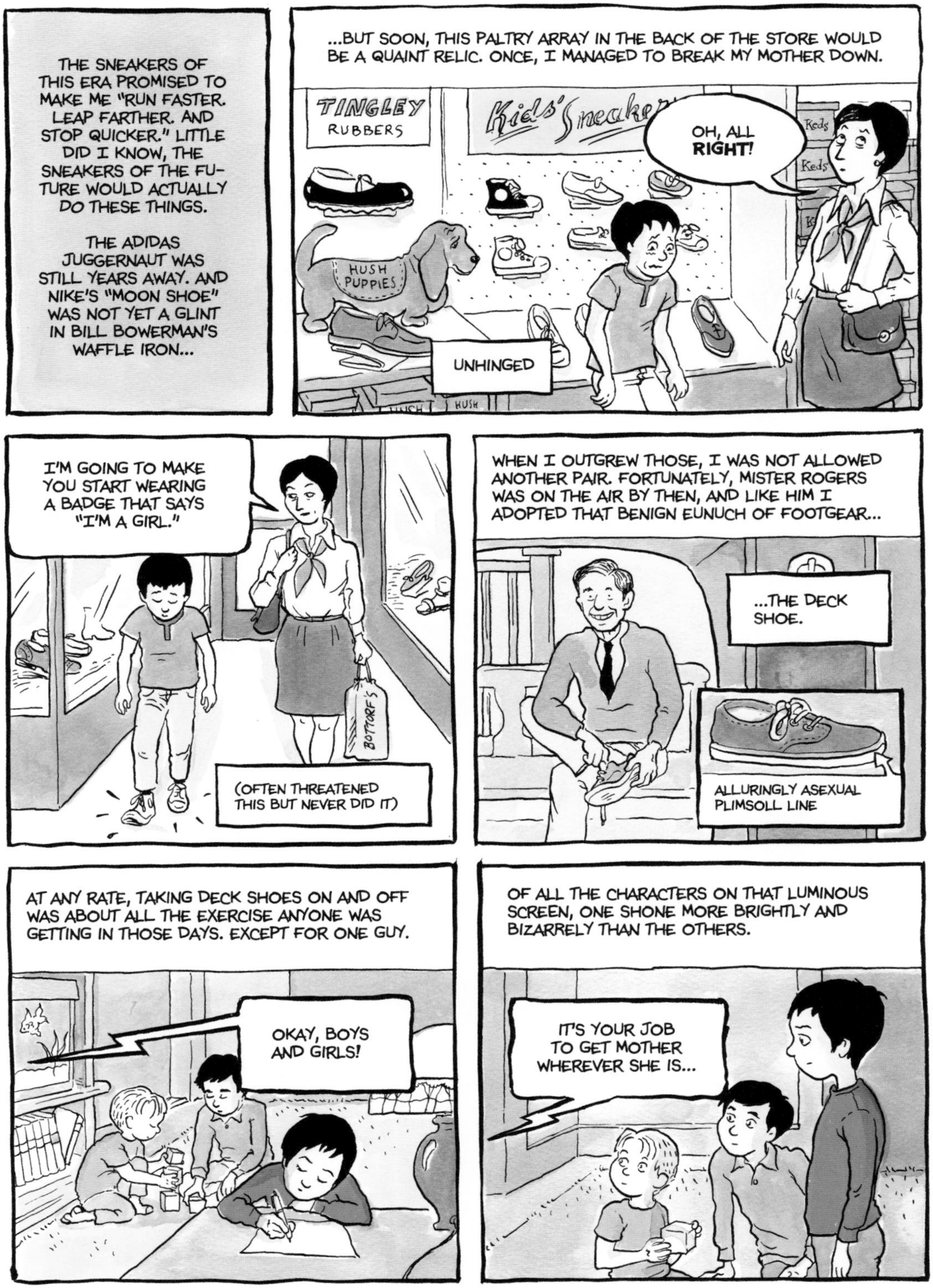
THE SNEAKERS OF THIS ERA PROMISED TO MAKE ME "RUN FASTER. LEAP FARTHER. AND STOP QUICKER." LITTLE DID I KNOW, THE SNEAKERS OF THE FUTURE WOULD ACTUALLY DO THESE THINGS.
THE ADIDAS JUGGERNAUT WAS STILL YEARS AWAY. AND NIKE'S "MOON SHOE" WAS NOT YET A GLINT IN BILL BOWERMAN'S WAFFLE IRON...
...BUT SOON, THIS PALTRY ARRAY IN THE BACK OF THE STORE WOULD BE A QUAINT RELIC. ONCE, I MANAGED TO BREAK MY MOTHER DOWN.
TINGLEY RUBBERS
HUSH PUPPIES
OH, ALL RIGHT!
Keds
Keds
UNHINGED
I'M GOING TO MAKE YOU START WEARING A BADGE THAT SAYS "I'M A GIRL."
BOTTORF'S
(OFTEN THREATENED THIS BUT NEVER DID IT)
WHEN I OUTGREW THOSE, I WAS NOT ALLOWED ANOTHER PAIR. FORTUNATELY, MISTER ROGERS WAS ON THE AIR BY THEN, AND LIKE HIM I ADOPTED THAT BENIGN EUNUCH OF FOOTGEAR...
...THE DECK SHOE.
ALLURINGLY ASEXUAL PLIMSOLL LINE
AT ANY RATE, TAKING DECK SHOES ON AND OFF WAS ABOUT ALL THE EXERCISE ANYONE WAS GETTING IN THOSE DAYS. EXCEPT FOR ONE GUY.
OKAY, BOYS AND GIRLS!
OF ALL THE CHARACTERS ON THAT LUMINOUS SCREEN, ONE SHONE MORE BRIGHTLY AND BIZARRELY THAN THE OTHERS.
IT'S YOUR JOB TO GET MOTHER WHEREVER SHE IS...

WHO COULD LOOK AWAY FROM JACK LALANNE?
...IF SHE'S BUSY AROUND THE HOUSE OR IF SHE'S DOIN' THE DISHES...
CANTALOUPE-SIZED GUNS
OUTLANDISH JUMPSUIT
JAUNTY ORGAN MUSIC
WASP WAIST
DELICATE SLIPPERS
LET'S FIRM UP YOUR BUSTLINE AND TAKE DOWN YOUR WAIST!
SERIOUS DÉCOLLETAGE
I WAS NOT INTERESTED IN MY BUSTLINE.
I WOULDN'T HAVE MINDED ARMS LIKE JACK'S, BUT HE DIDN'T EXPLAIN HOW TO GET THOSE.
WE'RE GONNA WORK THE BODY FROM THE BOTTOM OF THE FEET UP TO THE TOP OF YOUR CUTE LITTLE HEAD!
HOUSEWIVES IN THE '60S DID NOT WANT BULGING BICEPS. BUT FROM JACK I LEARNED THAT THE BODY WAS SOMETHING YOU COULD SHAPE. AND THAT EXERCISE GAVE YOU "ZEST" AND "PEP."
BOY, IS THAT A WONDERFUL ONE TO TRIM UP THE OL' ANKLE!
THAT'S PRETTY IMPORTANT TO YOU GALS, ISN'T IT?
I DIDN'T NOTICE HIS CONDESCENDING TONE. CASUAL MISOGYNY WAS THE AIR I BREATHED.

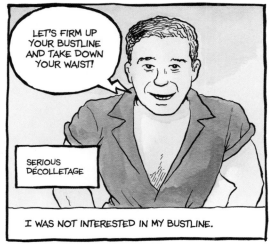

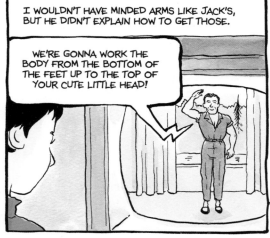

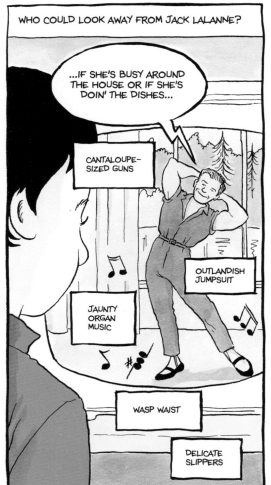

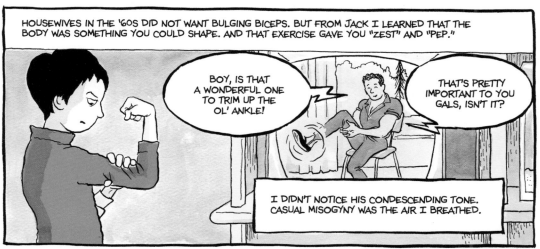

MY EARLY CHILDHOOD WAS A CONSTANT STREAM OF REMARKS ABOUT "DUMB BLONDES" AND "WOMEN DRIVERS" AND "THE WEAKER SEX."

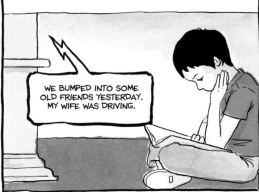

WE BUMPED INTO SOME OLD FRIENDS YESTERDAY. MY WIFE WAS DRIVING.

NOT BEING BLONDE OR OF LEGAL DRIVING AGE, I WAS ABLE TO LET THOSE TWO ROLL OFF MY BACK. BUT *WEAK*?

WEAK?!

I BECAME FASCINATED WITH THE BODYBUILDING ADS IN MY COMIC BOOKS. IT DIDN'T REALLY OCCUR TO ME--DESPITE THE ENDLESSLY REPEATED WORD "MAN"--THAT THESE WERE *MALE* BODIES.

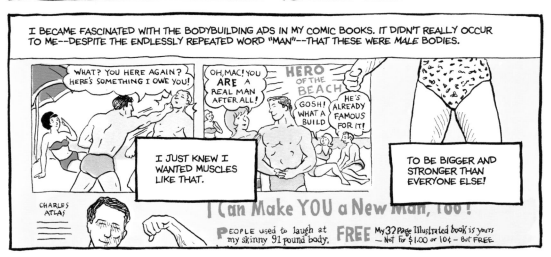

WHAT? YOU HERE AGAIN? HERE'S SOMETHING I OWE YOU!

OH, MAC! YOU *ARE* A REAL MAN AFTER ALL!

HERO OF THE BEACH

GOSH! WHAT A BUILD

HE'S ALREADY FAMOUS FOR IT!

I JUST KNEW I WANTED MUSCLES LIKE THAT.

TO BE BIGGER AND STRONGER THAN EVERYONE ELSE!

CHARLES ATLAS

I Can Make YOU a New Man, Too!

PEOPLE used to laugh at my skinny 91 pound body. FREE My 32 page Illustrated book is yours — Not for $1.00 or 10¢ – but FREE

BUT I DIDN'T HAVE THE NERVE TO SEND AWAY FOR THE CHARLES ATLAS BOOKLET, OR THE WEIGHT-GAIN DRINKS OR STRANGE DEVICES.

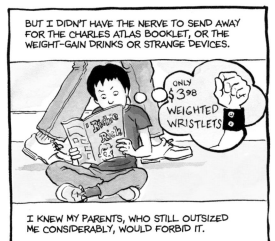

ONLY $3.98 WEIGHTED WRISTLETS

I KNEW MY PARENTS, WHO STILL OUTSIZED ME CONSIDERABLY, WOULD FORBID IT.

THERE WAS MUCH TALK OF "WEAKLINGS" IN THE ADS, IDENTIFIABLE BY THEIR PROTRUDING RIBS.

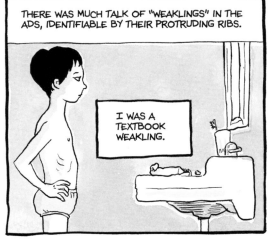

I WAS A TEXTBOOK WEAKLING.

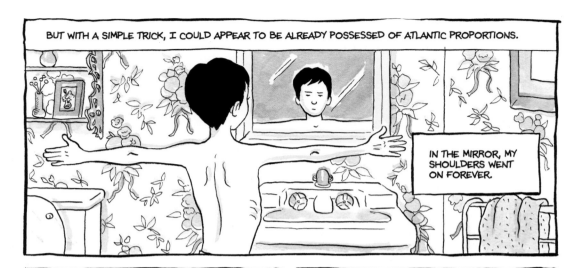

BUT WITH A SIMPLE TRICK, I COULD APPEAR TO BE ALREADY POSSESSED OF ATLANTIC PROPORTIONS.

IN THE MIRROR, MY SHOULDERS WENT ON FOREVER.

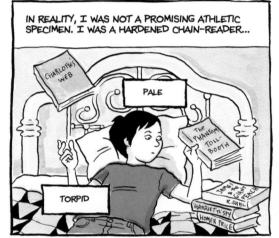

IN REALITY, I WAS NOT A PROMISING ATHLETIC SPECIMEN. I WAS A HARDENED CHAIN-READER...

CHARLOTTE'S WEB

PALE

The PHANTOM TOLL-BOOTH

TORPID

JAMES & the GIANT PEACH R. DAHL

HARRIET 'N' SPY

HOMER PRICE

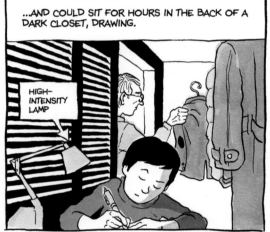

...AND COULD SIT FOR HOURS IN THE BACK OF A DARK CLOSET, DRAWING.

HIGH-INTENSITY LAMP

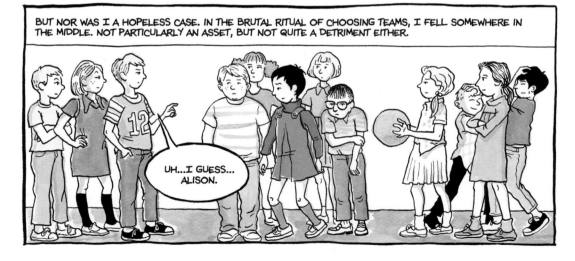

BUT NOR WAS I A HOPELESS CASE. IN THE BRUTAL RITUAL OF CHOOSING TEAMS, I FELL SOMEWHERE IN THE MIDDLE. NOT PARTICULARLY AN ASSET, BUT NOT QUITE A DETRIMENT EITHER.

UH...I GUESS... ALISON.

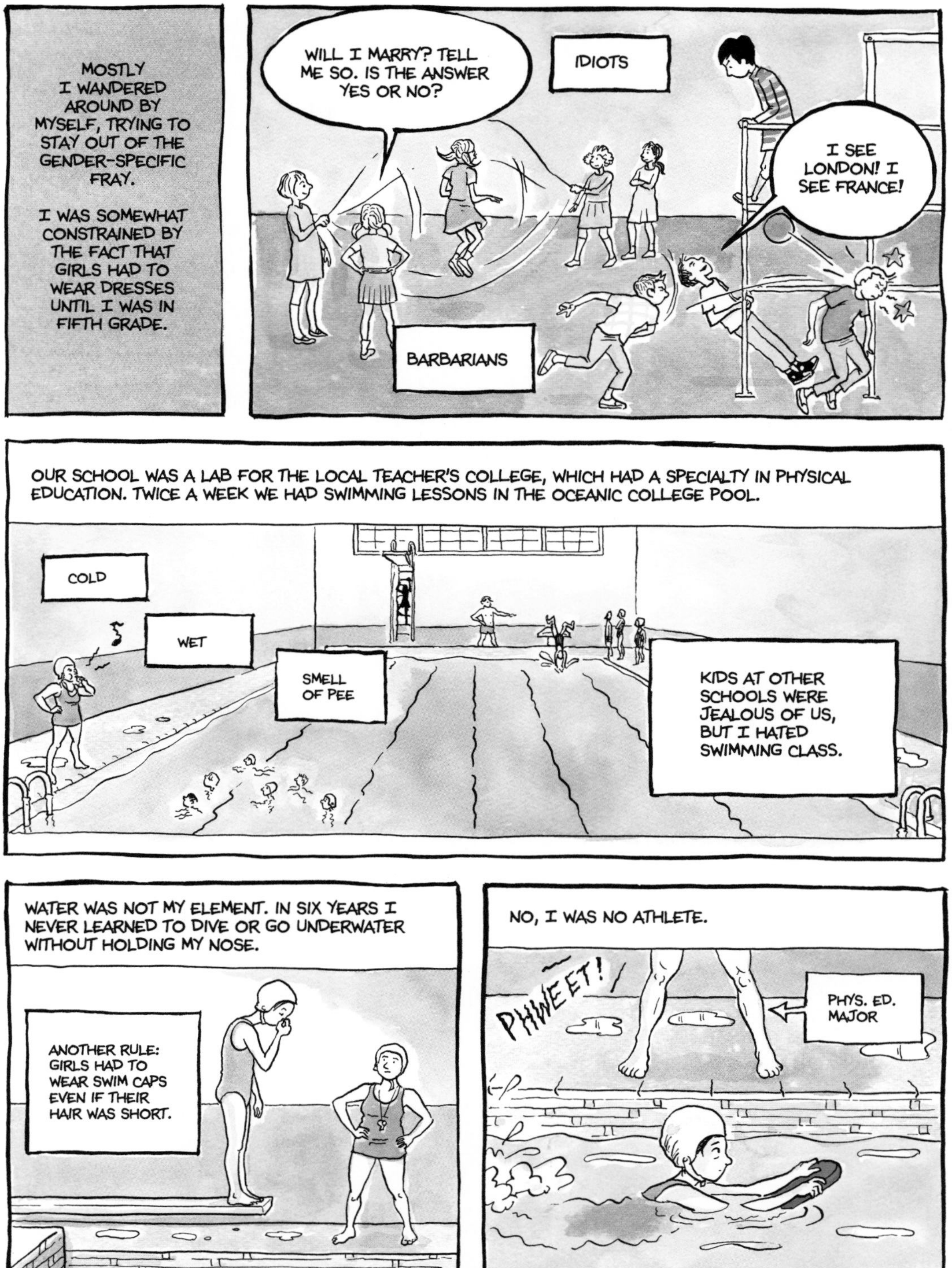
MOSTLY I WANDERED AROUND BY MYSELF, TRYING TO STAY OUT OF THE GENDER-SPECIFIC FRAY.
I WAS SOMEWHAT CONSTRAINED BY THE FACT THAT GIRLS HAD TO WEAR DRESSES UNTIL I WAS IN FIFTH GRADE.
WILL I MARRY? TELL ME SO. IS THE ANSWER YES OR NO?
IDIOTS
I SEE LONDON! I SEE FRANCE!
BARBARIANS
OUR SCHOOL WAS A LAB FOR THE LOCAL TEACHER'S COLLEGE, WHICH HAD A SPECIALTY IN PHYSICAL EDUCATION. TWICE A WEEK WE HAD SWIMMING LESSONS IN THE OCEANIC COLLEGE POOL.
COLD
WET
SMELL OF PEE
KIDS AT OTHER SCHOOLS WERE JEALOUS OF US, BUT I HATED SWIMMING CLASS.
WATER WAS NOT MY ELEMENT. IN SIX YEARS I NEVER LEARNED TO DIVE OR GO UNDERWATER WITHOUT HOLDING MY NOSE.
ANOTHER RULE: GIRLS HAD TO WEAR SWIM CAPS EVEN IF THEIR HAIR WAS SHORT.
NO, I WAS NO ATHLETE.
PHWEET!
PHYS. ED. MAJOR

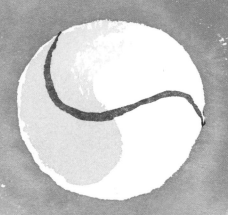

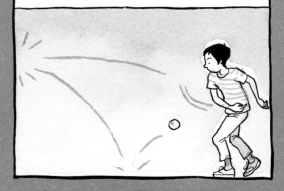

HOW MANY CATCHES COULD I MAKE WITHOUT MOVING MY FEET? THE HARDER I TRIED TO PERFORM A PARTICULAR TRICK, THE MORE ELUSIVE IT BECAME.

AT HOME, HOWEVER, AWAY FROM THE SOCIAL PRESS...

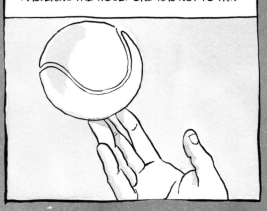

IN TIME I LEARNED THAT THE SECRET TO MASTERING THE WOOLY ORB WAS NOT TO TRY.

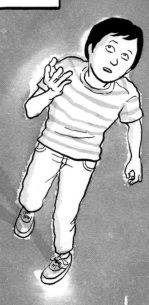

...I LOVED NOTHING MORE THAN TO WORK MYSELF INTO A TRANCE WITH AN OLD TENNIS BALL.

HOW HIGH COULD I THROW IT AND STILL MAKE THE CATCH?

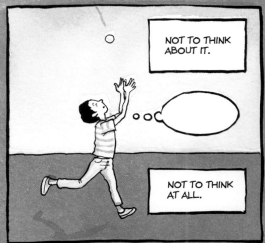

NOT TO THINK ABOUT IT.

NOT TO THINK AT ALL.

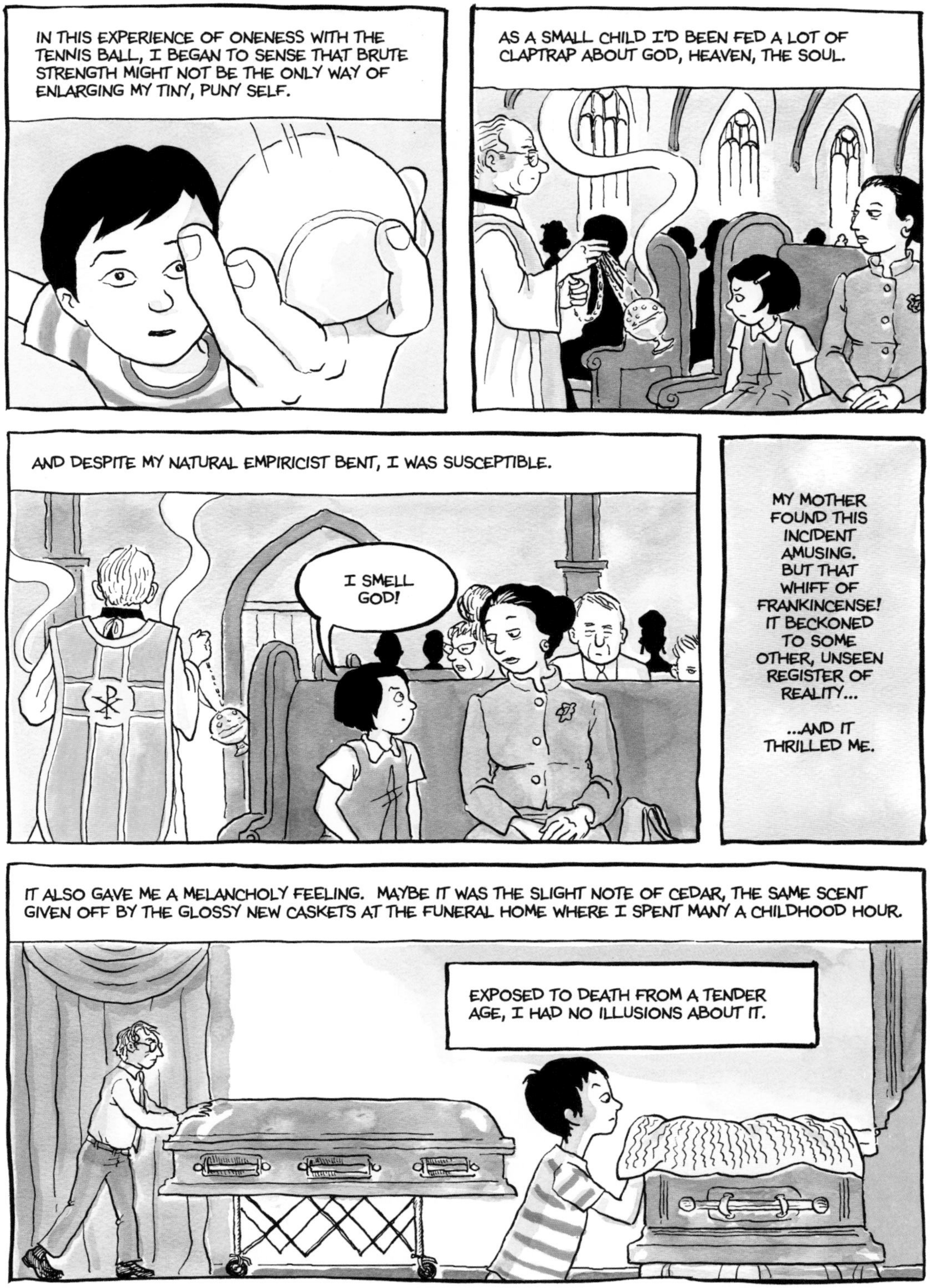
IN THIS EXPERIENCE OF ONENESS WITH THE TENNIS BALL, I BEGAN TO SENSE THAT BRUTE STRENGTH MIGHT NOT BE THE ONLY WAY OF ENLARGING MY TINY, PUNY SELF.
AS A SMALL CHILD I'D BEEN FED A LOT OF CLAPTRAP ABOUT GOD, HEAVEN, THE SOUL.
AND DESPITE MY NATURAL EMPIRICIST BENT, I WAS SUSCEPTIBLE.
I SMELL GOD!
MY MOTHER FOUND THIS INCIDENT AMUSING. BUT THAT WHIFF OF FRANKINCENSE! IT BECKONED TO SOME OTHER, UNSEEN REGISTER OF REALITY...
...AND IT THRILLED ME.
IT ALSO GAVE ME A MELANCHOLY FEELING. MAYBE IT WAS THE SLIGHT NOTE OF CEDAR, THE SAME SCENT GIVEN OFF BY THE GLOSSY NEW CASKETS AT THE FUNERAL HOME WHERE I SPENT MANY A CHILDHOOD HOUR.
EXPOSED TO DEATH FROM A TENDER AGE, I HAD NO ILLUSIONS ABOUT IT.

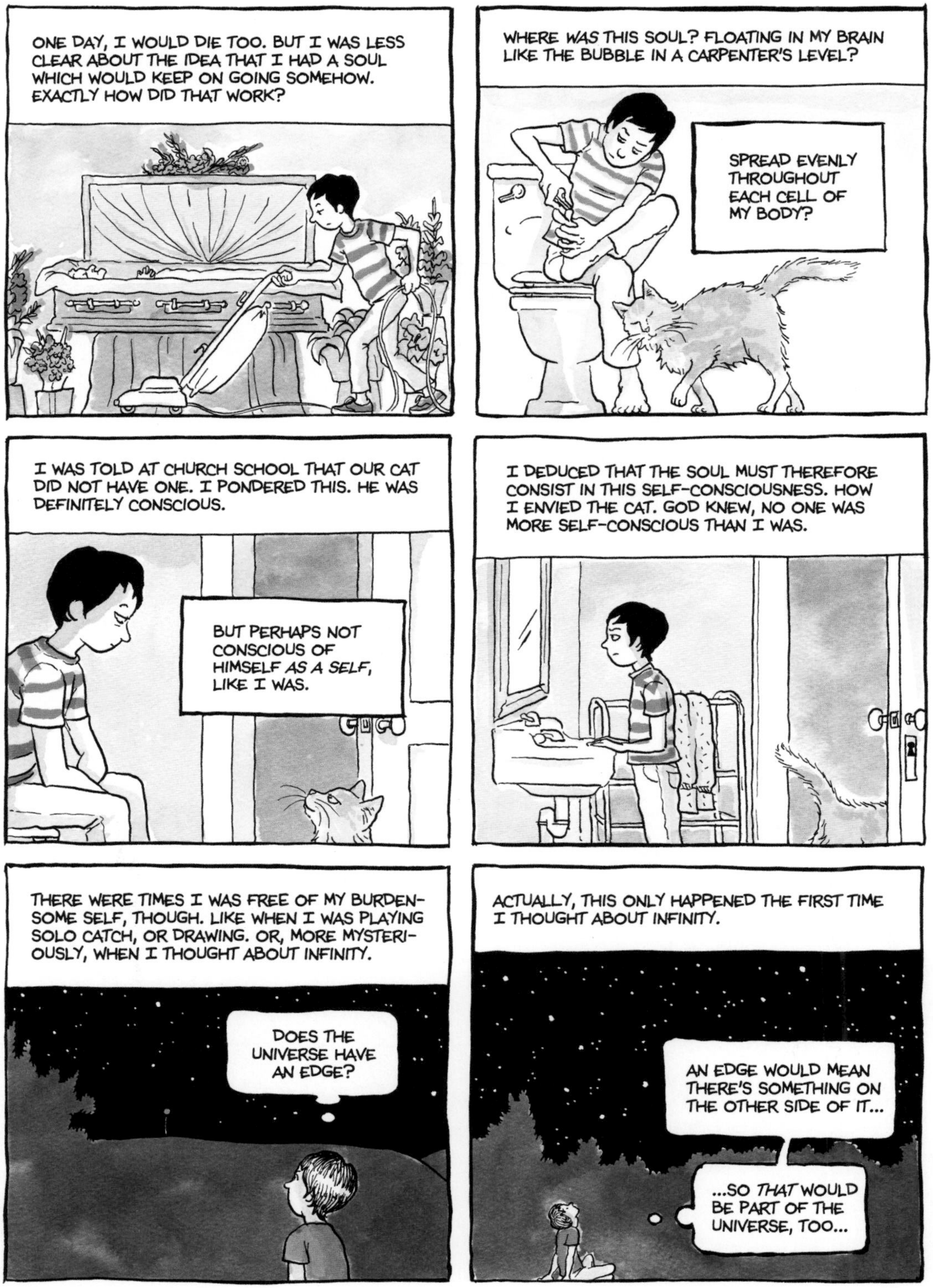
ONE DAY, I WOULD DIE TOO. BUT I WAS LESS CLEAR ABOUT THE IDEA THAT I HAD A SOUL WHICH WOULD KEEP ON GOING SOMEHOW. EXACTLY HOW DID THAT WORK?
WHERE *WAS* THIS SOUL? FLOATING IN MY BRAIN LIKE THE BUBBLE IN A CARPENTER'S LEVEL?
SPREAD EVENLY THROUGHOUT EACH CELL OF MY BODY?
I WAS TOLD AT CHURCH SCHOOL THAT OUR CAT DID NOT HAVE ONE. I PONDERED THIS. HE WAS DEFINITELY CONSCIOUS.
BUT PERHAPS NOT CONSCIOUS OF HIMSELF *AS A SELF*, LIKE I WAS.
I DEDUCED THAT THE SOUL MUST THEREFORE CONSIST IN THIS SELF-CONSCIOUSNESS. HOW I ENVIED THE CAT. GOD KNEW, NO ONE WAS MORE SELF-CONSCIOUS THAN I WAS.
THERE WERE TIMES I WAS FREE OF MY BURDENSOME SELF, THOUGH. LIKE WHEN I WAS PLAYING SOLO CATCH, OR DRAWING. OR, MORE MYSTERIOUSLY, WHEN I THOUGHT ABOUT INFINITY.
DOES THE UNIVERSE HAVE AN EDGE?
ACTUALLY, THIS ONLY HAPPENED THE FIRST TIME I THOUGHT ABOUT INFINITY.
AN EDGE WOULD MEAN THERE'S SOMETHING ON THE OTHER SIDE OF IT...
...SO *THAT* WOULD BE PART OF THE UNIVERSE, TOO...

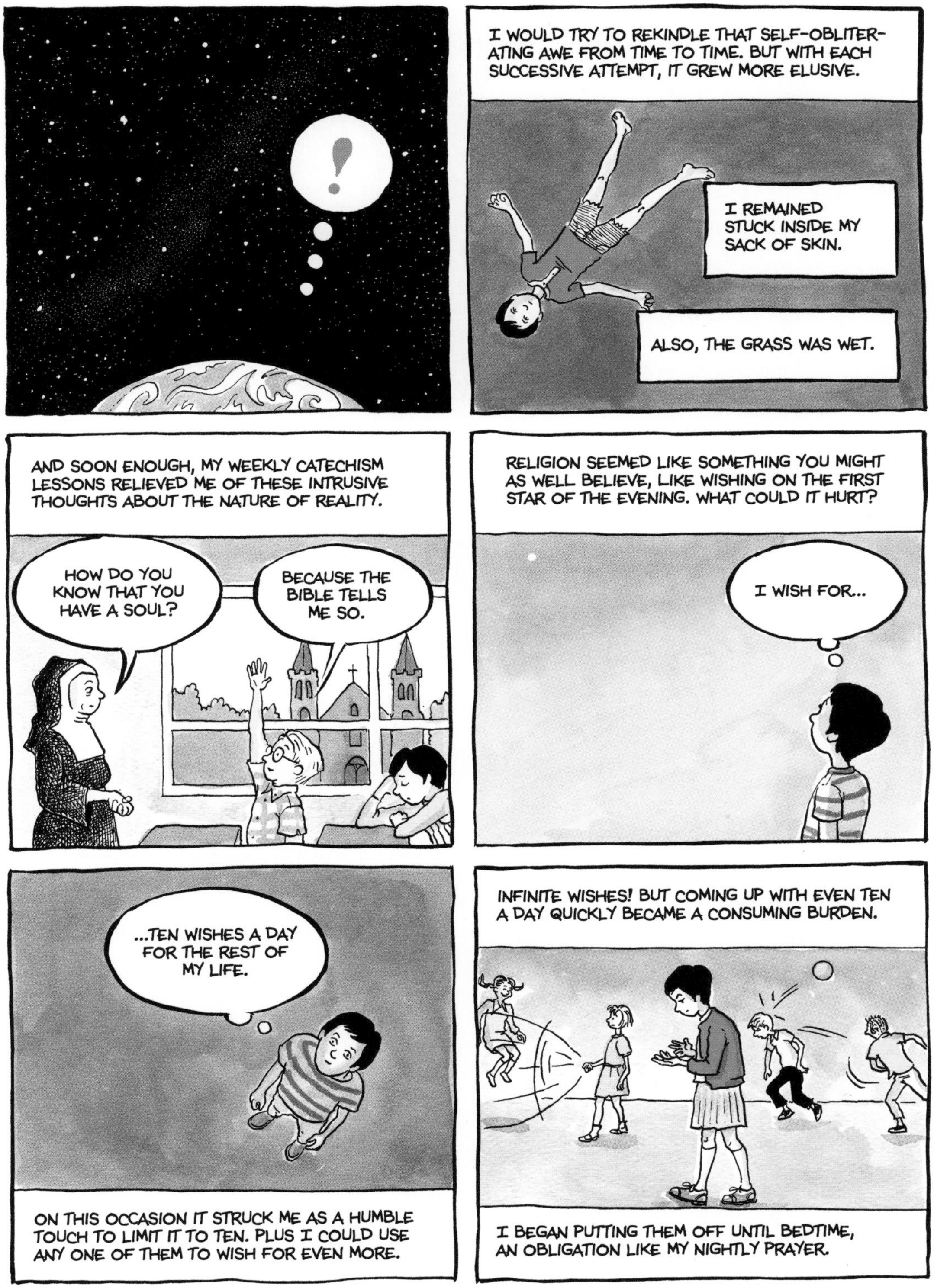
!
I WOULD TRY TO REKINDLE THAT SELF-OBLITERATING AWE FROM TIME TO TIME. BUT WITH EACH SUCCESSIVE ATTEMPT, IT GREW MORE ELUSIVE.
I REMAINED STUCK INSIDE MY SACK OF SKIN.
ALSO, THE GRASS WAS WET.
AND SOON ENOUGH, MY WEEKLY CATECHISM LESSONS RELIEVED ME OF THESE INTRUSIVE THOUGHTS ABOUT THE NATURE OF REALITY.
HOW DO YOU KNOW THAT YOU HAVE A SOUL?
BECAUSE THE BIBLE TELLS ME SO.
RELIGION SEEMED LIKE SOMETHING YOU MIGHT AS WELL BELIEVE, LIKE WISHING ON THE FIRST STAR OF THE EVENING. WHAT COULD IT HURT?
I WISH FOR...
...TEN WISHES A DAY FOR THE REST OF MY LIFE.
ON THIS OCCASION IT STRUCK ME AS A HUMBLE TOUCH TO LIMIT IT TO TEN. PLUS I COULD USE ANY ONE OF THEM TO WISH FOR EVEN MORE.
INFINITE WISHES! BUT COMING UP WITH EVEN TEN A DAY QUICKLY BECAME A CONSUMING BURDEN.
I BEGAN PUTTING THEM OFF UNTIL BEDTIME, AN OBLIGATION LIKE MY NIGHTLY PRAYER.

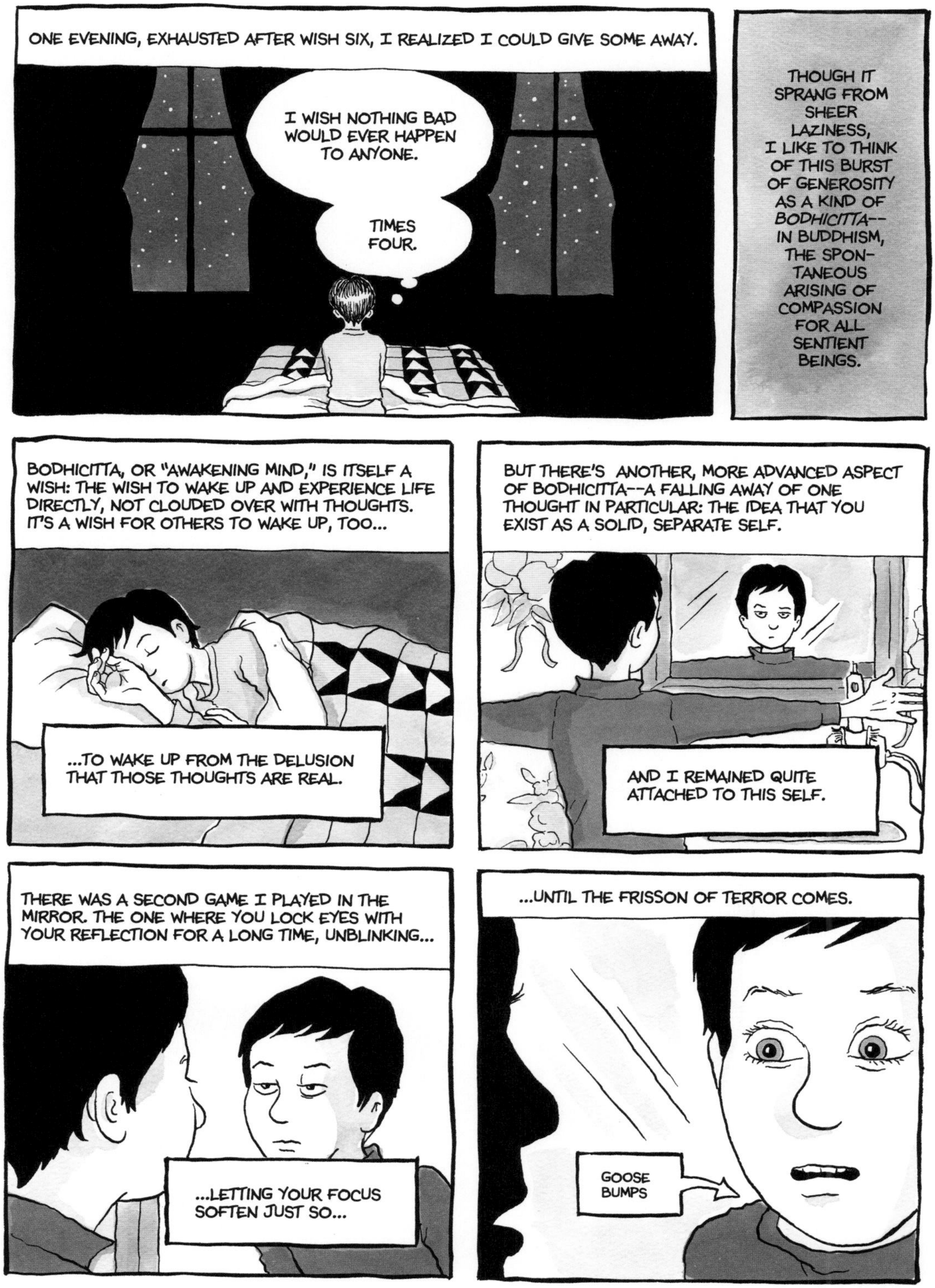
ONE EVENING, EXHAUSTED AFTER WISH SIX, I REALIZED I COULD GIVE SOME AWAY.
I WISH NOTHING BAD WOULD EVER HAPPEN TO ANYONE.
TIMES FOUR.
THOUGH IT SPRANG FROM SHEER LAZINESS, I LIKE TO THINK OF THIS BURST OF GENEROSITY AS A KIND OF *BODHICITTA*-- IN BUDDHISM, THE SPONTANEOUS ARISING OF COMPASSION FOR ALL SENTIENT BEINGS.
BODHICITTA, OR "AWAKENING MIND," IS ITSELF A WISH: THE WISH TO WAKE UP AND EXPERIENCE LIFE DIRECTLY, NOT CLOUDED OVER WITH THOUGHTS. IT'S A WISH FOR OTHERS TO WAKE UP, TOO...
...TO WAKE UP FROM THE DELUSION THAT THOSE THOUGHTS ARE REAL.
BUT THERE'S ANOTHER, MORE ADVANCED ASPECT OF BODHICITTA--A FALLING AWAY OF ONE THOUGHT IN PARTICULAR: THE IDEA THAT YOU EXIST AS A SOLID, SEPARATE SELF.
AND I REMAINED QUITE ATTACHED TO THIS SELF.
THERE WAS A SECOND GAME I PLAYED IN THE MIRROR. THE ONE WHERE YOU LOCK EYES WITH YOUR REFLECTION FOR A LONG TIME, UNBLINKING...
...LETTING YOUR FOCUS SOFTEN JUST SO...
...UNTIL THE FRISSON OF TERROR COMES.
GOOSE BUMPS

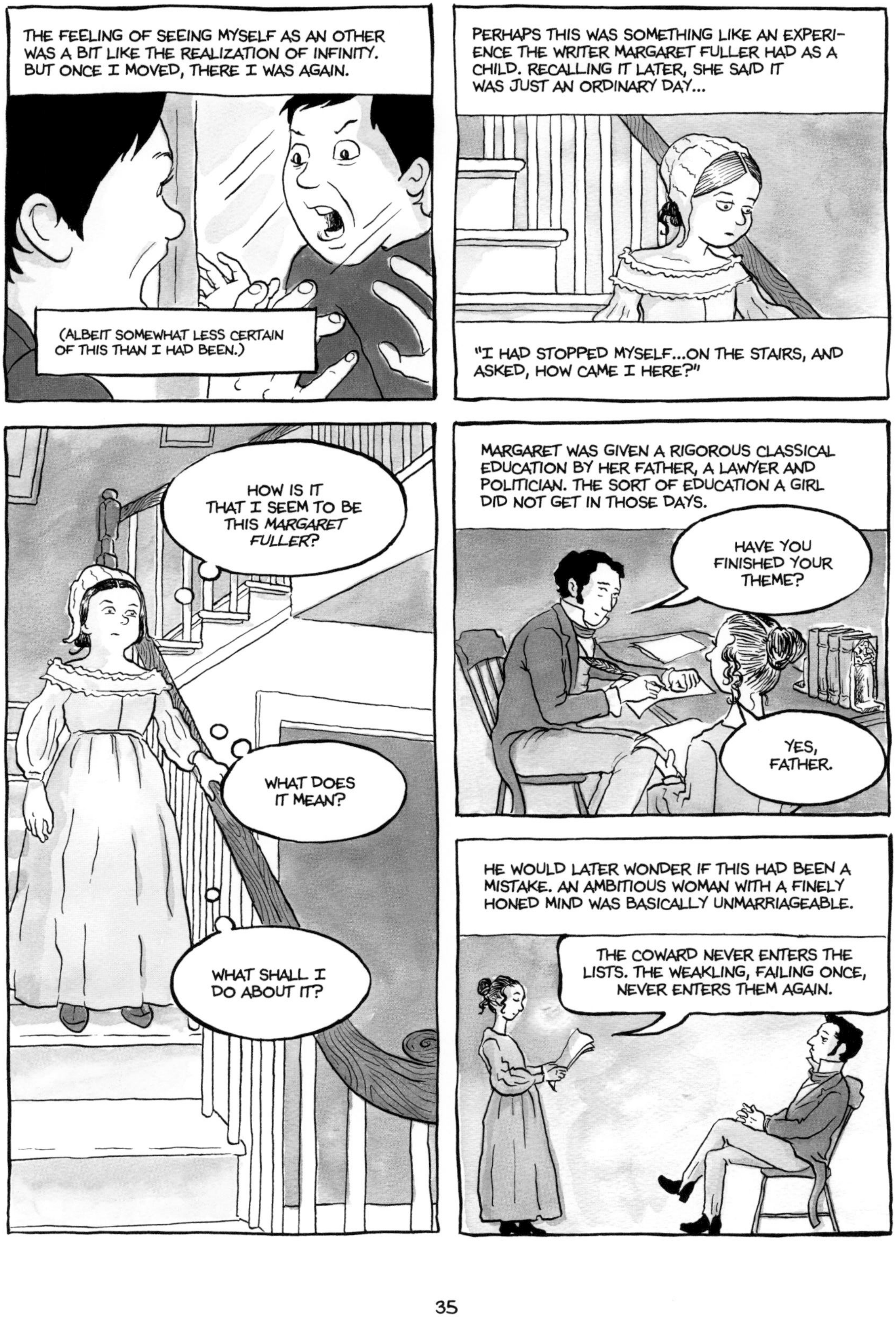
THE FEELING OF SEEING MYSELF AS AN OTHER WAS A BIT LIKE THE REALIZATION OF INFINITY. BUT ONCE I MOVED, THERE I WAS AGAIN.
(ALBEIT SOMEWHAT LESS CERTAIN OF THIS THAN I HAD BEEN.)
PERHAPS THIS WAS SOMETHING LIKE AN EXPERIENCE THE WRITER MARGARET FULLER HAD AS A CHILD. RECALLING IT LATER, SHE SAID IT WAS JUST AN ORDINARY DAY...
"I HAD STOPPED MYSELF...ON THE STAIRS, AND ASKED, HOW CAME I HERE?"
HOW IS IT THAT I SEEM TO BE THIS *MARGARET FULLER*?
WHAT DOES IT MEAN?
WHAT SHALL I DO ABOUT IT?
MARGARET WAS GIVEN A RIGOROUS CLASSICAL EDUCATION BY HER FATHER, A LAWYER AND POLITICIAN. THE SORT OF EDUCATION A GIRL DID NOT GET IN THOSE DAYS.
HAVE YOU FINISHED YOUR THEME?
YES, FATHER.
HE WOULD LATER WONDER IF THIS HAD BEEN A MISTAKE. AN AMBITIOUS WOMAN WITH A FINELY HONED MIND WAS BASICALLY UNMARRIAGEABLE.
THE COWARD NEVER ENTERS THE LISTS. THE WEAKLING, FAILING ONCE, NEVER ENTERS THEM AGAIN.

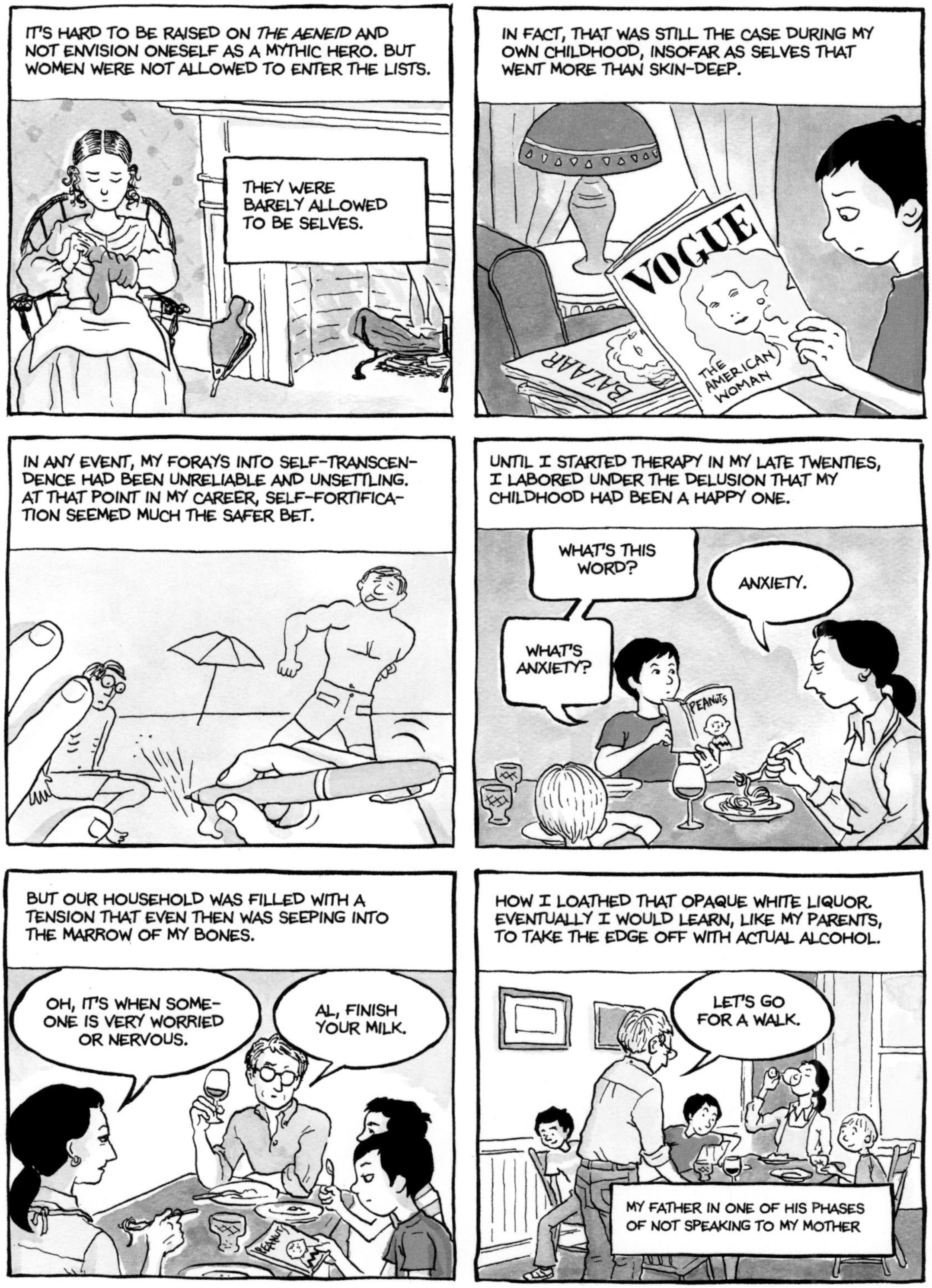
IT'S HARD TO BE RAISED ON THE AENEID AND NOT ENVISION ONESELF AS A MYTHIC HERO. BUT WOMEN WERE NOT ALLOWED TO ENTER THE LISTS.
THEY WERE BARELY ALLOWED TO BE SELVES.
IN FACT, THAT WAS STILL THE CASE DURING MY OWN CHILDHOOD, INSOFAR AS SELVES THAT WENT MORE THAN SKIN-DEEP.
VOGUE
THE AMERICAN WOMAN
BAZAAR
IN ANY EVENT, MY FORAYS INTO SELF-TRANSCENDENCE HAD BEEN UNRELIABLE AND UNSETTLING. AT THAT POINT IN MY CAREER, SELF-FORTIFICATION SEEMED MUCH THE SAFER BET.
UNTIL I STARTED THERAPY IN MY LATE TWENTIES, I LABORED UNDER THE DELUSION THAT MY CHILDHOOD HAD BEEN A HAPPY ONE.
WHAT'S THIS WORD?
ANXIETY.
WHAT'S ANXIETY?
PEANUTS
BUT OUR HOUSEHOLD WAS FILLED WITH A TENSION THAT EVEN THEN WAS SEEPING INTO THE MARROW OF MY BONES.
OH, IT'S WHEN SOMEONE IS VERY WORRIED OR NERVOUS.
AL, FINISH YOUR MILK.
PEANUTS
HOW I LOATHED THAT OPAQUE WHITE LIQUOR. EVENTUALLY I WOULD LEARN, LIKE MY PARENTS, TO TAKE THE EDGE OFF WITH ACTUAL ALCOHOL.
LET'S GO FOR A WALK.
MY FATHER IN ONE OF HIS PHASES OF NOT SPEAKING TO MY MOTHER

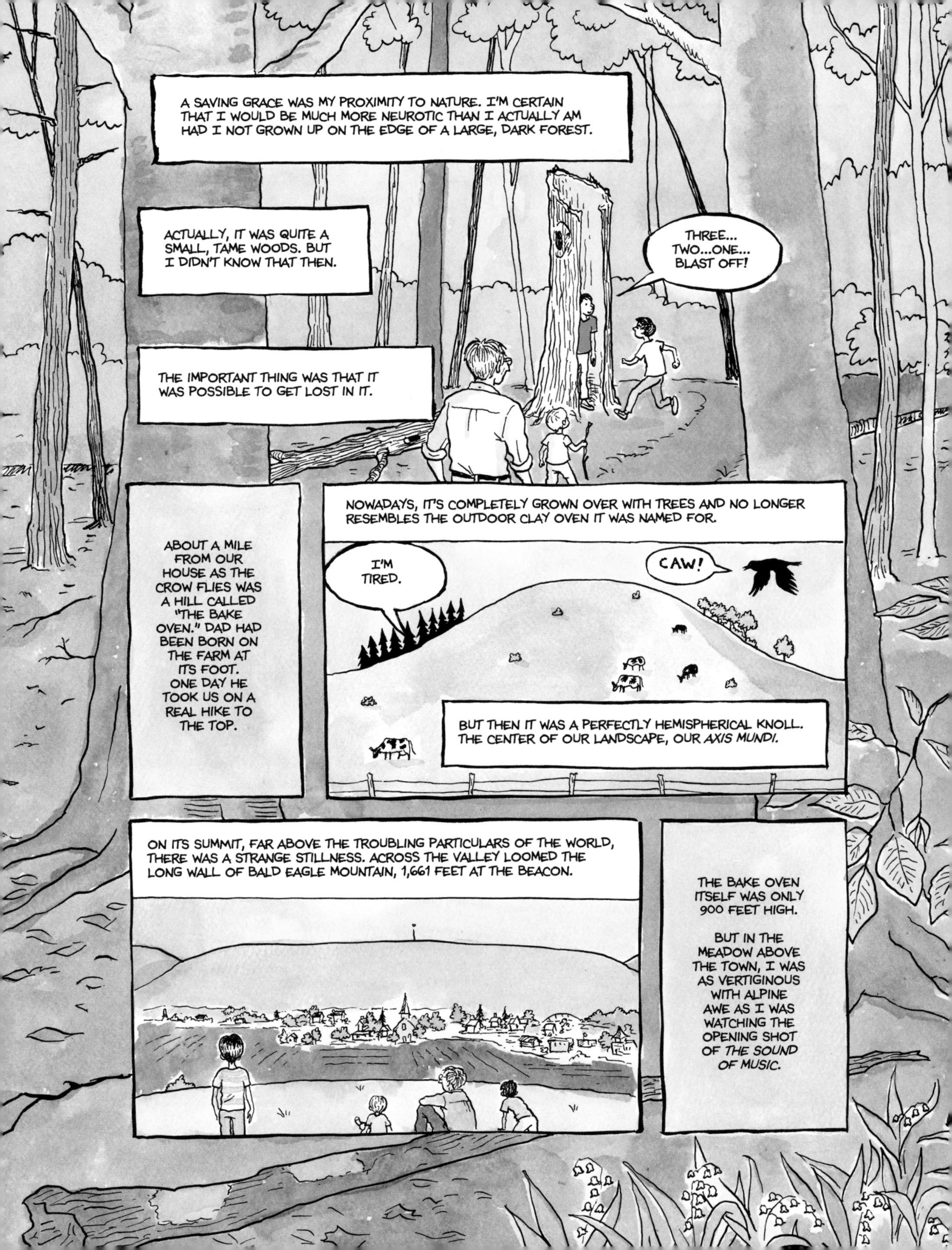
A SAVING GRACE WAS MY PROXIMITY TO NATURE. I'M CERTAIN THAT I WOULD BE MUCH MORE NEUROTIC THAN I ACTUALLY AM HAD I NOT GROWN UP ON THE EDGE OF A LARGE, DARK FOREST.
ACTUALLY, IT WAS QUITE A SMALL, TAME WOODS. BUT I DIDN'T KNOW THAT THEN.
THREE... TWO...ONE... BLAST OFF!
THE IMPORTANT THING WAS THAT IT WAS POSSIBLE TO GET LOST IN IT.
ABOUT A MILE FROM OUR HOUSE AS THE CROW FLIES WAS A HILL CALLED "THE BAKE OVEN." DAD HAD BEEN BORN ON THE FARM AT ITS FOOT. ONE DAY HE TOOK US ON A REAL HIKE TO THE TOP.
NOWADAYS, IT'S COMPLETELY GROWN OVER WITH TREES AND NO LONGER RESEMBLES THE OUTDOOR CLAY OVEN IT WAS NAMED FOR.
I'M TIRED.
CAW!
BUT THEN IT WAS A PERFECTLY HEMISPHERICAL KNOLL. THE CENTER OF OUR LANDSCAPE, OUR *AXIS MUNDI.*
ON ITS SUMMIT, FAR ABOVE THE TROUBLING PARTICULARS OF THE WORLD, THERE WAS A STRANGE STILLNESS. ACROSS THE VALLEY LOOMED THE LONG WALL OF BALD EAGLE MOUNTAIN, 1,661 FEET AT THE BEACON.
THE BAKE OVEN ITSELF WAS ONLY 900 FEET HIGH.
BUT IN THE MEADOW ABOVE THE TOWN, I WAS AS VERTIGINOUS WITH ALPINE AWE AS I WAS WATCHING THE OPENING SHOT OF *THE SOUND OF MUSIC.*

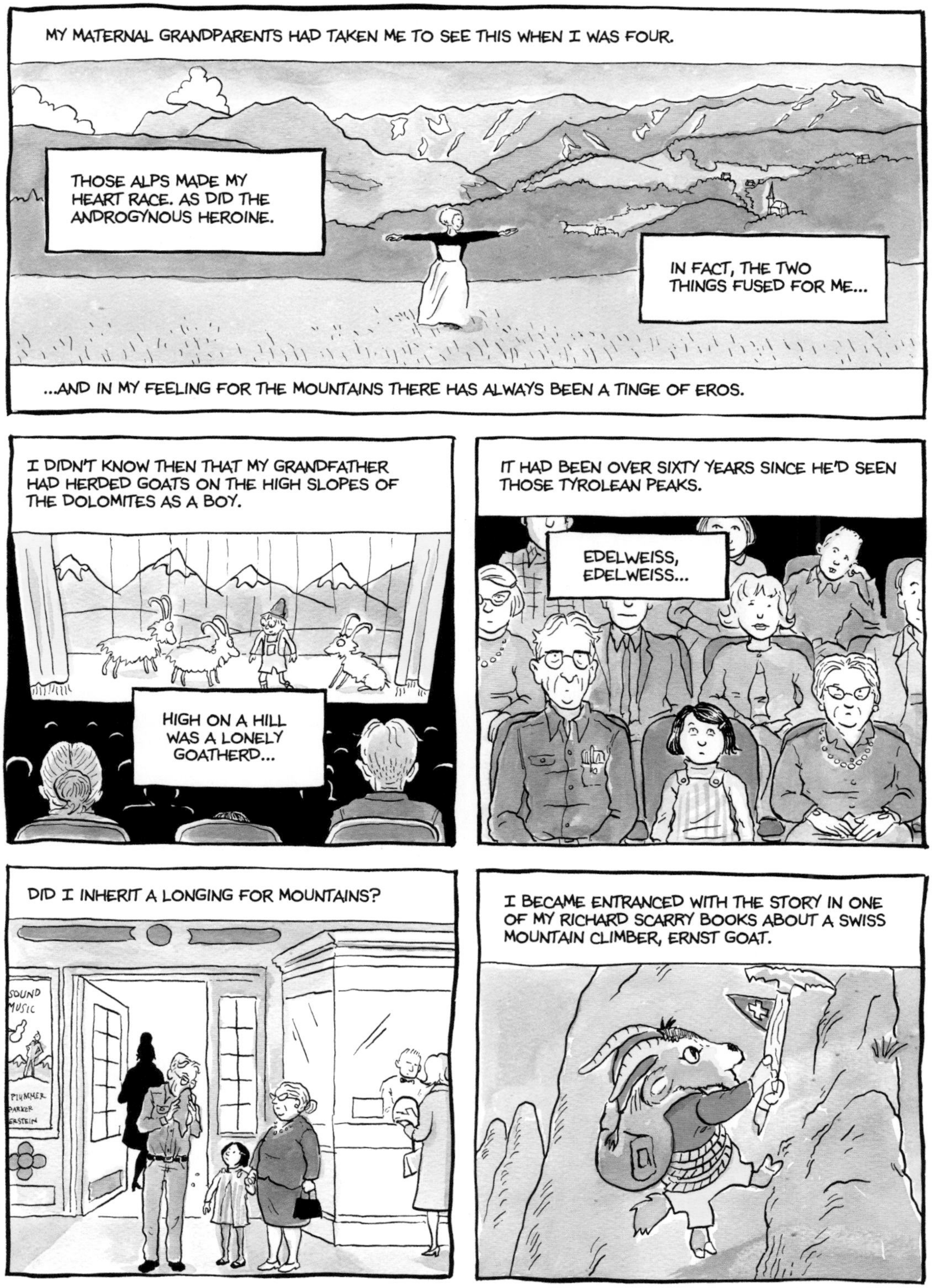
MY MATERNAL GRANDPARENTS HAD TAKEN ME TO SEE THIS WHEN I WAS FOUR.
THOSE ALPS MADE MY HEART RACE. AS DID THE ANDROGYNOUS HEROINE.
IN FACT, THE TWO THINGS FUSED FOR ME...
...AND IN MY FEELING FOR THE MOUNTAINS THERE HAS ALWAYS BEEN A TINGE OF EROS.
I DIDN'T KNOW THEN THAT MY GRANDFATHER HAD HERDED GOATS ON THE HIGH SLOPES OF THE DOLOMITES AS A BOY.
HIGH ON A HILL WAS A LONELY GOATHERD...
IT HAD BEEN OVER SIXTY YEARS SINCE HE'D SEEN THOSE TYROLEAN PEAKS.
EDELWEISS, EDELWEISS...
DID I INHERIT A LONGING FOR MOUNTAINS?
I BECAME ENTRANCED WITH THE STORY IN ONE OF MY RICHARD SCARRY BOOKS ABOUT A SWISS MOUNTAIN CLIMBER, ERNST GOAT.

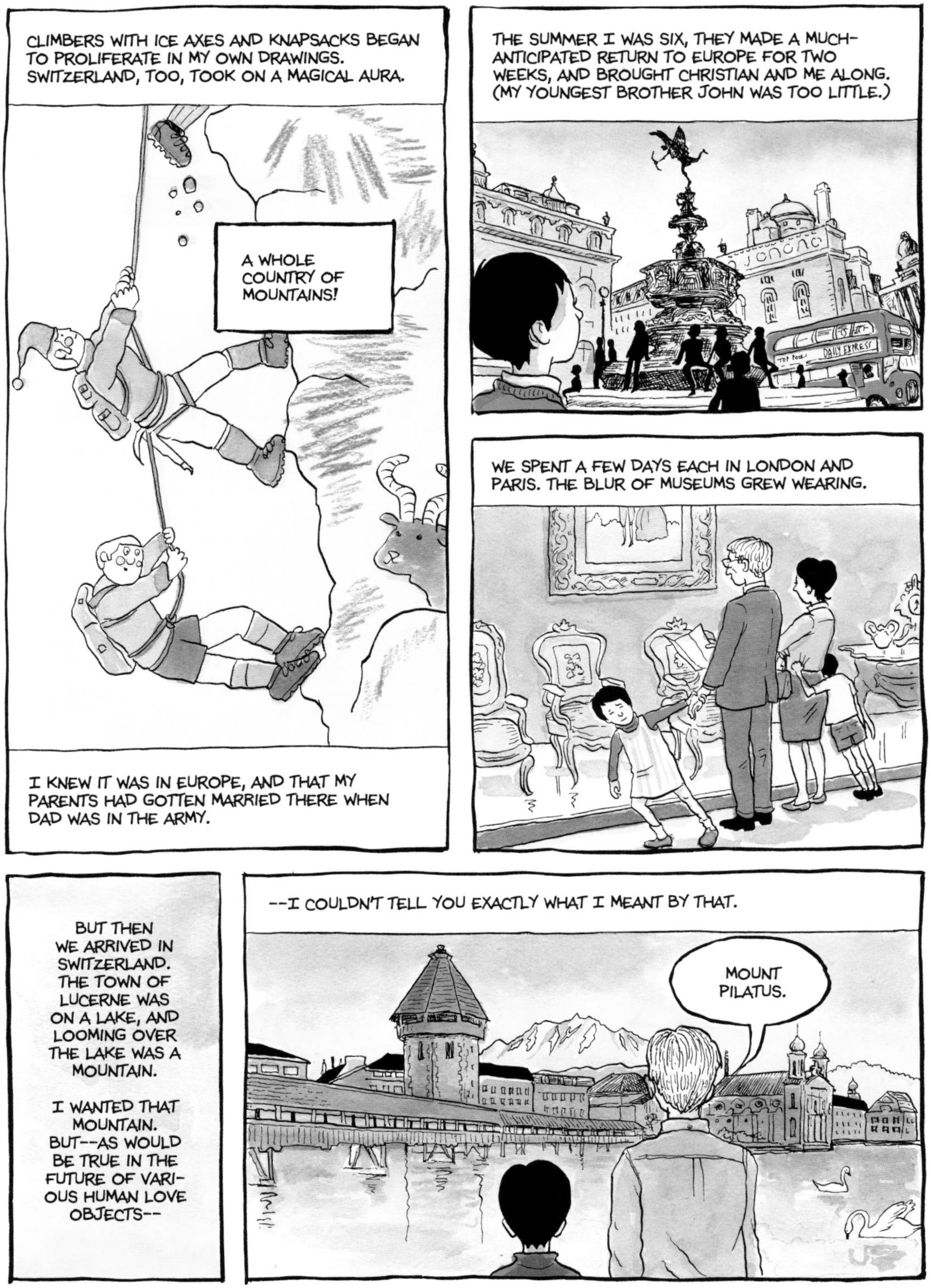
CLIMBERS WITH ICE AXES AND KNAPSACKS BEGAN TO PROLIFERATE IN MY OWN DRAWINGS. SWITZERLAND, TOO, TOOK ON A MAGICAL AURA.
A WHOLE COUNTRY OF MOUNTAINS!
I KNEW IT WAS IN EUROPE, AND THAT MY PARENTS HAD GOTTEN MARRIED THERE WHEN DAD WAS IN THE ARMY.
THE SUMMER I WAS SIX, THEY MADE A MUCH-ANTICIPATED RETURN TO EUROPE FOR TWO WEEKS, AND BROUGHT CHRISTIAN AND ME ALONG. (MY YOUNGEST BROTHER JOHN WAS TOO LITTLE.)
DAILY EXPRESS
WE SPENT A FEW DAYS EACH IN LONDON AND PARIS. THE BLUR OF MUSEUMS GREW WEARING.
BUT THEN WE ARRIVED IN SWITZERLAND. THE TOWN OF LUCERNE WAS ON A LAKE, AND LOOMING OVER THE LAKE WAS A MOUNTAIN.
I WANTED THAT MOUNTAIN. BUT--AS WOULD BE TRUE IN THE FUTURE OF VARIOUS HUMAN LOVE OBJECTS--
--I COULDN'T TELL YOU EXACTLY WHAT I MEANT BY THAT.
MOUNT PILATUS.

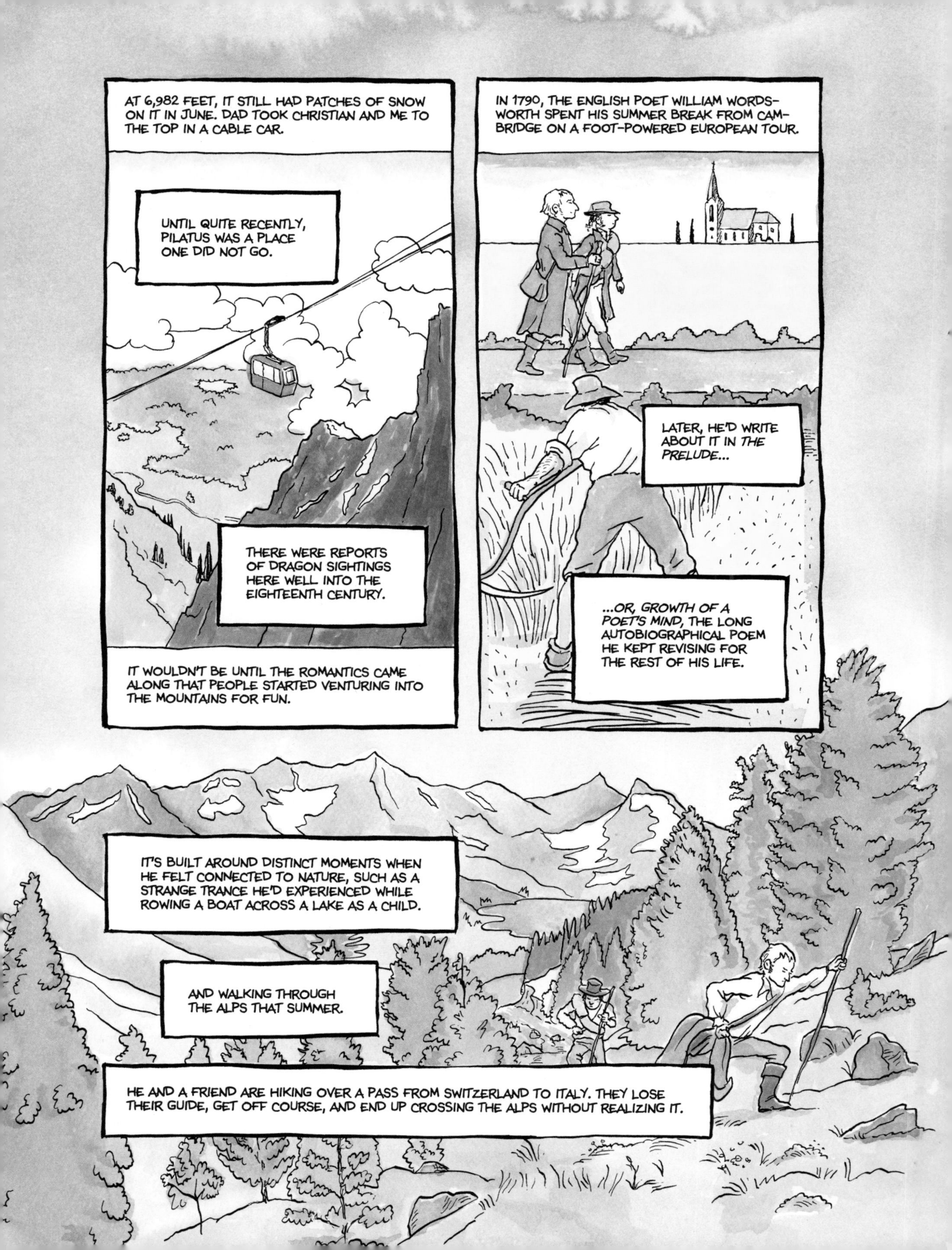
AT 6,982 FEET, IT STILL HAD PATCHES OF SNOW ON IT IN JUNE. DAD TOOK CHRISTIAN AND ME TO THE TOP IN A CABLE CAR.
UNTIL QUITE RECENTLY, PILATUS WAS A PLACE ONE DID NOT GO.
THERE WERE REPORTS OF DRAGON SIGHTINGS HERE WELL INTO THE EIGHTEENTH CENTURY.
IT WOULDN'T BE UNTIL THE ROMANTICS CAME ALONG THAT PEOPLE STARTED VENTURING INTO THE MOUNTAINS FOR FUN.
IN 1790, THE ENGLISH POET WILLIAM WORDS-WORTH SPENT HIS SUMMER BREAK FROM CAM-BRIDGE ON A FOOT-POWERED EUROPEAN TOUR.
LATER, HE'D WRITE ABOUT IT IN *THE PRELUDE*...
...*OR, GROWTH OF A POET'S MIND*, THE LONG AUTOBIOGRAPHICAL POEM HE KEPT REVISING FOR THE REST OF HIS LIFE.
IT'S BUILT AROUND DISTINCT MOMENTS WHEN HE FELT CONNECTED TO NATURE, SUCH AS A STRANGE TRANCE HE'D EXPERIENCED WHILE ROWING A BOAT ACROSS A LAKE AS A CHILD.
AND WALKING THROUGH THE ALPS THAT SUMMER.
HE AND A FRIEND ARE HIKING OVER A PASS FROM SWITZERLAND TO ITALY. THEY LOSE THEIR GUIDE, GET OFF COURSE, AND END UP CROSSING THE ALPS WITHOUT REALIZING IT.

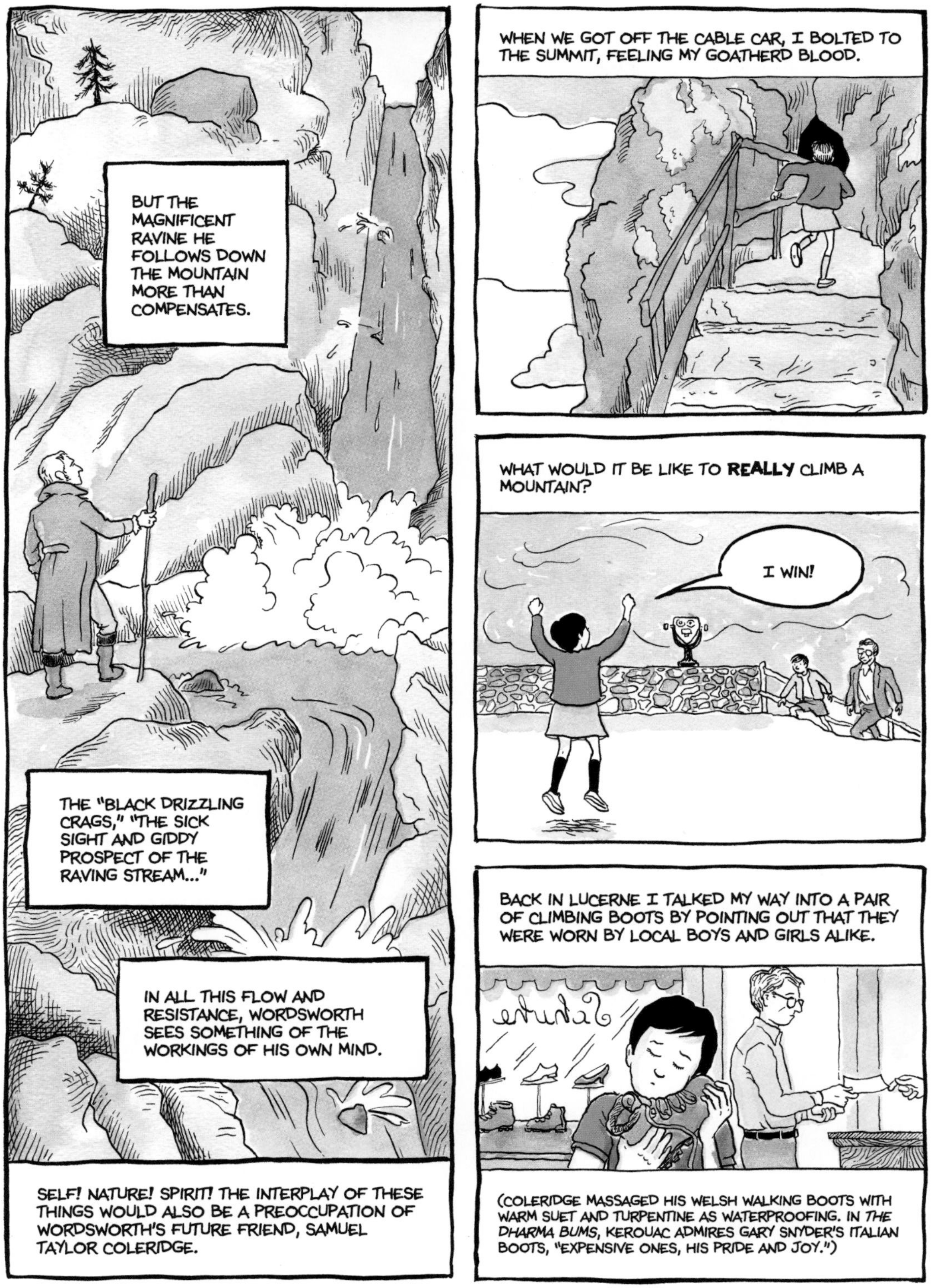

BUT THE MAGNIFICENT RAVINE HE FOLLOWS DOWN THE MOUNTAIN MORE THAN COMPENSATES.
THE "BLACK DRIZZLING CRAGS," "THE SICK SIGHT AND GIDDY PROSPECT OF THE RAVING STREAM..."
IN ALL THIS FLOW AND RESISTANCE, WORDSWORTH SEES SOMETHING OF THE WORKINGS OF HIS OWN MIND.
SELF! NATURE! SPIRIT! THE INTERPLAY OF THESE THINGS WOULD ALSO BE A PREOCCUPATION OF WORDSWORTH'S FUTURE FRIEND, SAMUEL TAYLOR COLERIDGE.
WHEN WE GOT OFF THE CABLE CAR, I BOLTED TO THE SUMMIT, FEELING MY GOATHERD BLOOD.
WHAT WOULD IT BE LIKE TO **REALLY** CLIMB A MOUNTAIN?
I WIN!
BACK IN LUCERNE I TALKED MY WAY INTO A PAIR OF CLIMBING BOOTS BY POINTING OUT THAT THEY WERE WORN BY LOCAL BOYS AND GIRLS ALIKE.
(COLERIDGE MASSAGED HIS WELSH WALKING BOOTS WITH WARM SUET AND TURPENTINE AS WATERPROOFING. IN *THE DHARMA BUMS*, KEROUAC ADMIRES GARY SNYDER'S ITALIAN BOOTS, "EXPENSIVE ONES, HIS PRIDE AND JOY.")

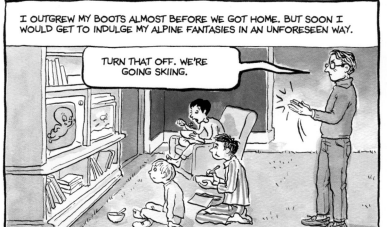

I OUTGREW MY BOOTS ALMOST BEFORE WE GOT HOME. BUT SOON I WOULD GET TO INDULGE MY ALPINE FANTASIES IN AN UNFORESEEN WAY.

TURN THAT OFF. WE'RE GOING SKIING.

UNTIL MIDCENTURY, SKIING HAD BEEN MOSTLY A SPORT FOR THE WEALTHY. BUT NOW THE MIDDLE CLASS WAS TAKING TO THE SLOPES. SMALL SKI AREAS WERE POPPING UP ALL OVER THE PLACE.

WE DROVE DEEP INTO THE WILDS OF PENNSYLVANIA.

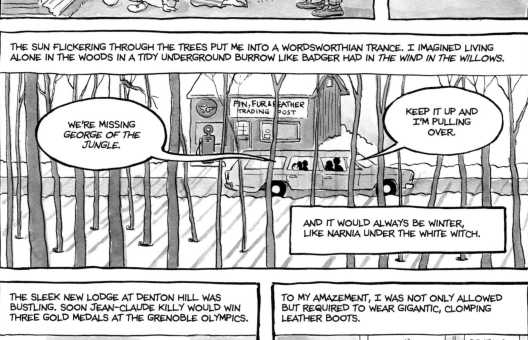

THE SUN FLICKERING THROUGH THE TREES PUT ME INTO A WORDSWORTHIAN TRANCE. I IMAGINED LIVING ALONE IN THE WOODS IN A TIDY UNDERGROUND BURROW LIKE BADGER HAD IN *THE WIND IN THE WILLOWS*.

WE'RE MISSING *GEORGE OF THE JUNGLE*.

KEEP IT UP AND I'M PULLING OVER.

FIN, FUR & FEATHER TRADING POST

AND IT WOULD ALWAYS BE WINTER, LIKE NARNIA UNDER THE WHITE WITCH.

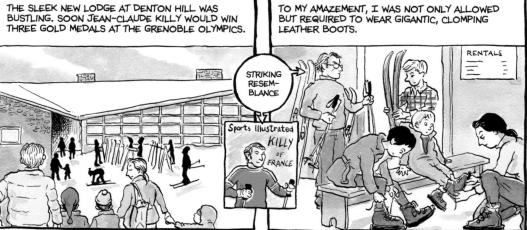

THE SLEEK NEW LODGE AT DENTON HILL WAS BUSTLING. SOON JEAN-CLAUDE KILLY WOULD WIN THREE GOLD MEDALS AT THE GRENOBLE OLYMPICS.

STRIKING RESEM-BLANCE

Sports Illustrated
KILLY OF FRANCE

TO MY AMAZEMENT, I WAS NOT ONLY ALLOWED BUT REQUIRED TO WEAR GIGANTIC, CLOMPING LEATHER BOOTS.

RENTALS

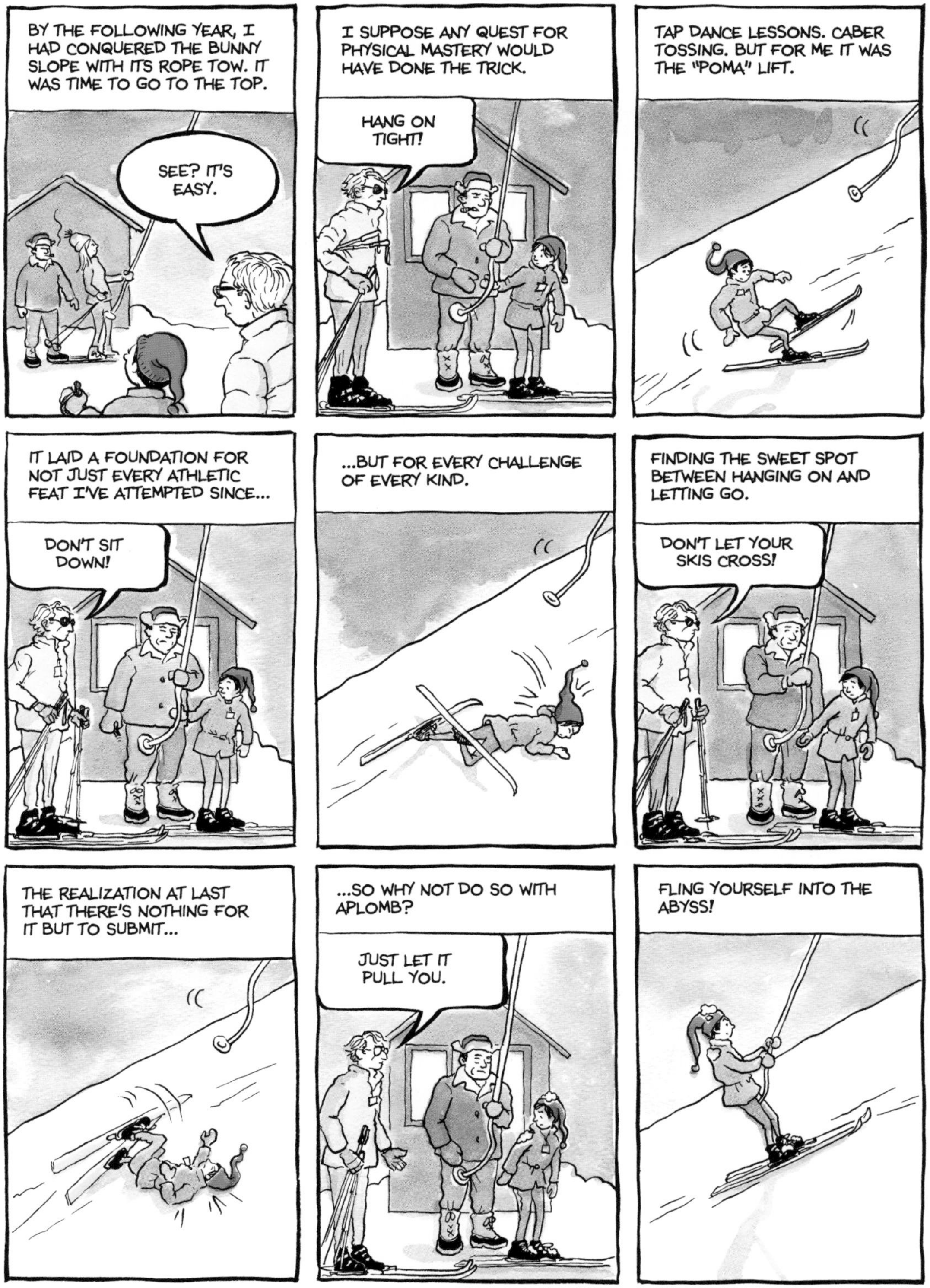
BY THE FOLLOWING YEAR, I HAD CONQUERED THE BUNNY SLOPE WITH ITS ROPE TOW. IT WAS TIME TO GO TO THE TOP.
SEE? IT'S EASY.
I SUPPOSE ANY QUEST FOR PHYSICAL MASTERY WOULD HAVE DONE THE TRICK.
HANG ON TIGHT!
TAP DANCE LESSONS. CABER TOSSING. BUT FOR ME IT WAS THE "POMA" LIFT.
IT LAID A FOUNDATION FOR NOT JUST EVERY ATHLETIC FEAT I'VE ATTEMPTED SINCE...
DON'T SIT DOWN!
...BUT FOR EVERY CHALLENGE OF EVERY KIND.
FINDING THE SWEET SPOT BETWEEN HANGING ON AND LETTING GO.
DON'T LET YOUR SKIS CROSS!
THE REALIZATION AT LAST THAT THERE'S NOTHING FOR IT BUT TO SUBMIT...
...SO WHY NOT DO SO WITH APLOMB?
JUST LET IT PULL YOU.
FLING YOURSELF INTO THE ABYSS!

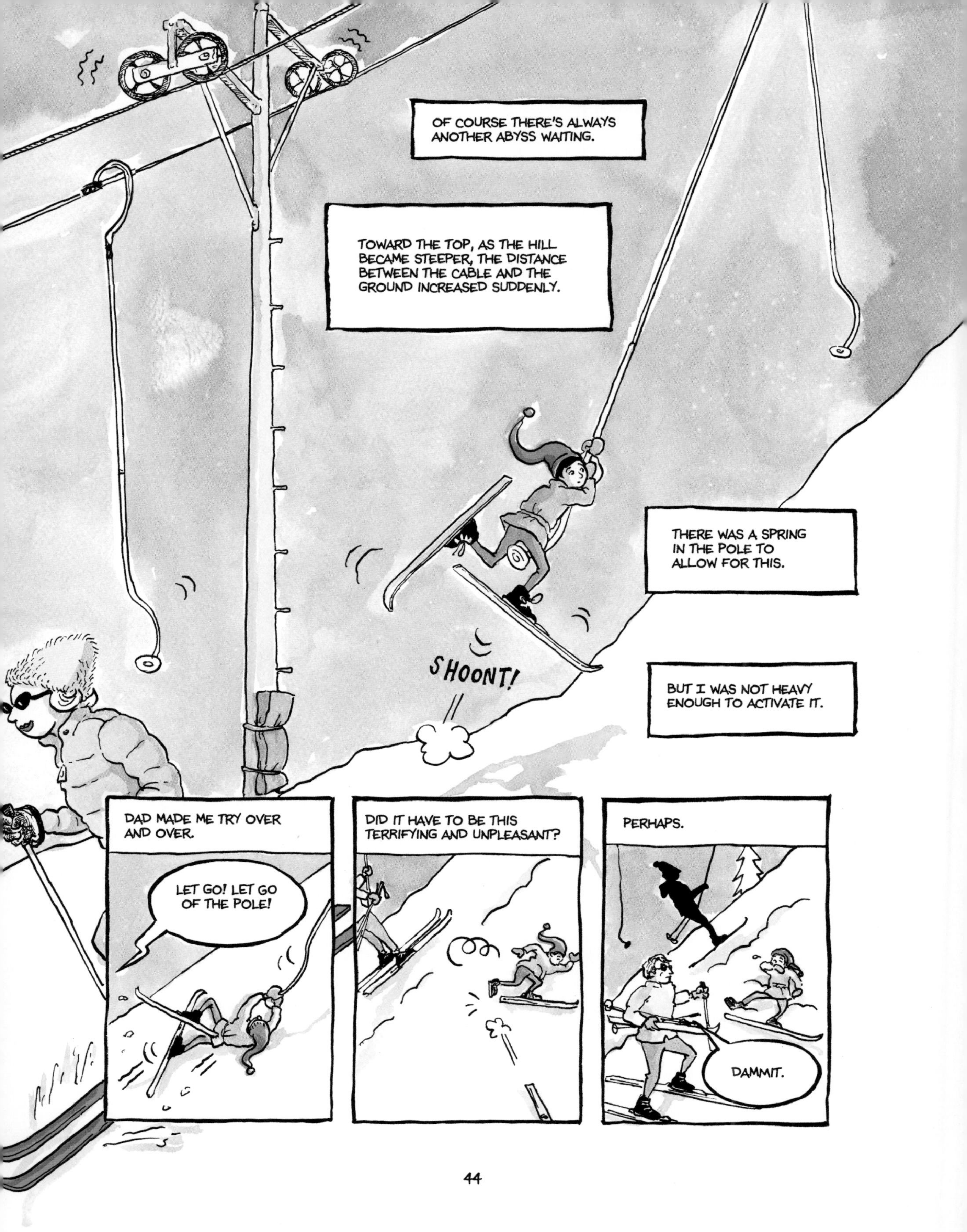
OF COURSE THERE'S ALWAYS ANOTHER ABYSS WAITING.
TOWARD THE TOP, AS THE HILL BECAME STEEPER, THE DISTANCE BETWEEN THE CABLE AND THE GROUND INCREASED SUDDENLY.
THERE WAS A SPRING IN THE POLE TO ALLOW FOR THIS.
SHOONT!
BUT I WAS NOT HEAVY ENOUGH TO ACTIVATE IT.
DAD MADE ME TRY OVER AND OVER.
LET GO! LET GO OF THE POLE!
DID IT HAVE TO BE THIS TERRIFYING AND UNPLEASANT?
PERHAPS.
DAMMIT.

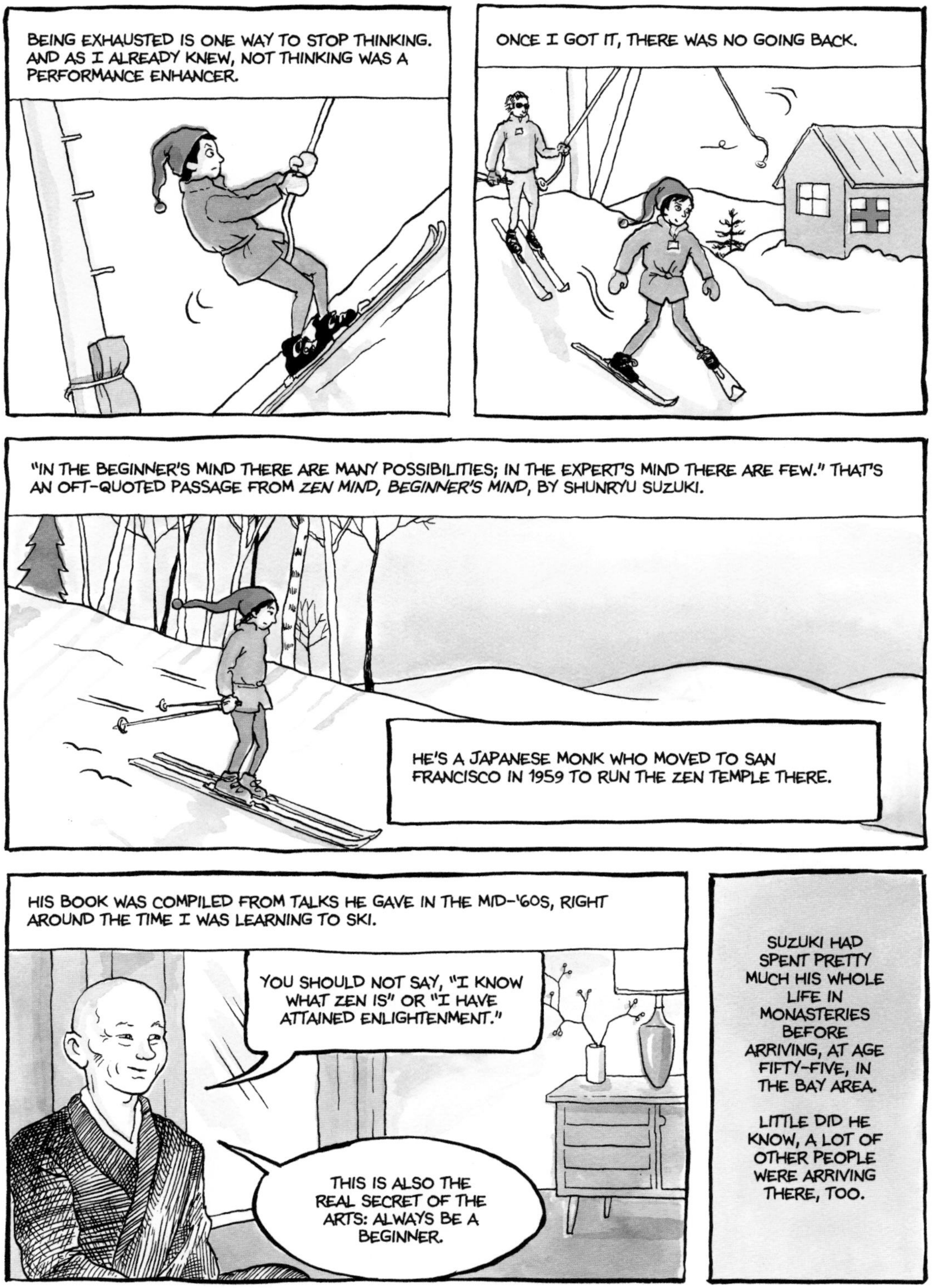
BEING EXHAUSTED IS ONE WAY TO STOP THINKING. AND AS I ALREADY KNEW, NOT THINKING WAS A PERFORMANCE ENHANCER.
ONCE I GOT IT, THERE WAS NO GOING BACK.
"IN THE BEGINNER'S MIND THERE ARE MANY POSSIBILITIES; IN THE EXPERT'S MIND THERE ARE FEW." THAT'S AN OFT-QUOTED PASSAGE FROM *ZEN MIND, BEGINNER'S MIND*, BY SHUNRYU SUZUKI.
HE'S A JAPANESE MONK WHO MOVED TO SAN FRANCISCO IN 1959 TO RUN THE ZEN TEMPLE THERE.
HIS BOOK WAS COMPILED FROM TALKS HE GAVE IN THE MID-'60S, RIGHT AROUND THE TIME I WAS LEARNING TO SKI.
YOU SHOULD NOT SAY, "I KNOW WHAT ZEN IS" OR "I HAVE ATTAINED ENLIGHTENMENT."
THIS IS ALSO THE REAL SECRET OF THE ARTS: ALWAYS BE A BEGINNER.
SUZUKI HAD SPENT PRETTY MUCH HIS WHOLE LIFE IN MONASTERIES BEFORE ARRIVING, AT AGE FIFTY-FIVE, IN THE BAY AREA.
LITTLE DID HE KNOW, A LOT OF OTHER PEOPLE WERE ARRIVING THERE, TOO.

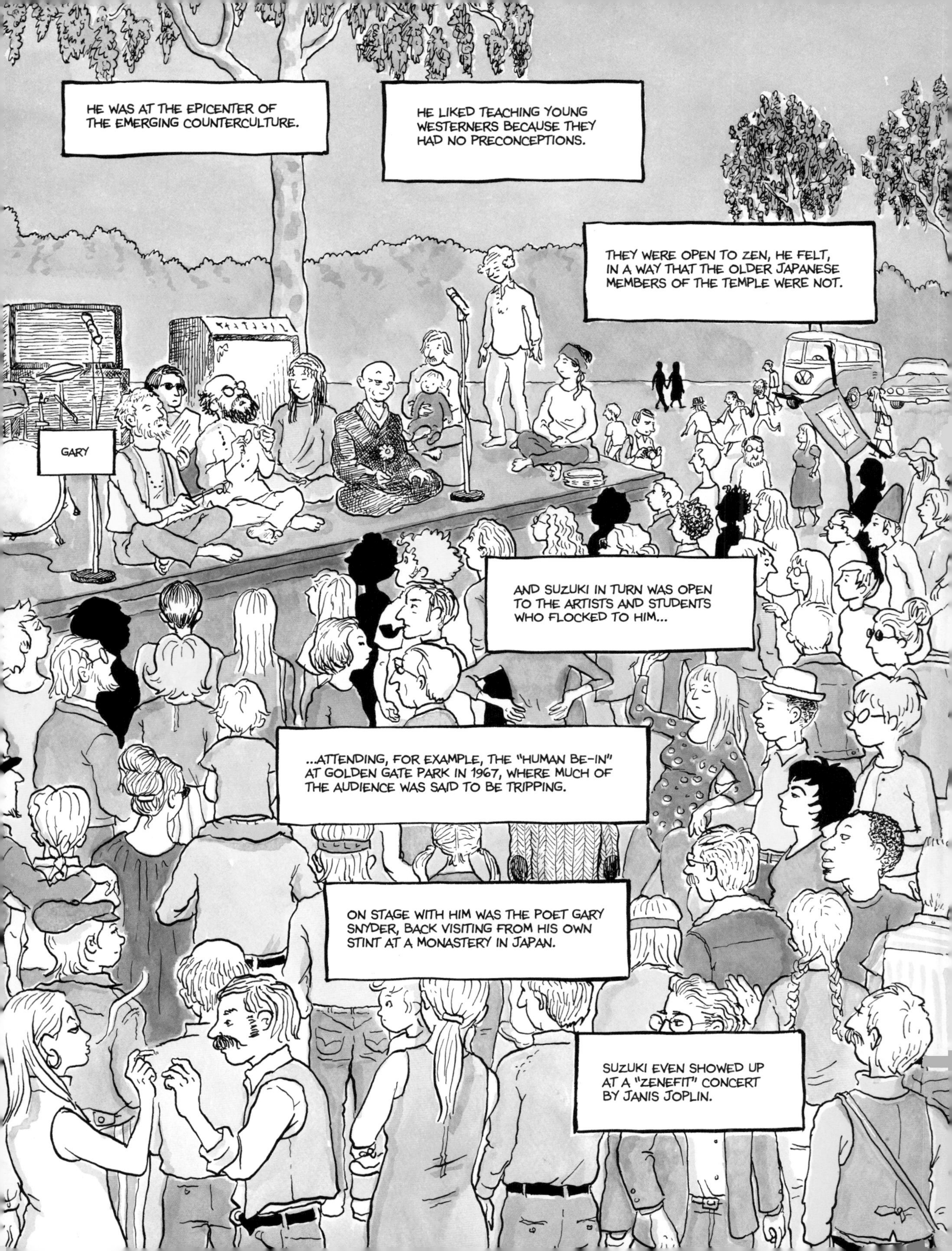
HE WAS AT THE EPICENTER OF THE EMERGING COUNTERCULTURE.
HE LIKED TEACHING YOUNG WESTERNERS BECAUSE THEY HAD NO PRECONCEPTIONS.
THEY WERE OPEN TO ZEN, HE FELT, IN A WAY THAT THE OLDER JAPANESE MEMBERS OF THE TEMPLE WERE NOT.
GARY
AND SUZUKI IN TURN WAS OPEN TO THE ARTISTS AND STUDENTS WHO FLOCKED TO HIM...
...ATTENDING, FOR EXAMPLE, THE "HUMAN BE-IN" AT GOLDEN GATE PARK IN 1967, WHERE MUCH OF THE AUDIENCE WAS SAID TO BE TRIPPING.
ON STAGE WITH HIM WAS THE POET GARY SNYDER, BACK VISITING FROM HIS OWN STINT AT A MONASTERY IN JAPAN.
SUZUKI EVEN SHOWED UP AT A "ZENEFIT" CONCERT BY JANIS JOPLIN.

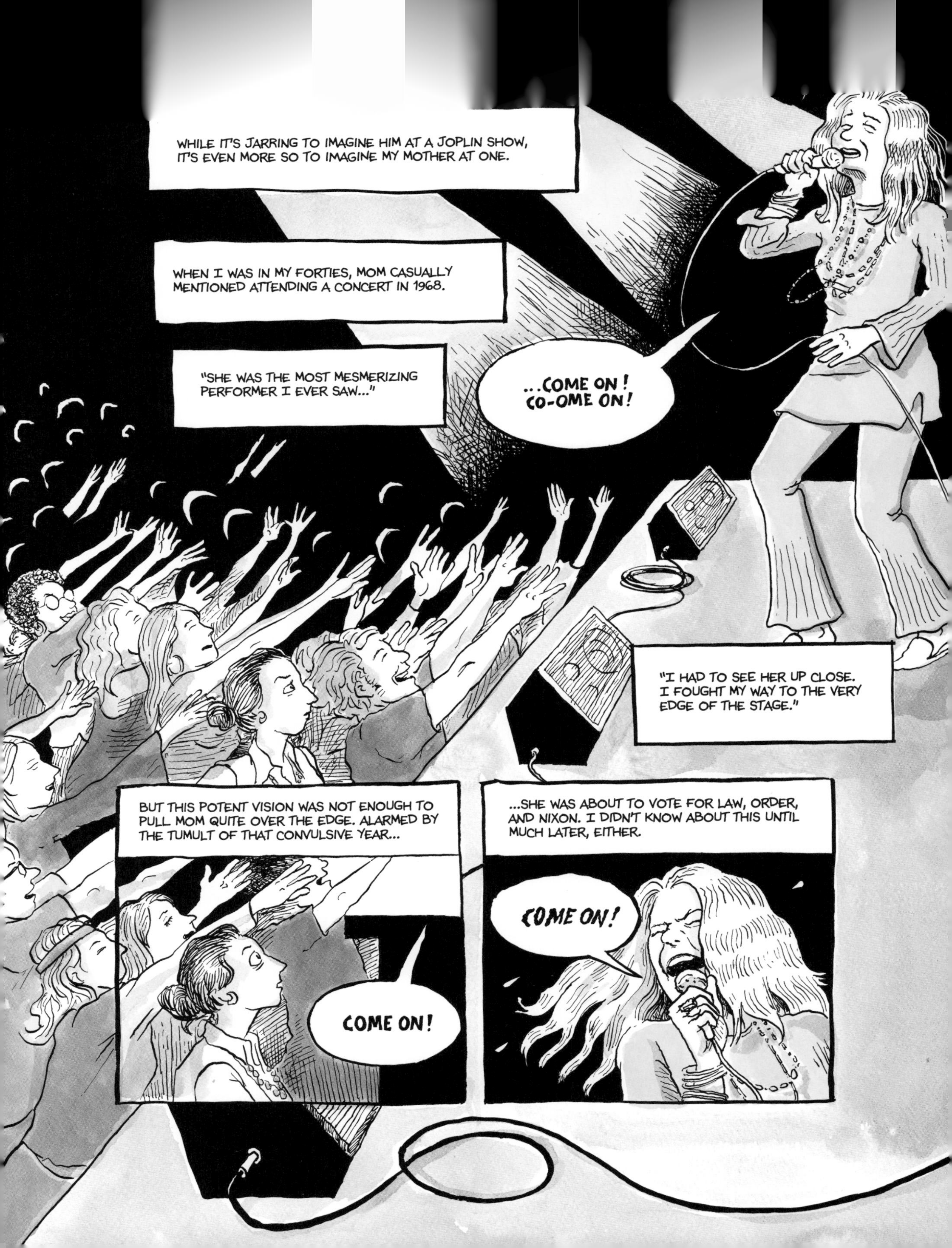
WHILE IT'S JARRING TO IMAGINE HIM AT A JOPLIN SHOW, IT'S EVEN MORE SO TO IMAGINE MY MOTHER AT ONE.
WHEN I WAS IN MY FORTIES, MOM CASUALLY MENTIONED ATTENDING A CONCERT IN 1968.
"SHE WAS THE MOST MESMERIZING PERFORMER I EVER SAW..."
...COME ON! CO-OME ON!
"I HAD TO SEE HER UP CLOSE. I FOUGHT MY WAY TO THE VERY EDGE OF THE STAGE."
BUT THIS POTENT VISION WAS NOT ENOUGH TO PULL MOM QUITE OVER THE EDGE. ALARMED BY THE TUMULT OF THAT CONVULSIVE YEAR...
COME ON!
...SHE WAS ABOUT TO VOTE FOR LAW, ORDER, AND NIXON. I DIDN'T KNOW ABOUT THIS UNTIL MUCH LATER, EITHER.
COME ON!

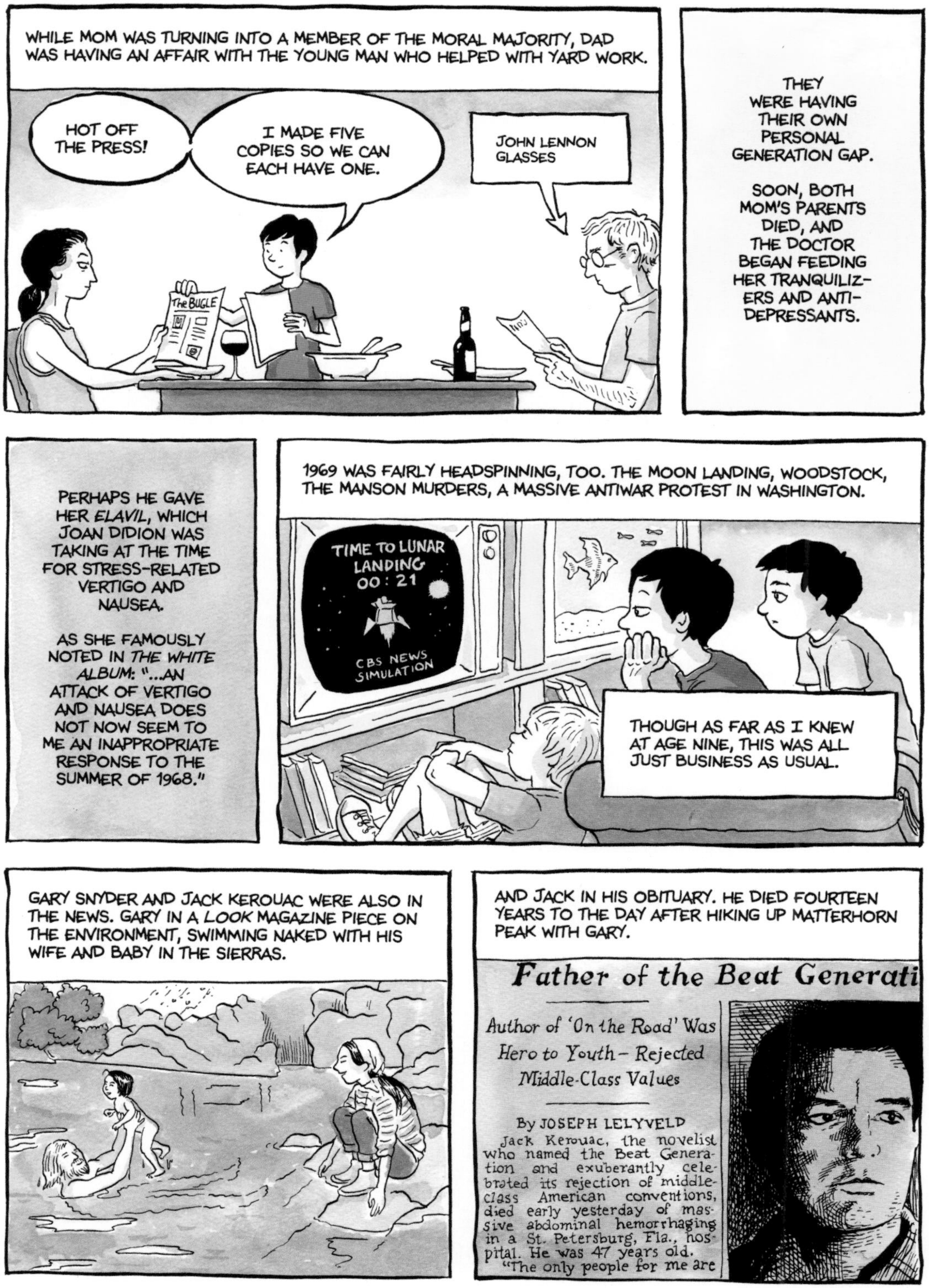
WHILE MOM WAS TURNING INTO A MEMBER OF THE MORAL MAJORITY, DAD WAS HAVING AN AFFAIR WITH THE YOUNG MAN WHO HELPED WITH YARD WORK.
HOT OFF THE PRESS!
I MADE FIVE COPIES SO WE CAN EACH HAVE ONE.
JOHN LENNON GLASSES
The BUGLE
THEY WERE HAVING THEIR OWN PERSONAL GENERATION GAP.
SOON, BOTH MOM'S PARENTS DIED, AND THE DOCTOR BEGAN FEEDING HER TRANQUILIZERS AND ANTI-DEPRESSANTS.
PERHAPS HE GAVE HER *ELAVIL*, WHICH JOAN DIDION WAS TAKING AT THE TIME FOR STRESS-RELATED VERTIGO AND NAUSEA.
AS SHE FAMOUSLY NOTED IN *THE WHITE ALBUM*: "...AN ATTACK OF VERTIGO AND NAUSEA DOES NOT NOW SEEM TO ME AN INAPPROPRIATE RESPONSE TO THE SUMMER OF 1968."
1969 WAS FAIRLY HEADSPINNING, TOO. THE MOON LANDING, WOODSTOCK, THE MANSON MURDERS, A MASSIVE ANTIWAR PROTEST IN WASHINGTON.
TIME TO LUNAR LANDING 00 : 21
CBS NEWS SIMULATION
THOUGH AS FAR AS I KNEW AT AGE NINE, THIS WAS ALL JUST BUSINESS AS USUAL.
GARY SNYDER AND JACK KEROUAC WERE ALSO IN THE NEWS. GARY IN A *LOOK* MAGAZINE PIECE ON THE ENVIRONMENT, SWIMMING NAKED WITH HIS WIFE AND BABY IN THE SIERRAS.
AND JACK IN HIS OBITUARY. HE DIED FOURTEEN YEARS TO THE DAY AFTER HIKING UP MATTERHORN PEAK WITH GARY.
Father of the Beat Generati
Author of 'On the Road' Was Hero to Youth—Rejected Middle-Class Values
By JOSEPH LELYVELD
Jack Kerouac, the novelist who named the Beat Generation and exuberantly celebrated its rejection of middle-class American conventions, died early yesterday of massive abdominal hemorrhaging in a St. Petersburg, Fla., hospital. He was 47 years old.
"The only people for me are

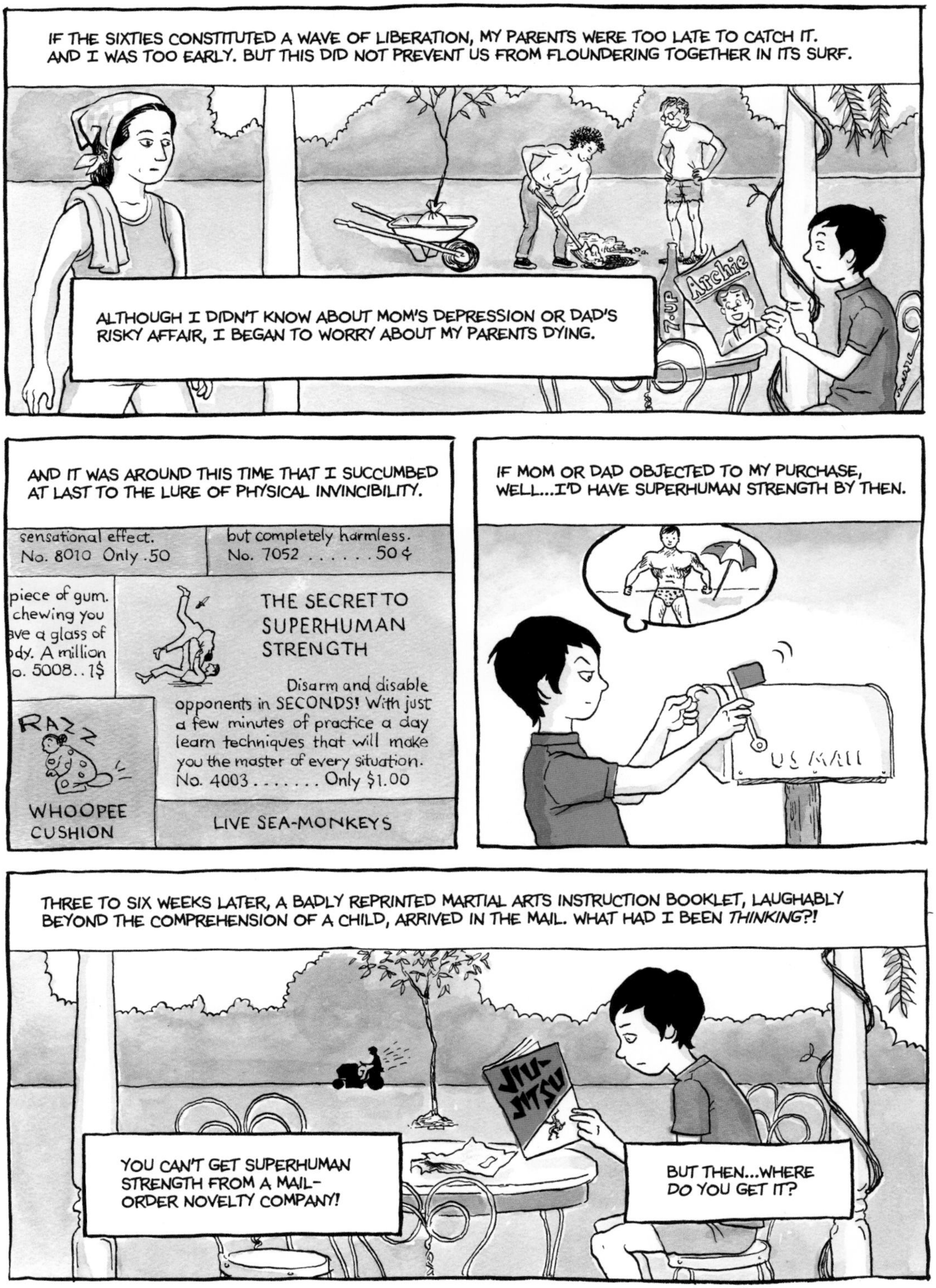

IF THE SIXTIES CONSTITUTED A WAVE OF LIBERATION, MY PARENTS WERE TOO LATE TO CATCH IT. AND I WAS TOO EARLY. BUT THIS DID NOT PREVENT US FROM FLOUNDERING TOGETHER IN ITS SURF.
7-UP
Archie
ALTHOUGH I DIDN'T KNOW ABOUT MOM'S DEPRESSION OR DAD'S RISKY AFFAIR, I BEGAN TO WORRY ABOUT MY PARENTS DYING.
AND IT WAS AROUND THIS TIME THAT I SUCCUMBED AT LAST TO THE LURE OF PHYSICAL INVINCIBILITY.
sensational effect. No. 8010 Only .50
but completely harmless. No. 7052 . . . . . . 50¢
piece of gum. chewing you ave a glass of ody. A million o. 5008. . 1$
THE SECRET TO SUPERHUMAN STRENGTH
Disarm and disable opponents in SECONDS! With just a few minutes of practice a day learn techniques that will make you the master of every situation. No. 4003 . . . . Only $1.00
RAZZ
WHOOPEE CUSHION
LIVE SEA-MONKEYS
IF MOM OR DAD OBJECTED TO MY PURCHASE, WELL...I'D HAVE SUPERHUMAN STRENGTH BY THEN.
US MAIL
THREE TO SIX WEEKS LATER, A BADLY REPRINTED MARTIAL ARTS INSTRUCTION BOOKLET, LAUGHABLY BEYOND THE COMPREHENSION OF A CHILD, ARRIVED IN THE MAIL. WHAT HAD I BEEN *THINKING*?!
JIU-JITSU
YOU CAN'T GET SUPERHUMAN STRENGTH FROM A MAIL-ORDER NOVELTY COMPANY!
BUT THEN...WHERE DO YOU GET IT?

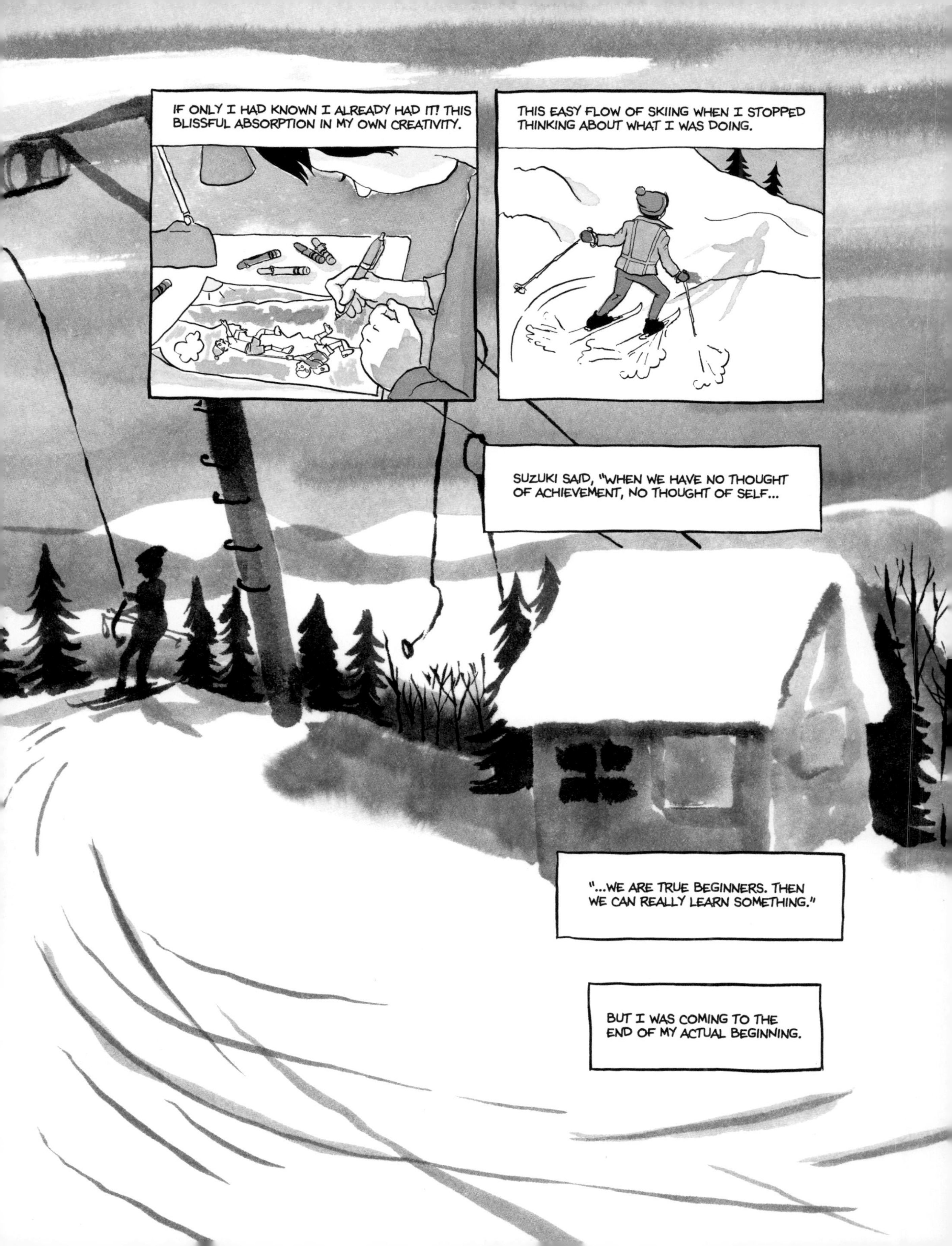
IF ONLY I HAD KNOWN I ALREADY HAD IT! THIS BLISSFUL ABSORPTION IN MY OWN CREATIVITY.
THIS EASY FLOW OF SKIING WHEN I STOPPED THINKING ABOUT WHAT I WAS DOING.
SUZUKI SAID, "WHEN WE HAVE NO THOUGHT OF ACHIEVEMENT, NO THOUGHT OF SELF...
"...WE ARE TRUE BEGINNERS. THEN WE CAN REALLY LEARN SOMETHING."
BUT I WAS COMING TO THE END OF MY ACTUAL BEGINNING.

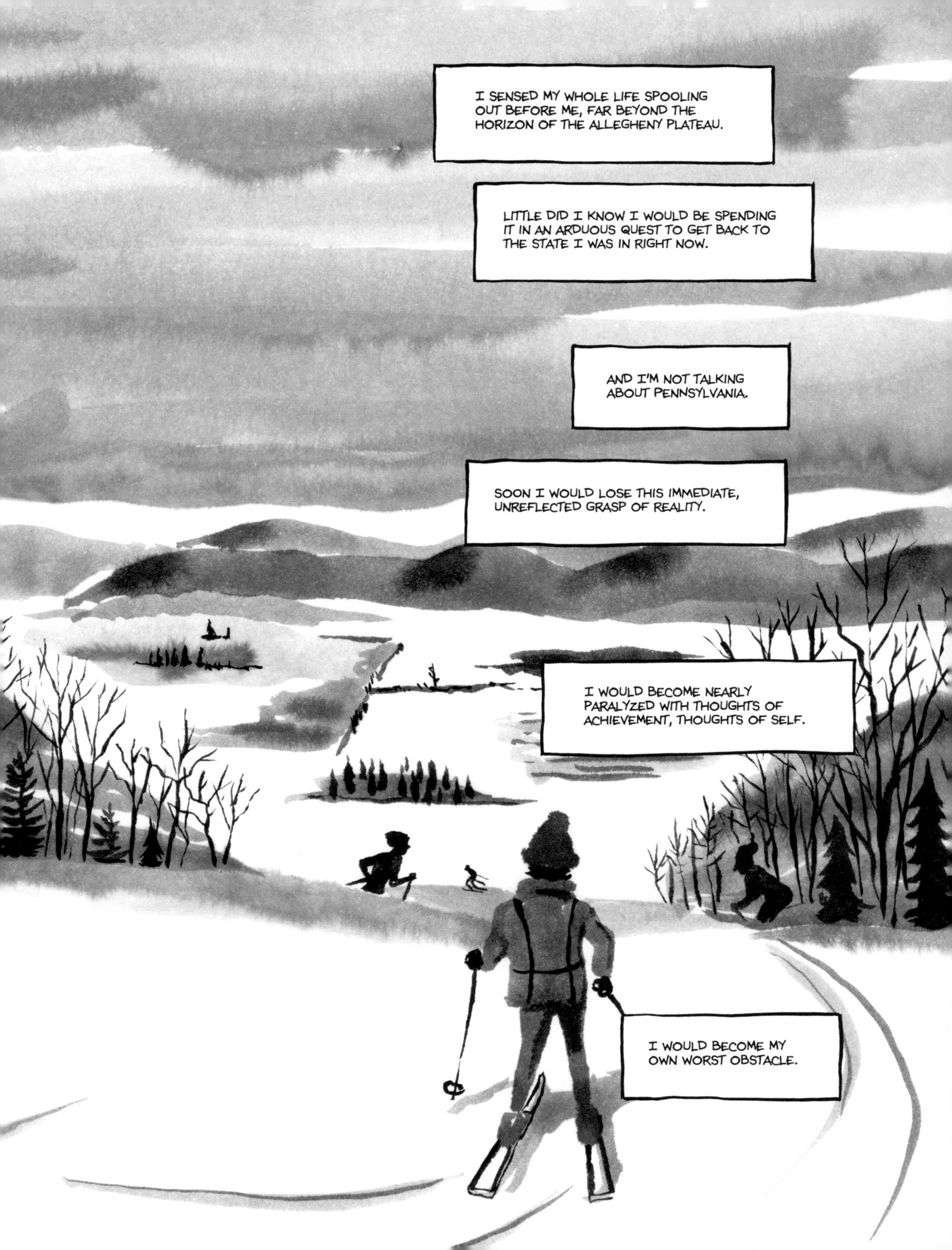
I SENSED MY WHOLE LIFE SPOOLING OUT BEFORE ME, FAR BEYOND THE HORIZON OF THE ALLEGHENY PLATEAU.
LITTLE DID I KNOW I WOULD BE SPENDING IT IN AN ARDUOUS QUEST TO GET BACK TO THE STATE I WAS IN RIGHT NOW.
AND I'M NOT TALKING ABOUT PENNSYLVANIA.
SOON I WOULD LOSE THIS IMMEDIATE, UNREFLECTED GRASP OF REALITY.
I WOULD BECOME NEARLY PARALYZED WITH THOUGHTS OF ACHIEVEMENT, THOUGHTS OF SELF.
I WOULD BECOME MY OWN WORST OBSTACLE.

1970s

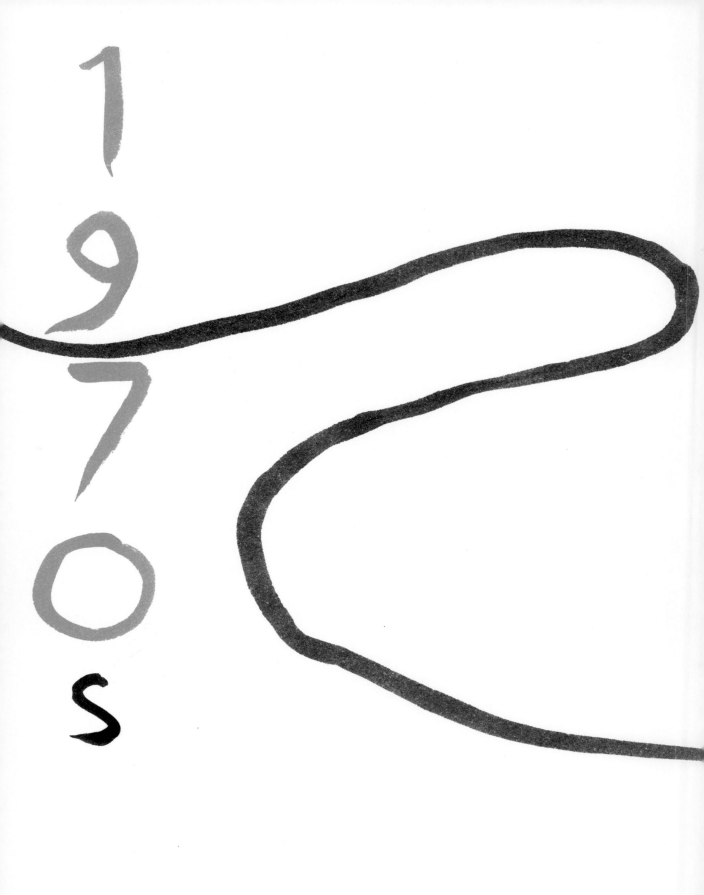

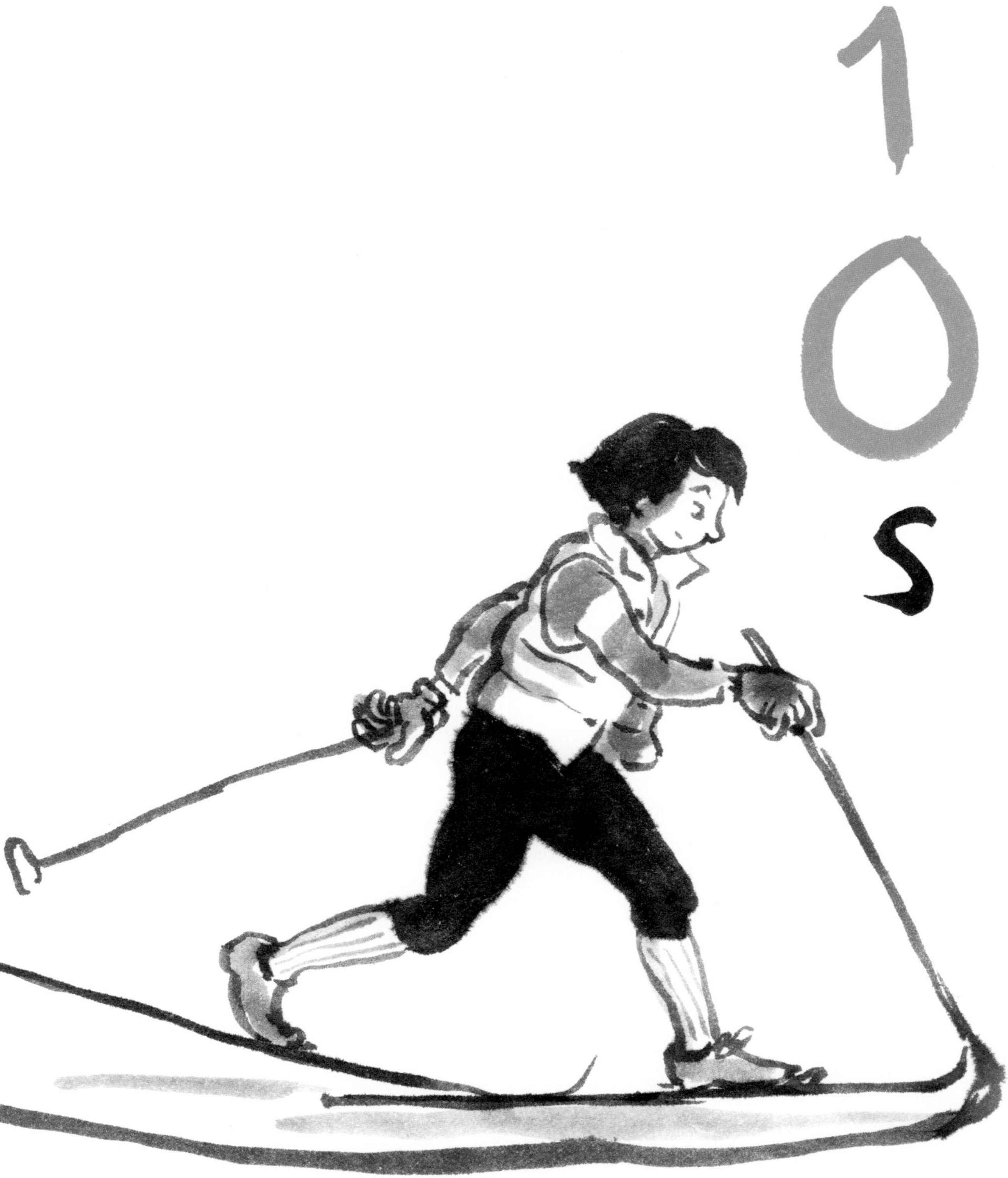
10s

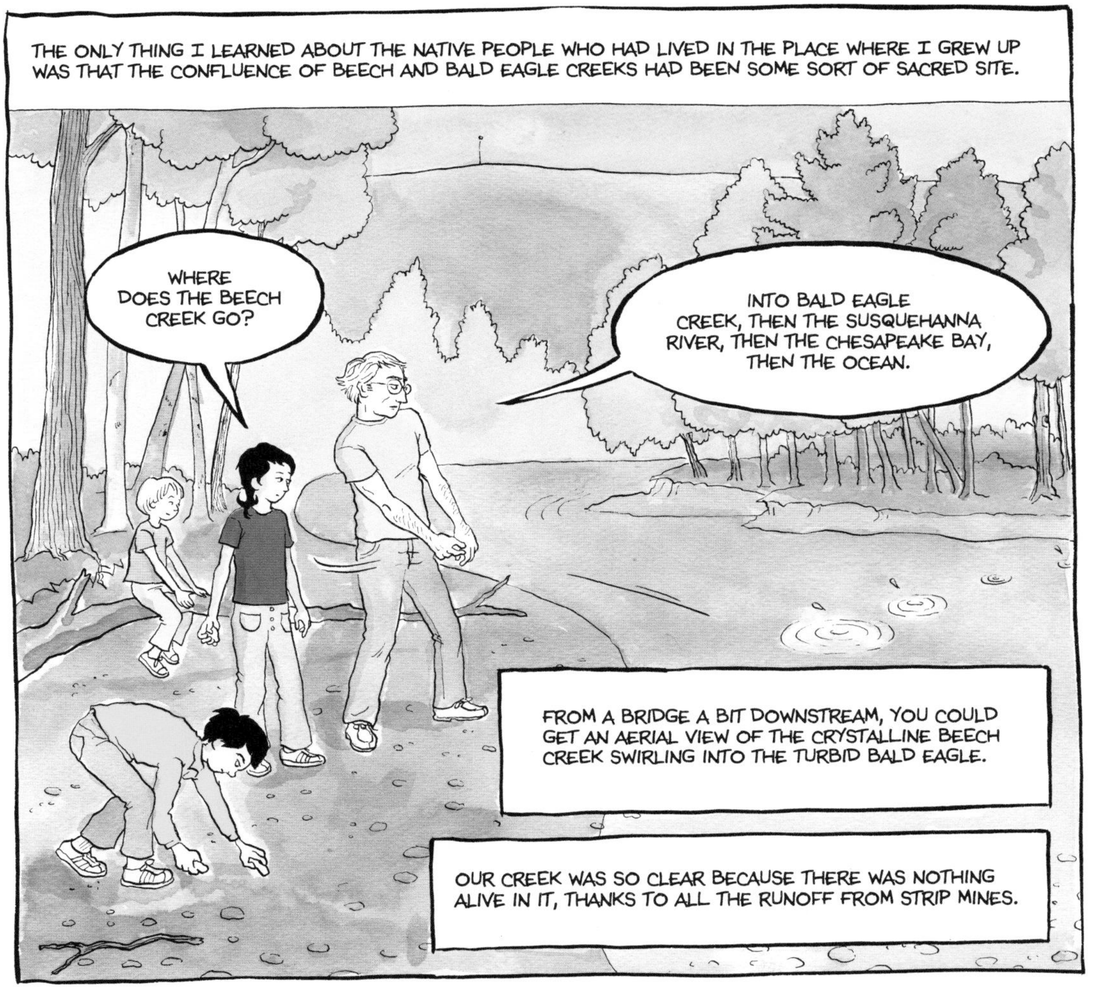
THE ONLY THING I LEARNED ABOUT THE NATIVE PEOPLE WHO HAD LIVED IN THE PLACE WHERE I GREW UP WAS THAT THE CONFLUENCE OF BEECH AND BALD EAGLE CREEKS HAD BEEN SOME SORT OF SACRED SITE.
WHERE DOES THE BEECH CREEK GO?
INTO BALD EAGLE CREEK, THEN THE SUSQUEHANNA RIVER, THEN THE CHESAPEAKE BAY, THEN THE OCEAN.
FROM A BRIDGE A BIT DOWNSTREAM, YOU COULD GET AN AERIAL VIEW OF THE CRYSTALLINE BEECH CREEK SWIRLING INTO THE TURBID BALD EAGLE.
OUR CREEK WAS SO CLEAR BECAUSE THERE WAS NOTHING ALIVE IN IT, THANKS TO ALL THE RUNOFF FROM STRIP MINES.

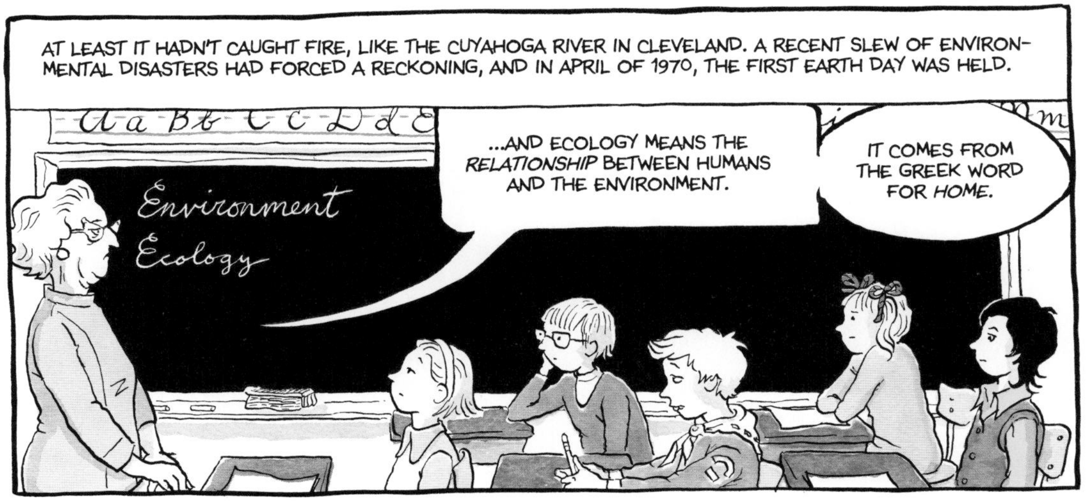
AT LEAST IT HADN'T CAUGHT FIRE, LIKE THE CUYAHOGA RIVER IN CLEVELAND. A RECENT SLEW OF ENVIRONMENTAL DISASTERS HAD FORCED A RECKONING, AND IN APRIL OF 1970, THE FIRST EARTH DAY WAS HELD.
Environment
Ecology
...AND ECOLOGY MEANS THE *RELATIONSHIP* BETWEEN HUMANS AND THE ENVIRONMENT.
IT COMES FROM THE GREEK WORD FOR *HOME*.

OIL SPILLS, SMOG, GARBAGE, LOST WETLANDS. IF THINGS WENT ON LIKE THIS, I LEARNED, THE PLANET WOULD SOON BE UNINHABITABLE.

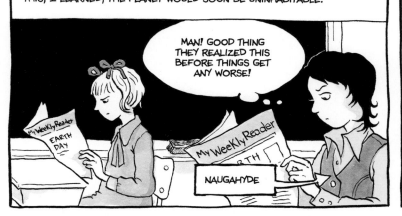

MAN! GOOD THING THEY REALIZED THIS BEFORE THINGS GET ANY WORSE!

My Weekly Reader
EARTH DAY

My Weekly Reader
RTH

NAUGAHYDE

ALTHOUGH THE ROMANTICS HAD EXPRESSED ALARM ABOUT THE ENVIRONMENT AS SOON AS THE FIRST FACTORIES STARTED SPEWING PARTICULATES, IT HAD TAKEN A COUPLE HUNDRED YEARS FOR THAT SENTIMENT TO REALLY GAIN TRACTION.

BUT NOW PEOPLE WERE STARTING TO UNDERSTAND THAT WE LIVE IN AN ECOSYSTEM. IN THE SUMMER OF 1971, DAD BROUGHT A CURIOUS BOOK HOME.

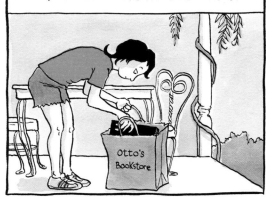

Otto's Bookstore

IT WAS LIKE THE SEARS "WISH BOOK" ON LSD.* STEWART BRAND, THE GUY BEHIND IT, WAS OBSESSED WITH THE SATELLITE PHOTOS NASA HAD BEEN TAKING OF THE PLANET.

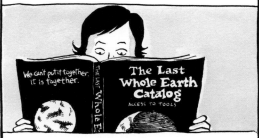

We can't put it together. It is together.

THE LAST WHOLE EARTH CATALOG

The Last Whole Earth Catalog
ACCESS TO TOOLS

*NOT THAT I KNEW ANYTHING ABOUT LSD YET, BUT IF I'D READ CLOSELY ENOUGH I MIGHT HAVE FOUND A RECIPE FOR IT IN HERE.

IF PEOPLE COULD ACTUALLY SEE IMAGES OF THE WHOLE EARTH, HE REASONED, WE'D UNDERSTAND IT WAS NOT AN UNLIMITED RESOURCE THERE FOR THE PILLAGING.

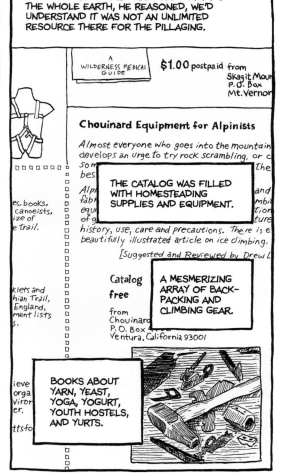

A WILDERNESS MEDICAL GUIDE
$1.00 postpaid from
Skagit Moun
P. O. Box
Mt. Vernor

Chouinard Equipment for Alpinists

Almost everyone who goes into the mountain develops an urge to try rock scrambling, or c som   The
bes

THE CATALOG WAS FILLED WITH HOMESTEADING SUPPLIES AND EQUIPMENT.

Alp   and
fab   mbi
equi   tion
of g   ture
history, use, care and precautions. There is e
beautifully illustrated article on ice climbing.

[Suggested and Reviewed by Drew L

Catalog
free

A MESMERIZING ARRAY OF BACK-PACKING AND CLIMBING GEAR.

from
Chouinard
P. O. Box 4
Ventura, California 93001

es, books, canoeists, ize of e trail.

klets and hian Trail, England, ment lists s.

ieve orga viror er.

ttsfo

BOOKS ABOUT YARN, YEAST, YOGA, YOGURT, YOUTH HOSTELS, AND YURTS.

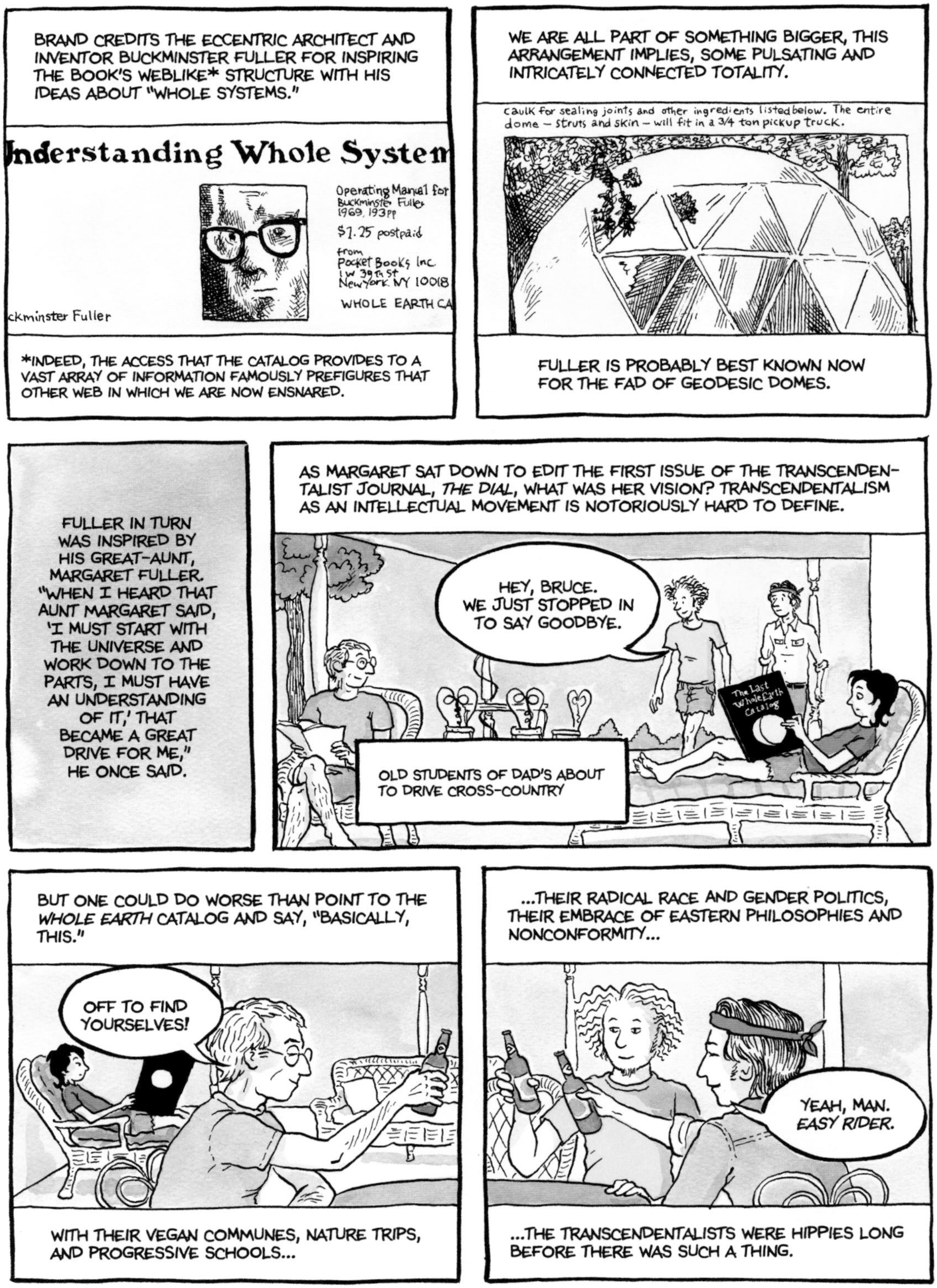
BRAND CREDITS THE ECCENTRIC ARCHITECT AND INVENTOR BUCKMINSTER FULLER FOR INSPIRING THE BOOK'S WEBLIKE* STRUCTURE WITH HIS IDEAS ABOUT "WHOLE SYSTEMS."
Inderstanding Whole System
Operating Manual for Buckminster Fuller 1969, 193pp
$1.25 postpaid
from Pocket Books Inc. 1 W 39th St New York, NY 10018
WHOLE EARTH CA
ckminster Fuller
*INDEED, THE ACCESS THAT THE CATALOG PROVIDES TO A VAST ARRAY OF INFORMATION FAMOUSLY PREFIGURES THAT OTHER WEB IN WHICH WE ARE NOW ENSNARED.
WE ARE ALL PART OF SOMETHING BIGGER, THIS ARRANGEMENT IMPLIES, SOME PULSATING AND INTRICATELY CONNECTED TOTALITY.
caulk for sealing joints and other ingredients listed below. The entire dome – struts and skin – will fit in a 3/4 ton pickup truck.
FULLER IS PROBABLY BEST KNOWN NOW FOR THE FAD OF GEODESIC DOMES.
FULLER IN TURN WAS INSPIRED BY HIS GREAT-AUNT, MARGARET FULLER. "WHEN I HEARD THAT AUNT MARGARET SAID, 'I MUST START WITH THE UNIVERSE AND WORK DOWN TO THE PARTS, I MUST HAVE AN UNDERSTANDING OF IT,' THAT BECAME A GREAT DRIVE FOR ME," HE ONCE SAID.
AS MARGARET SAT DOWN TO EDIT THE FIRST ISSUE OF THE TRANSCENDENTALIST JOURNAL, *THE DIAL*, WHAT WAS HER VISION? TRANSCENDENTALISM AS AN INTELLECTUAL MOVEMENT IS NOTORIOUSLY HARD TO DEFINE.
HEY, BRUCE. WE JUST STOPPED IN TO SAY GOODBYE.
The Last Whole Earth Catalog
OLD STUDENTS OF DAD'S ABOUT TO DRIVE CROSS-COUNTRY
BUT ONE COULD DO WORSE THAN POINT TO THE *WHOLE EARTH* CATALOG AND SAY, "BASICALLY, THIS."
OFF TO FIND YOURSELVES!
WITH THEIR VEGAN COMMUNES, NATURE TRIPS, AND PROGRESSIVE SCHOOLS...
...THEIR RADICAL RACE AND GENDER POLITICS, THEIR EMBRACE OF EASTERN PHILOSOPHIES AND NONCONFORMITY...
YEAH, MAN. *EASY RIDER.*
...THE TRANSCENDENTALISTS WERE HIPPIES LONG BEFORE THERE WAS SUCH A THING.

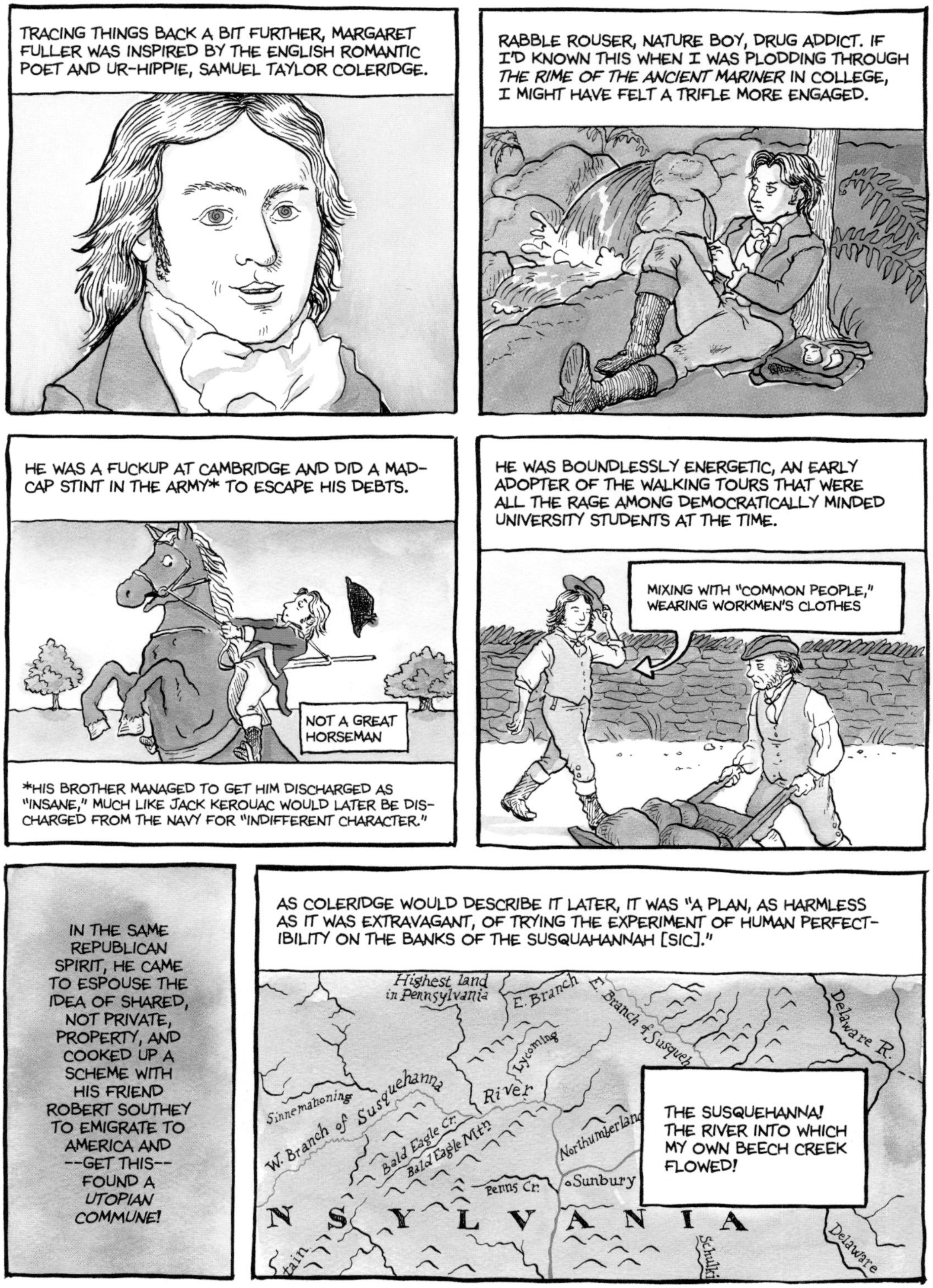
TRACING THINGS BACK A BIT FURTHER, MARGARET FULLER WAS INSPIRED BY THE ENGLISH ROMANTIC POET AND UR-HIPPIE, SAMUEL TAYLOR COLERIDGE.
RABBLE ROUSER, NATURE BOY, DRUG ADDICT. IF I'D KNOWN THIS WHEN I WAS PLODDING THROUGH *THE RIME OF THE ANCIENT MARINER* IN COLLEGE, I MIGHT HAVE FELT A TRIFLE MORE ENGAGED.
HE WAS A FUCKUP AT CAMBRIDGE AND DID A MAD-CAP STINT IN THE ARMY* TO ESCAPE HIS DEBTS.
NOT A GREAT HORSEMAN
*HIS BROTHER MANAGED TO GET HIM DISCHARGED AS "INSANE," MUCH LIKE JACK KEROUAC WOULD LATER BE DISCHARGED FROM THE NAVY FOR "INDIFFERENT CHARACTER."
HE WAS BOUNDLESSLY ENERGETIC, AN EARLY ADOPTER OF THE WALKING TOURS THAT WERE ALL THE RAGE AMONG DEMOCRATICALLY MINDED UNIVERSITY STUDENTS AT THE TIME.
MIXING WITH "COMMON PEOPLE," WEARING WORKMEN'S CLOTHES
IN THE SAME REPUBLICAN SPIRIT, HE CAME TO ESPOUSE THE IDEA OF SHARED, NOT PRIVATE, PROPERTY, AND COOKED UP A SCHEME WITH HIS FRIEND ROBERT SOUTHEY TO EMIGRATE TO AMERICA AND --GET THIS-- FOUND A *UTOPIAN COMMUNE!*
AS COLERIDGE WOULD DESCRIBE IT LATER, IT WAS "A PLAN, AS HARMLESS AS IT WAS EXTRAVAGANT, OF TRYING THE EXPERIMENT OF HUMAN PERFECTIBILITY ON THE BANKS OF THE SUSQUAHANNAH [SIC]."
Highest land in Pennsylvania
E. Branch
E. Branch of Susqueh
Delaware R.
Lycoming
W. Branch of Susquehanna
River
Sinnemahoning
Bald Eagle Cr.
Bald Eagle Mtn
Northumberland
Penns Cr.
Sunbury
NSYLVANIA
Schulki
Delaware
THE SUSQUEHANNA! THE RIVER INTO WHICH MY OWN BEECH CREEK FLOWED!

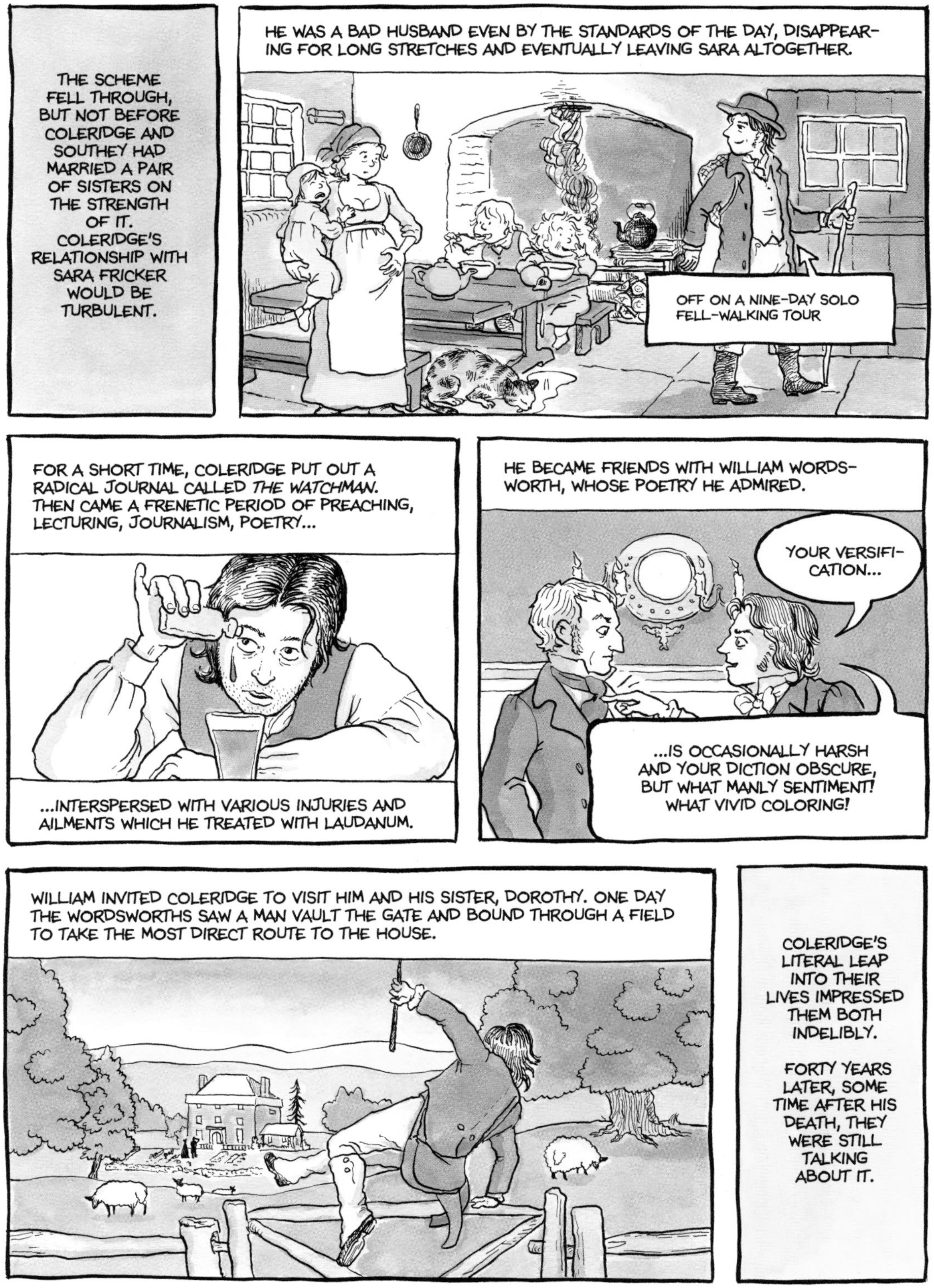
THE SCHEME FELL THROUGH, BUT NOT BEFORE COLERIDGE AND SOUTHEY HAD MARRIED A PAIR OF SISTERS ON THE STRENGTH OF IT. COLERIDGE'S RELATIONSHIP WITH SARA FRICKER WOULD BE TURBULENT.
HE WAS A BAD HUSBAND EVEN BY THE STANDARDS OF THE DAY, DISAPPEARING FOR LONG STRETCHES AND EVENTUALLY LEAVING SARA ALTOGETHER.
OFF ON A NINE-DAY SOLO FELL-WALKING TOUR
FOR A SHORT TIME, COLERIDGE PUT OUT A RADICAL JOURNAL CALLED *THE WATCHMAN*. THEN CAME A FRENETIC PERIOD OF PREACHING, LECTURING, JOURNALISM, POETRY...
...INTERSPERSED WITH VARIOUS INJURIES AND AILMENTS WHICH HE TREATED WITH LAUDANUM.
HE BECAME FRIENDS WITH WILLIAM WORDSWORTH, WHOSE POETRY HE ADMIRED.
YOUR VERSIFICATION...
...IS OCCASIONALLY HARSH AND YOUR DICTION OBSCURE, BUT WHAT MANLY SENTIMENT! WHAT VIVID COLORING!
WILLIAM INVITED COLERIDGE TO VISIT HIM AND HIS SISTER, DOROTHY. ONE DAY THE WORDSWORTHS SAW A MAN VAULT THE GATE AND BOUND THROUGH A FIELD TO TAKE THE MOST DIRECT ROUTE TO THE HOUSE.
COLERIDGE'S LITERAL LEAP INTO THEIR LIVES IMPRESSED THEM BOTH INDELIBLY.
FORTY YEARS LATER, SOME TIME AFTER HIS DEATH, THEY WERE STILL TALKING ABOUT IT.

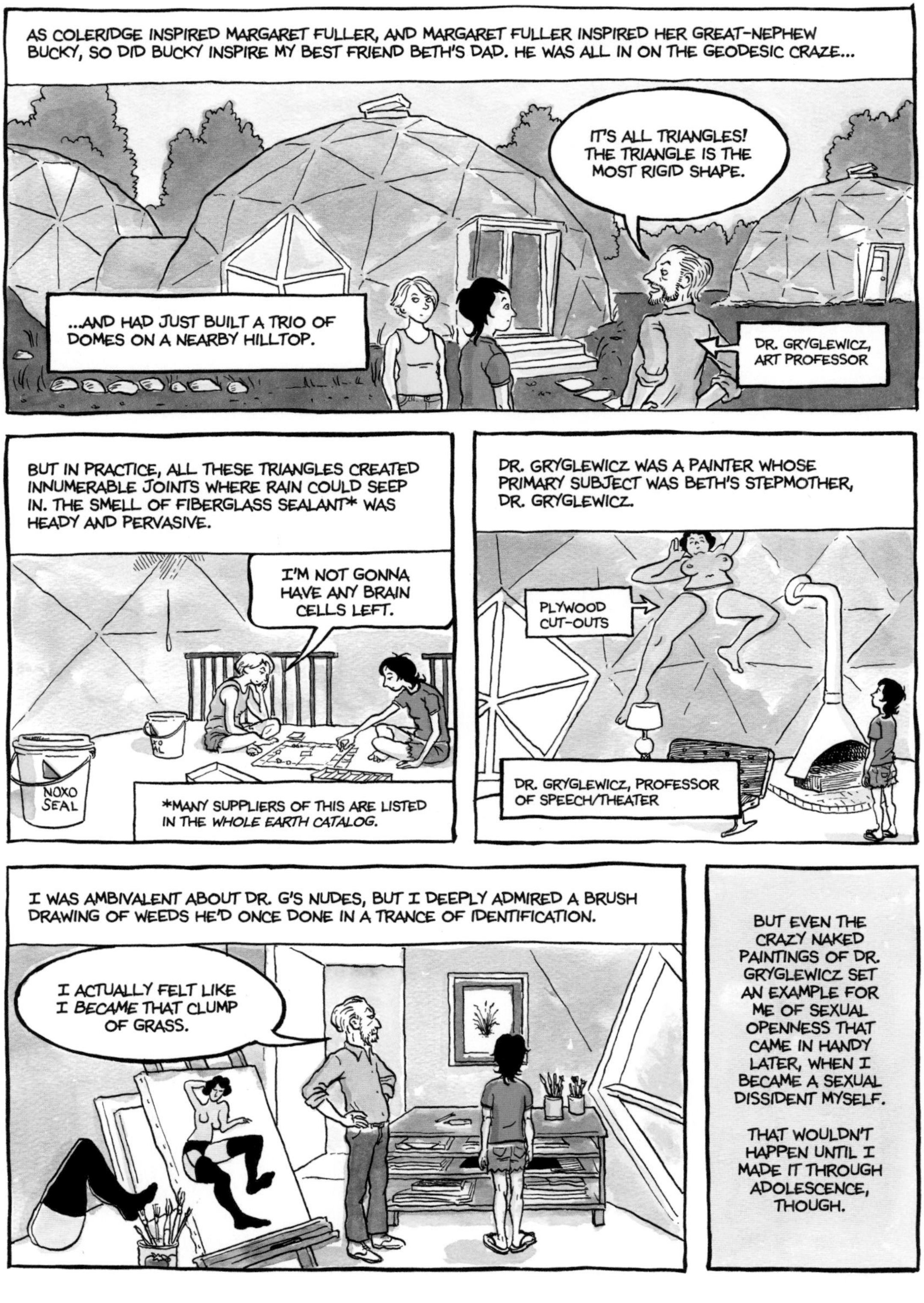
AS COLERIDGE INSPIRED MARGARET FULLER, AND MARGARET FULLER INSPIRED HER GREAT-NEPHEW BUCKY, SO DID BUCKY INSPIRE MY BEST FRIEND BETH'S DAD. HE WAS ALL IN ON THE GEODESIC CRAZE...
IT'S ALL TRIANGLES! THE TRIANGLE IS THE MOST RIGID SHAPE.
...AND HAD JUST BUILT A TRIO OF DOMES ON A NEARBY HILLTOP.
DR. GRYGLEWICZ, ART PROFESSOR
BUT IN PRACTICE, ALL THESE TRIANGLES CREATED INNUMERABLE JOINTS WHERE RAIN COULD SEEP IN. THE SMELL OF FIBERGLASS SEALANT* WAS HEADY AND PERVASIVE.
I'M NOT GONNA HAVE ANY BRAIN CELLS LEFT.
NOXO SEAL
*MANY SUPPLIERS OF THIS ARE LISTED IN THE *WHOLE EARTH CATALOG*.
DR. GRYGLEWICZ WAS A PAINTER WHOSE PRIMARY SUBJECT WAS BETH'S STEPMOTHER, DR. GRYGLEWICZ.
PLYWOOD CUT-OUTS
DR. GRYGLEWICZ, PROFESSOR OF SPEECH/THEATER
I WAS AMBIVALENT ABOUT DR. G'S NUDES, BUT I DEEPLY ADMIRED A BRUSH DRAWING OF WEEDS HE'D ONCE DONE IN A TRANCE OF IDENTIFICATION.
I ACTUALLY FELT LIKE I *BECAME* THAT CLUMP OF GRASS.
BUT EVEN THE CRAZY NAKED PAINTINGS OF DR. GRYGLEWICZ SET AN EXAMPLE FOR ME OF SEXUAL OPENNESS THAT CAME IN HANDY LATER, WHEN I BECAME A SEXUAL DISSIDENT MYSELF.
THAT WOULDN'T HAPPEN UNTIL I MADE IT THROUGH ADOLESCENCE, THOUGH.

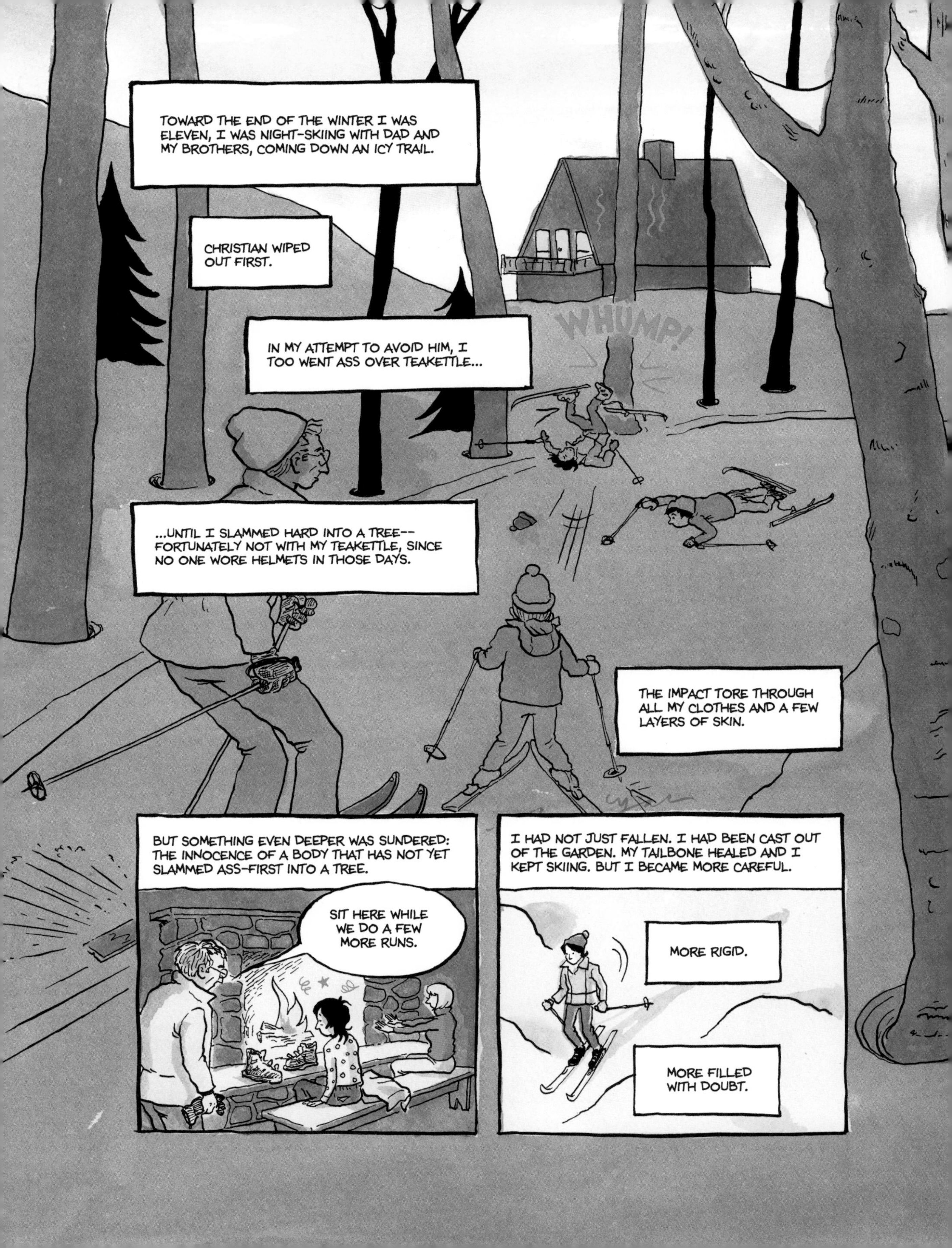
TOWARD THE END OF THE WINTER I WAS ELEVEN, I WAS NIGHT-SKIING WITH DAD AND MY BROTHERS, COMING DOWN AN ICY TRAIL.
CHRISTIAN WIPED OUT FIRST.
IN MY ATTEMPT TO AVOID HIM, I TOO WENT ASS OVER TEAKETTLE...
WHUMP!
...UNTIL I SLAMMED HARD INTO A TREE--FORTUNATELY NOT WITH MY TEAKETTLE, SINCE NO ONE WORE HELMETS IN THOSE DAYS.
THE IMPACT TORE THROUGH ALL MY CLOTHES AND A FEW LAYERS OF SKIN.
BUT SOMETHING EVEN DEEPER WAS SUNDERED: THE INNOCENCE OF A BODY THAT HAS NOT YET SLAMMED ASS-FIRST INTO A TREE.
SIT HERE WHILE WE DO A FEW MORE RUNS.
I HAD NOT JUST FALLEN. I HAD BEEN CAST OUT OF THE GARDEN. MY TAILBONE HEALED AND I KEPT SKIING. BUT I BECAME MORE CAREFUL.
MORE RIGID.
MORE FILLED WITH DOUBT.

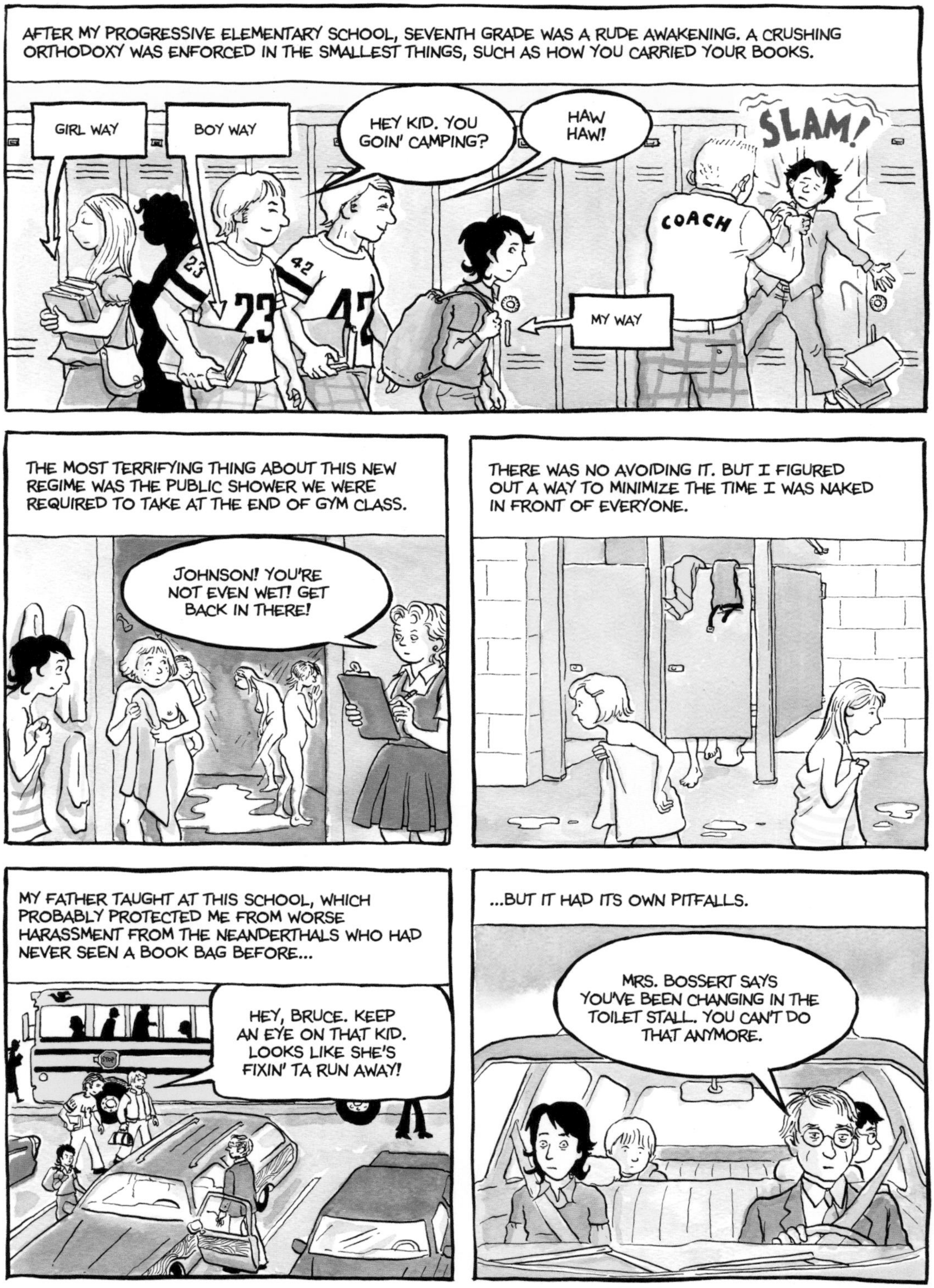
AFTER MY PROGRESSIVE ELEMENTARY SCHOOL, SEVENTH GRADE WAS A RUDE AWAKENING. A CRUSHING ORTHODOXY WAS ENFORCED IN THE SMALLEST THINGS, SUCH AS HOW YOU CARRIED YOUR BOOKS.
GIRL WAY
BOY WAY
HEY KID. YOU GOIN' CAMPING?
HAW HAW!
SLAM!
COACH
MY WAY
THE MOST TERRIFYING THING ABOUT THIS NEW REGIME WAS THE PUBLIC SHOWER WE WERE REQUIRED TO TAKE AT THE END OF GYM CLASS.
JOHNSON! YOU'RE NOT EVEN WET! GET BACK IN THERE!
THERE WAS NO AVOIDING IT. BUT I FIGURED OUT A WAY TO MINIMIZE THE TIME I WAS NAKED IN FRONT OF EVERYONE.
MY FATHER TAUGHT AT THIS SCHOOL, WHICH PROBABLY PROTECTED ME FROM WORSE HARASSMENT FROM THE NEANDERTHALS WHO HAD NEVER SEEN A BOOK BAG BEFORE...
HEY, BRUCE. KEEP AN EYE ON THAT KID. LOOKS LIKE SHE'S FIXIN' TA RUN AWAY!
...BUT IT HAD ITS OWN PITFALLS.
MRS. BOSSERT SAYS YOU'VE BEEN CHANGING IN THE TOILET STALL. YOU CAN'T DO THAT ANYMORE.

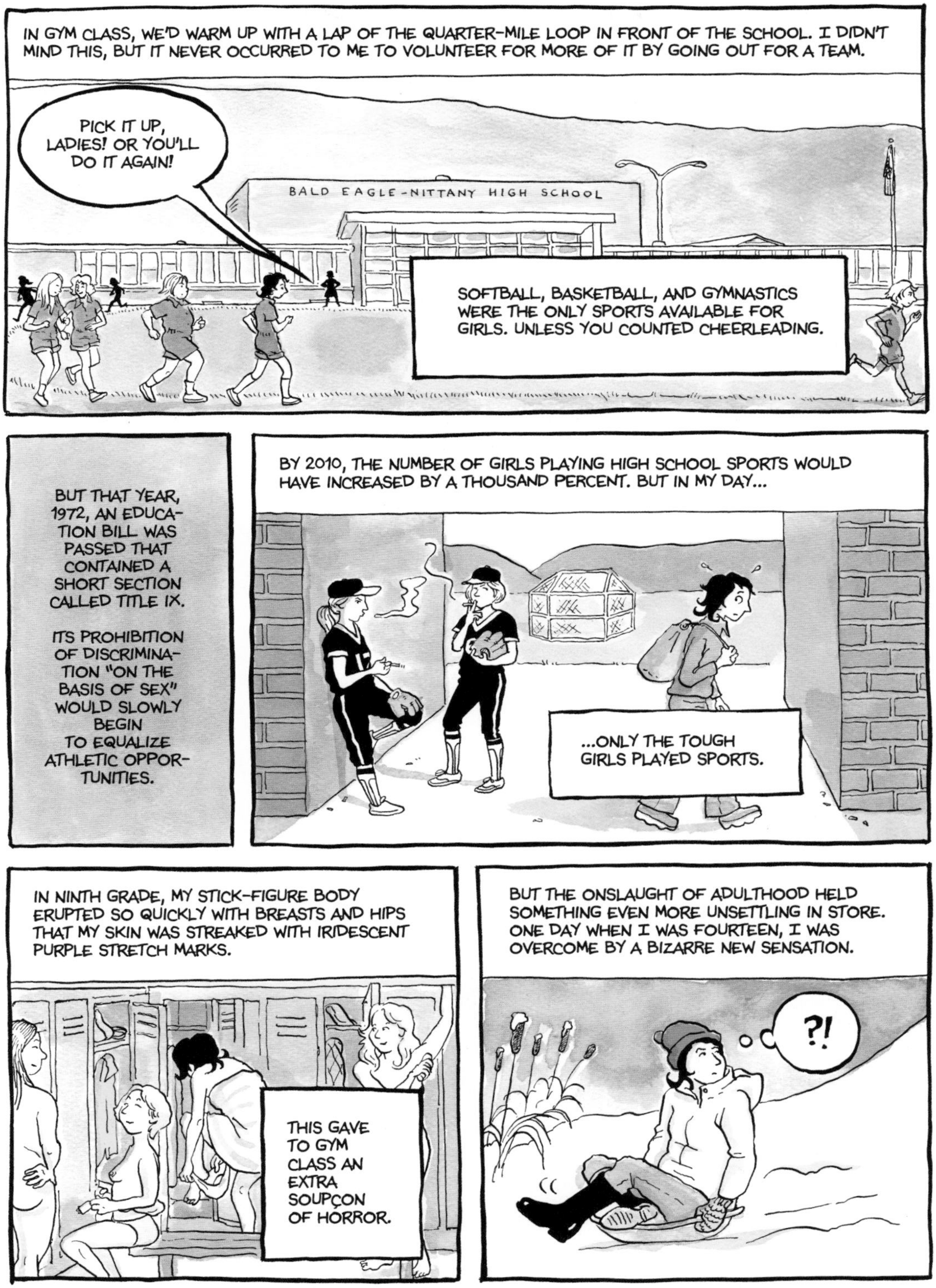
IN GYM CLASS, WE'D WARM UP WITH A LAP OF THE QUARTER-MILE LOOP IN FRONT OF THE SCHOOL. I DIDN'T MIND THIS, BUT IT NEVER OCCURRED TO ME TO VOLUNTEER FOR MORE OF IT BY GOING OUT FOR A TEAM.
PICK IT UP, LADIES! OR YOU'LL DO IT AGAIN!
BALD EAGLE-NITTANY HIGH SCHOOL
SOFTBALL, BASKETBALL, AND GYMNASTICS WERE THE ONLY SPORTS AVAILABLE FOR GIRLS. UNLESS YOU COUNTED CHEERLEADING.
BUT THAT YEAR, 1972, AN EDUCATION BILL WAS PASSED THAT CONTAINED A SHORT SECTION CALLED TITLE IX.
ITS PROHIBITION OF DISCRIMINATION "ON THE BASIS OF SEX" WOULD SLOWLY BEGIN TO EQUALIZE ATHLETIC OPPORTUNITIES.
BY 2010, THE NUMBER OF GIRLS PLAYING HIGH SCHOOL SPORTS WOULD HAVE INCREASED BY A THOUSAND PERCENT. BUT IN MY DAY...
...ONLY THE TOUGH GIRLS PLAYED SPORTS.
IN NINTH GRADE, MY STICK-FIGURE BODY ERUPTED SO QUICKLY WITH BREASTS AND HIPS THAT MY SKIN WAS STREAKED WITH IRIDESCENT PURPLE STRETCH MARKS.
THIS GAVE TO GYM CLASS AN EXTRA SOUPÇON OF HORROR.
BUT THE ONSLAUGHT OF ADULTHOOD HELD SOMETHING EVEN MORE UNSETTLING IN STORE. ONE DAY WHEN I WAS FOURTEEN, I WAS OVERCOME BY A BIZARRE NEW SENSATION.
?!

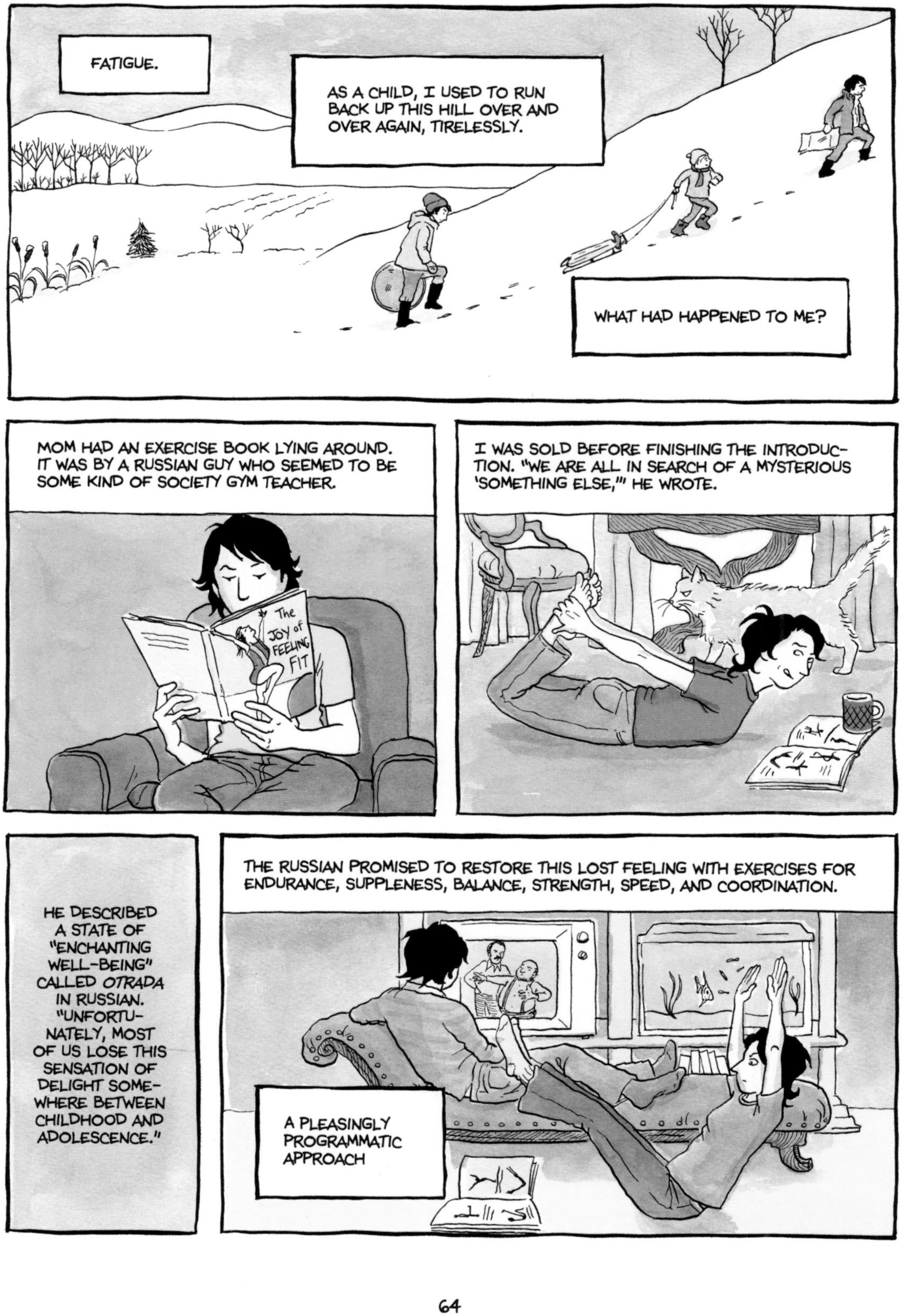
FATIGUE.
AS A CHILD, I USED TO RUN BACK UP THIS HILL OVER AND OVER AGAIN, TIRELESSLY.
WHAT HAD HAPPENED TO ME?
MOM HAD AN EXERCISE BOOK LYING AROUND. IT WAS BY A RUSSIAN GUY WHO SEEMED TO BE SOME KIND OF SOCIETY GYM TEACHER.
The Joy of FEELING FIT
I WAS SOLD BEFORE FINISHING THE INTRODUCTION. "WE ARE ALL IN SEARCH OF A MYSTERIOUS 'SOMETHING ELSE,'" HE WROTE.
HE DESCRIBED A STATE OF "ENCHANTING WELL-BEING" CALLED *OTRADA* IN RUSSIAN. "UNFORTUNATELY, MOST OF US LOSE THIS SENSATION OF DELIGHT SOMEWHERE BETWEEN CHILDHOOD AND ADOLESCENCE."
THE RUSSIAN PROMISED TO RESTORE THIS LOST FEELING WITH EXERCISES FOR ENDURANCE, SUPPLENESS, BALANCE, STRENGTH, SPEED, AND COORDINATION.
A PLEASINGLY PROGRAMMATIC APPROACH

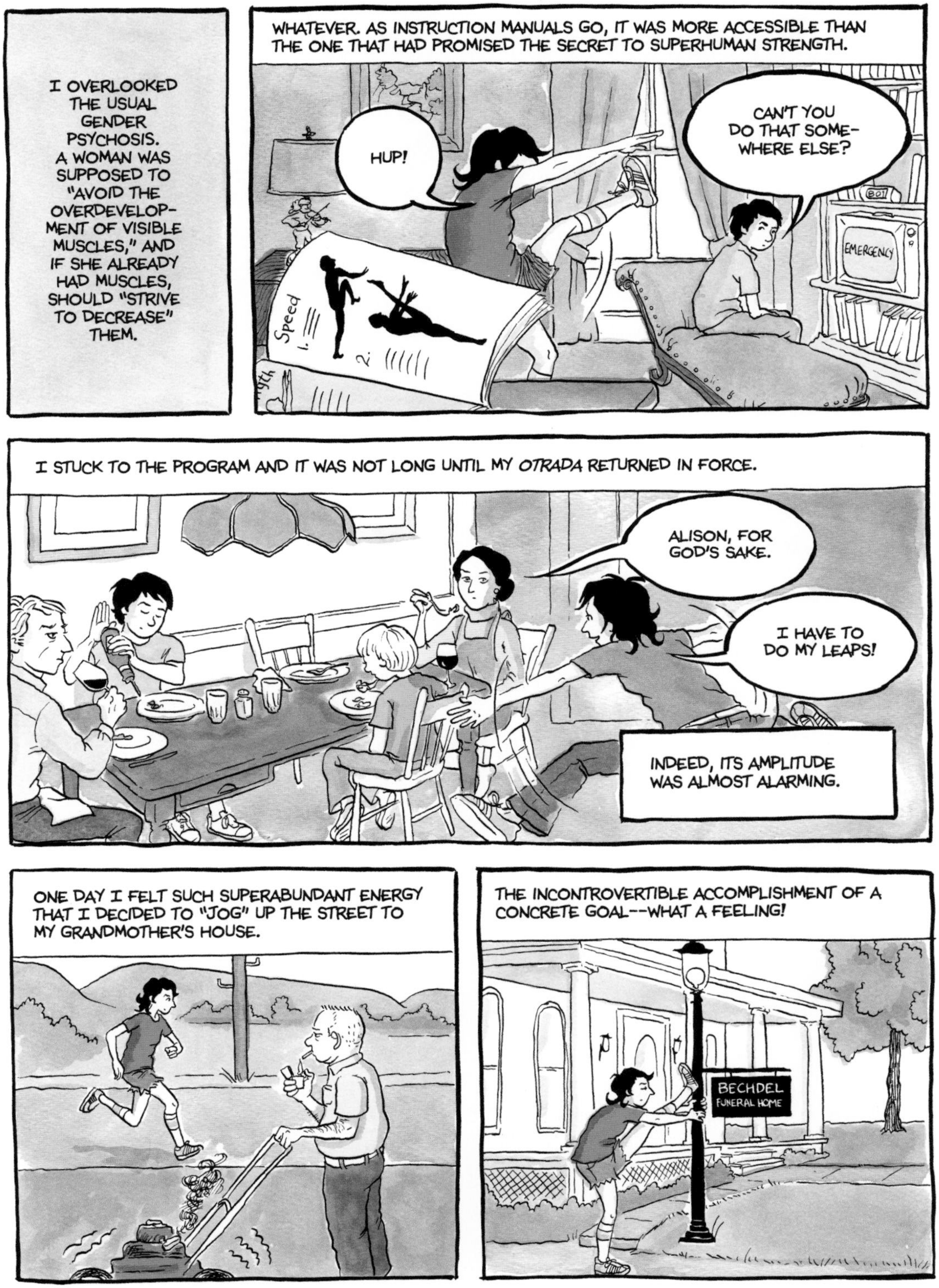
I OVERLOOKED THE USUAL GENDER PSYCHOSIS. A WOMAN WAS SUPPOSED TO "AVOID THE OVERDEVELOPMENT OF VISIBLE MUSCLES," AND IF SHE ALREADY HAD MUSCLES, SHOULD "STRIVE TO DECREASE" THEM.
WHATEVER. AS INSTRUCTION MANUALS GO, IT WAS MORE ACCESSIBLE THAN THE ONE THAT HAD PROMISED THE SECRET TO SUPERHUMAN STRENGTH.
HUP!
CAN'T YOU DO THAT SOMEWHERE ELSE?
EMERGENCY
I STUCK TO THE PROGRAM AND IT WAS NOT LONG UNTIL MY *OTRADA* RETURNED IN FORCE.
ALISON, FOR GOD'S SAKE.
I HAVE TO DO MY LEAPS!
INDEED, ITS AMPLITUDE WAS ALMOST ALARMING.
ONE DAY I FELT SUCH SUPERABUNDANT ENERGY THAT I DECIDED TO "JOG" UP THE STREET TO MY GRANDMOTHER'S HOUSE.
THE INCONTROVERTIBLE ACCOMPLISHMENT OF A CONCRETE GOAL--WHAT A FEELING!
BECHDEL
FUNERAL HOME

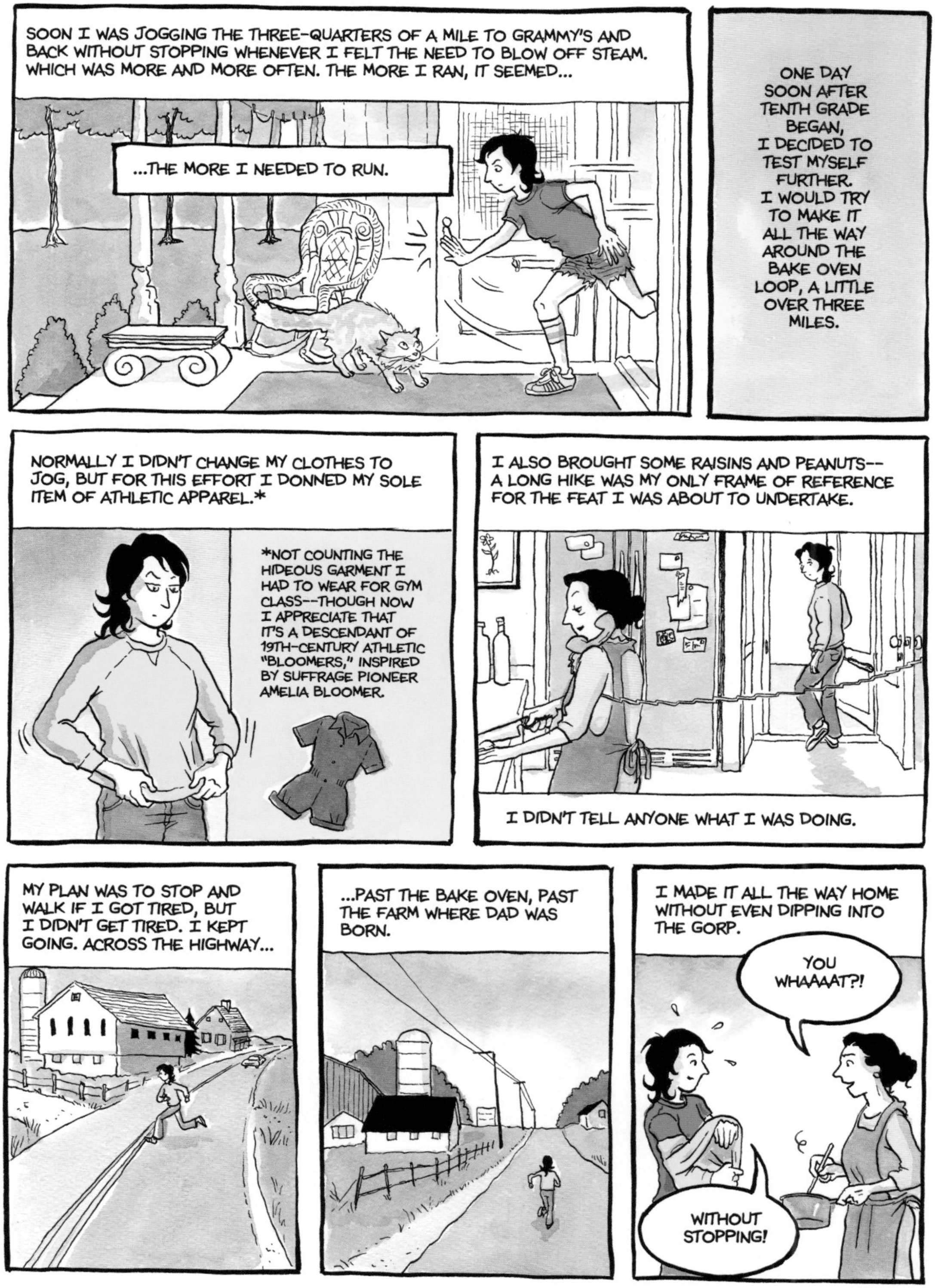
SOON I WAS JOGGING THE THREE-QUARTERS OF A MILE TO GRAMMY'S AND BACK WITHOUT STOPPING WHENEVER I FELT THE NEED TO BLOW OFF STEAM. WHICH WAS MORE AND MORE OFTEN. THE MORE I RAN, IT SEEMED...
...THE MORE I NEEDED TO RUN.
ONE DAY SOON AFTER TENTH GRADE BEGAN, I DECIDED TO TEST MYSELF FURTHER. I WOULD TRY TO MAKE IT ALL THE WAY AROUND THE BAKE OVEN LOOP, A LITTLE OVER THREE MILES.
NORMALLY I DIDN'T CHANGE MY CLOTHES TO JOG, BUT FOR THIS EFFORT I DONNED MY SOLE ITEM OF ATHLETIC APPAREL.*
*NOT COUNTING THE HIDEOUS GARMENT I HAD TO WEAR FOR GYM CLASS--THOUGH NOW I APPRECIATE THAT IT'S A DESCENDANT OF 19TH-CENTURY ATHLETIC "BLOOMERS," INSPIRED BY SUFFRAGE PIONEER AMELIA BLOOMER.
I ALSO BROUGHT SOME RAISINS AND PEANUTS-- A LONG HIKE WAS MY ONLY FRAME OF REFERENCE FOR THE FEAT I WAS ABOUT TO UNDERTAKE.
I DIDN'T TELL ANYONE WHAT I WAS DOING.
MY PLAN WAS TO STOP AND WALK IF I GOT TIRED, BUT I DIDN'T GET TIRED. I KEPT GOING. ACROSS THE HIGHWAY...
...PAST THE BAKE OVEN, PAST THE FARM WHERE DAD WAS BORN.
I MADE IT ALL THE WAY HOME WITHOUT EVEN DIPPING INTO THE GORP.
YOU WHAAAAT?!
WITHOUT STOPPING!

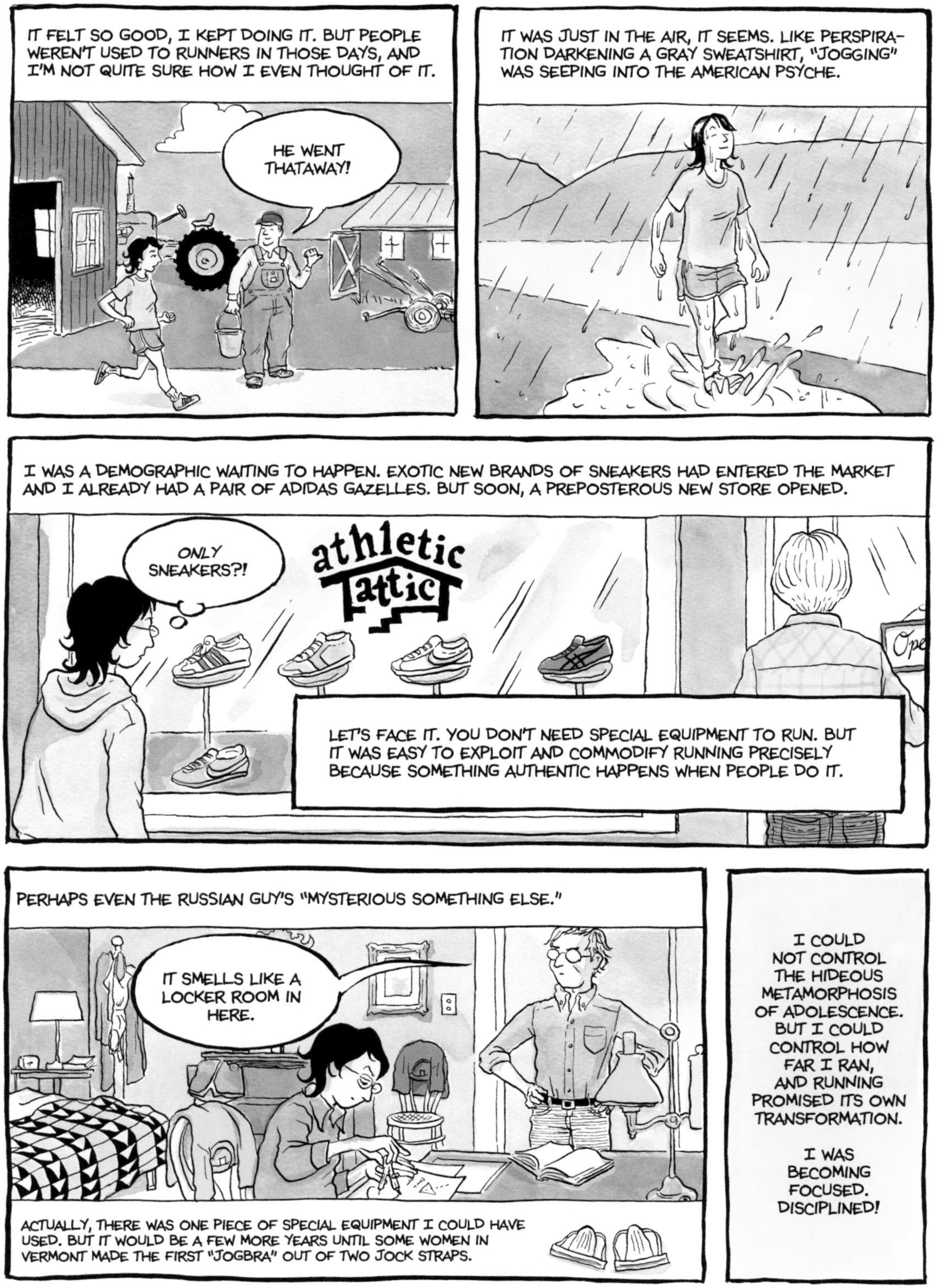
IT FELT SO GOOD, I KEPT DOING IT. BUT PEOPLE WEREN'T USED TO RUNNERS IN THOSE DAYS, AND I'M NOT QUITE SURE HOW I EVEN THOUGHT OF IT.
HE WENT THATAWAY!
IT WAS JUST IN THE AIR, IT SEEMS. LIKE PERSPIRATION DARKENING A GRAY SWEATSHIRT, "JOGGING" WAS SEEPING INTO THE AMERICAN PSYCHE.
I WAS A DEMOGRAPHIC WAITING TO HAPPEN. EXOTIC NEW BRANDS OF SNEAKERS HAD ENTERED THE MARKET AND I ALREADY HAD A PAIR OF ADIDAS GAZELLES. BUT SOON, A PREPOSTEROUS NEW STORE OPENED.
ONLY SNEAKERS?!
athletic attic
LET'S FACE IT. YOU DON'T NEED SPECIAL EQUIPMENT TO RUN. BUT IT WAS EASY TO EXPLOIT AND COMMODIFY RUNNING PRECISELY BECAUSE SOMETHING AUTHENTIC HAPPENS WHEN PEOPLE DO IT.
PERHAPS EVEN THE RUSSIAN GUY'S "MYSTERIOUS SOMETHING ELSE."
IT SMELLS LIKE A LOCKER ROOM IN HERE.
ACTUALLY, THERE WAS ONE PIECE OF SPECIAL EQUIPMENT I COULD HAVE USED. BUT IT WOULD BE A FEW MORE YEARS UNTIL SOME WOMEN IN VERMONT MADE THE FIRST "JOGBRA" OUT OF TWO JOCK STRAPS.
I COULD NOT CONTROL THE HIDEOUS METAMORPHOSIS OF ADOLESCENCE. BUT I COULD CONTROL HOW FAR I RAN, AND RUNNING PROMISED ITS OWN TRANSFORMATION.
I WAS BECOMING FOCUSED. DISCIPLINED!

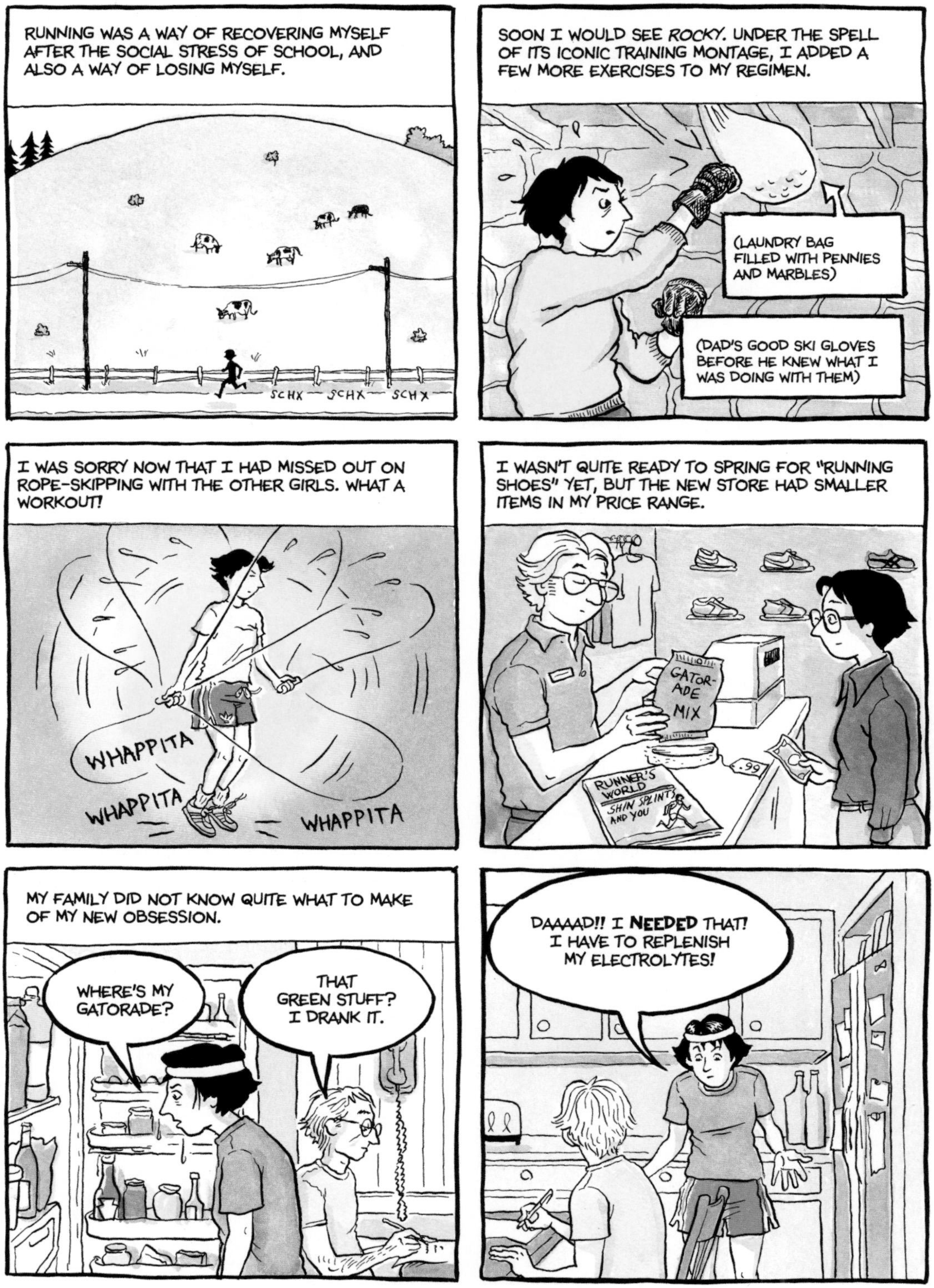
RUNNING WAS A WAY OF RECOVERING MYSELF AFTER THE SOCIAL STRESS OF SCHOOL, AND ALSO A WAY OF LOSING MYSELF.
SCHX SCHX SCHX
SOON I WOULD SEE *ROCKY*. UNDER THE SPELL OF ITS ICONIC TRAINING MONTAGE, I ADDED A FEW MORE EXERCISES TO MY REGIMEN.
(LAUNDRY BAG FILLED WITH PENNIES AND MARBLES)
(DAD'S GOOD SKI GLOVES BEFORE HE KNEW WHAT I WAS DOING WITH THEM)
I WAS SORRY NOW THAT I HAD MISSED OUT ON ROPE-SKIPPING WITH THE OTHER GIRLS. WHAT A WORKOUT!
WHAPPITA
WHAPPITA
WHAPPITA
I WASN'T QUITE READY TO SPRING FOR "RUNNING SHOES" YET, BUT THE NEW STORE HAD SMALLER ITEMS IN MY PRICE RANGE.
GATOR-ADE MIX
.99
RUNNER'S WORLD
SHIN SPLINTS AND YOU
MY FAMILY DID NOT KNOW QUITE WHAT TO MAKE OF MY NEW OBSESSION.
WHERE'S MY GATORADE?
THAT GREEN STUFF? I DRANK IT.
DAAAAD!! I **NEEDED** THAT! I HAVE TO REPLENISH MY ELECTROLYTES!

WHEN I STARTED GETTING SHIN SPLINTS, I TOSSED MY CUSHIONLESS GAZELLES* AND BOUGHT A PAIR OF THE PURPOSE-BUILT RUNNING SHOES.

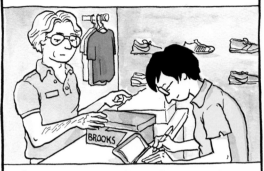

*DESPITE THE NAME, NOT DESIGNED FOR RUNNING

I FELT A KIND OF LUST FOR THOSE BROOKS VILLANOVAS. THERE'S SOMETHING INHERENTLY EROTIC ABOUT RUNNING. THE INCREASED AWARENESS OF YOUR OWN BODY...

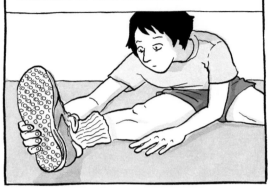

...BUT ALSO SOMETHING ABOUT DESIRE THAT'S HARDER TO QUANTIFY. RUNNING IS A CHASE. EARLY HUMANS RAN TO TIRE OUT THEIR PREY OVER LONG DISTANCES.

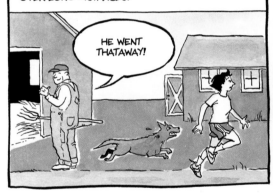

HE WENT THATAWAY!

THE MILD EUPHORIA THAT WOULD OFTEN COME OVER ME WHILE RUNNING WAS AN EVOLUTIONARY REWARD TO ENCOURAGE A BEHAVIOR THAT AIDED SURVIVAL.

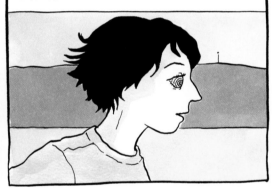

BUT AT THE TIME, I CONSIDERED MY ALTERED STATE MORE MYSTICAL THAN CHEMICAL. A BOOKLET AT THE SNEAKER STORE CAUGHT MY EYE.

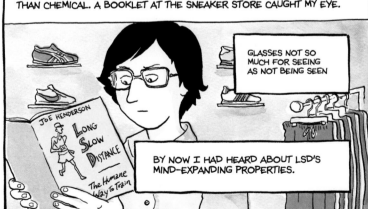

JOE HENDERSON
LONG SLOW DISTANCE
The Humane Way to Train

GLASSES NOT SO MUCH FOR SEEING AS NOT BEING SEEN

BY NOW I HAD HEARD ABOUT LSD'S MIND-EXPANDING PROPERTIES.

ALAS, IT WAS YET ANOTHER BAFFLING TRAINING MANUAL, WHICH DULY JOINED THE ONE ON JIUJITSU IN THE BACK OF MY CLOSET.

BUT THE IDEA OF LONG, SLOW DIS-TANCE STUCK WITH ME. ONE DAY I FINISHED MY LOOP AND JUST KEPT GOING, PAST OUR HOUSE, AND RAN THE WHOLE THING AGAIN.

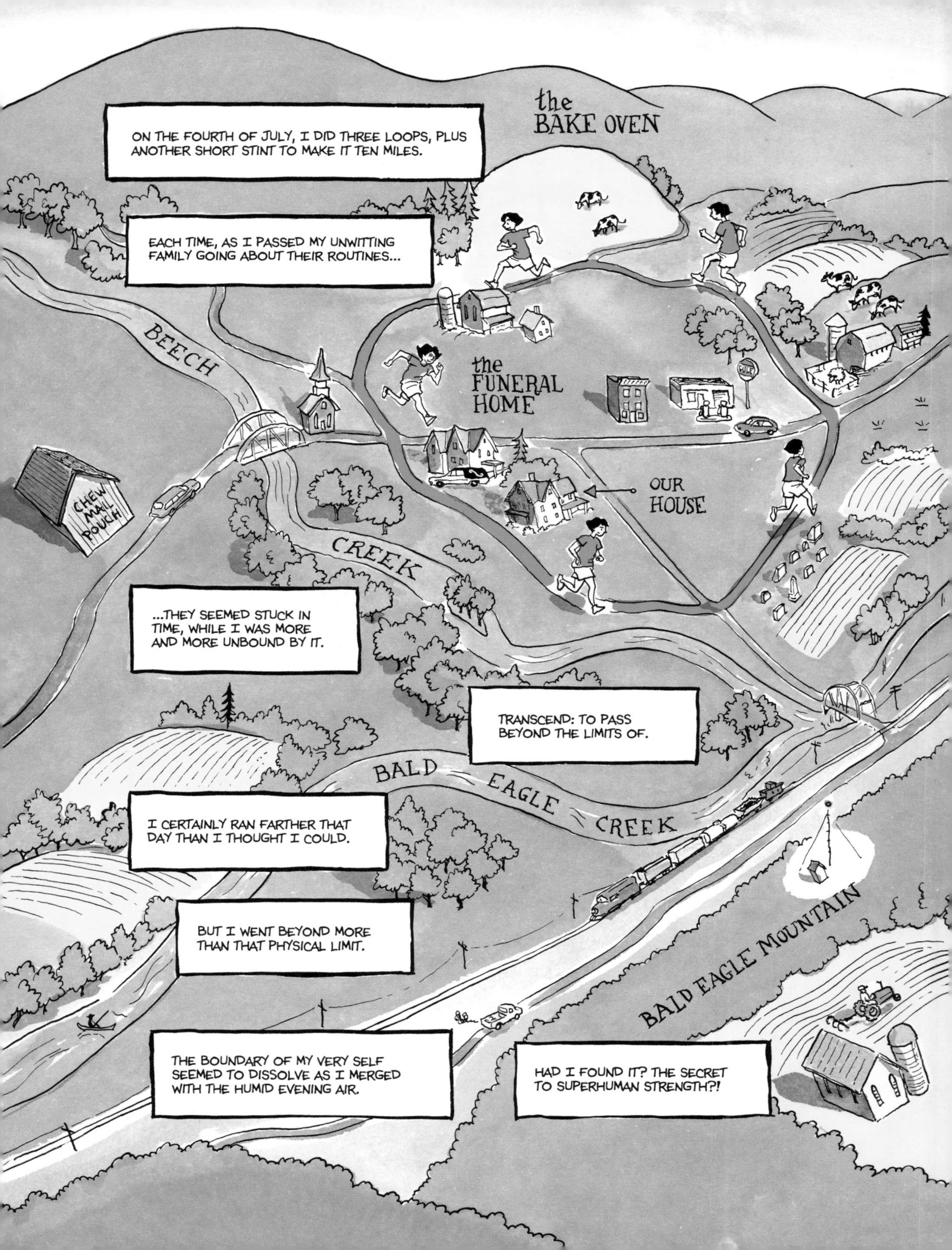
ON THE FOURTH OF JULY, I DID THREE LOOPS, PLUS ANOTHER SHORT STINT TO MAKE IT TEN MILES.
the BAKE OVEN
EACH TIME, AS I PASSED MY UNWITTING FAMILY GOING ABOUT THEIR ROUTINES...
BEECH
the FUNERAL HOME
GULF
CHEW MAIL POUCH
OUR HOUSE
CREEK
...THEY SEEMED STUCK IN TIME, WHILE I WAS MORE AND MORE UNBOUND BY IT.
TRANSCEND: TO PASS BEYOND THE LIMITS OF.
BALD EAGLE CREEK
I CERTAINLY RAN FARTHER THAT DAY THAN I THOUGHT I COULD.
BUT I WENT BEYOND MORE THAN THAT PHYSICAL LIMIT.
BALD EAGLE MOUNTAIN
THE BOUNDARY OF MY VERY SELF SEEMED TO DISSOLVE AS I MERGED WITH THE HUMID EVENING AIR.
HAD I FOUND IT? THE SECRET TO SUPERHUMAN STRENGTH?!

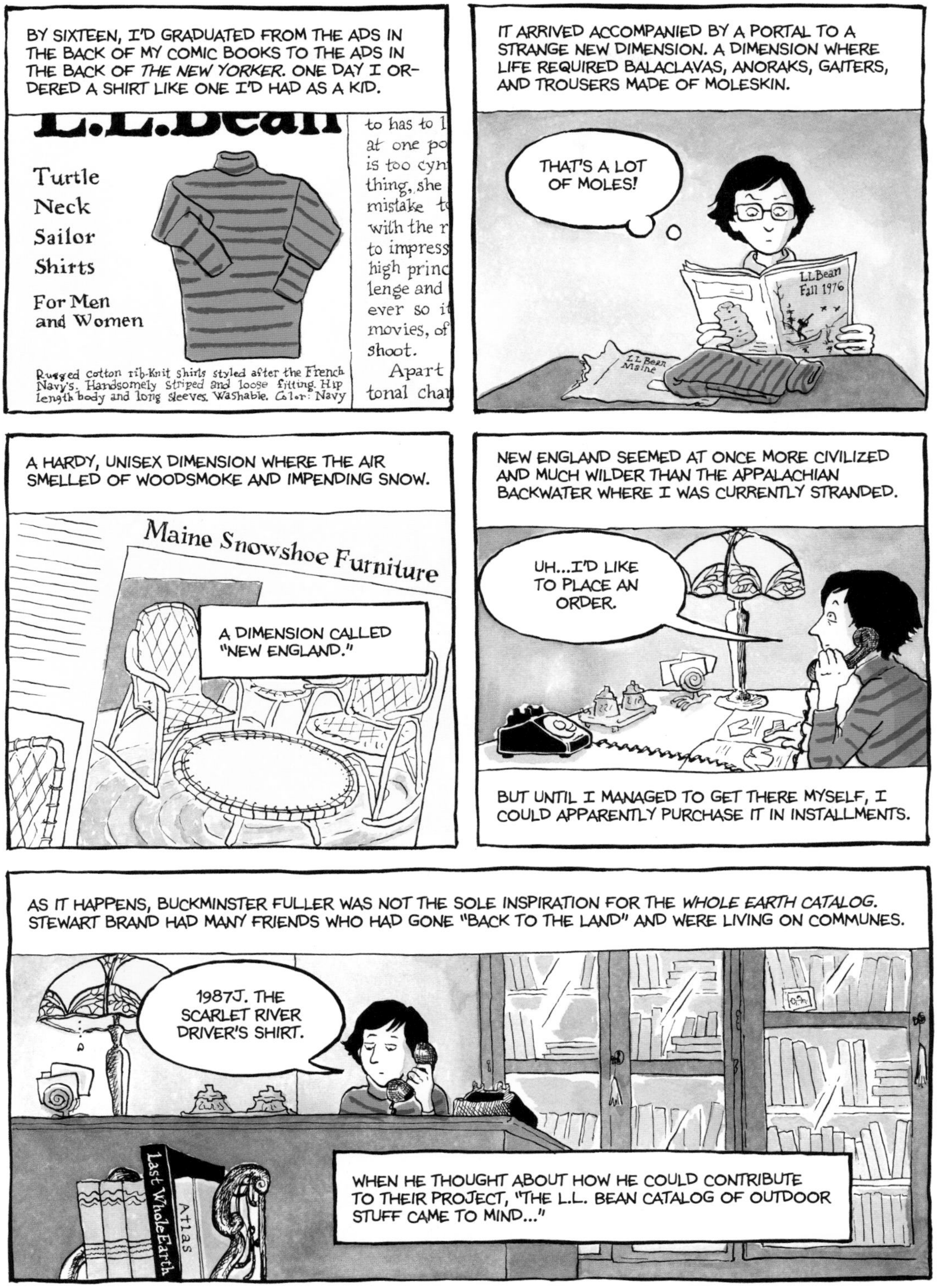

BY SIXTEEN, I'D GRADUATED FROM THE ADS IN THE BACK OF MY COMIC BOOKS TO THE ADS IN THE BACK OF *THE NEW YORKER*. ONE DAY I ORDERED A SHIRT LIKE ONE I'D HAD AS A KID.

L.L.Bean

Turtle
Neck
Sailor
Shirts

For Men
and Women

Rugged cotton rib-knit shirts styled after the French Navy's. Handsomely striped and loose fitting. Hip length body and long sleeves. Washable. Color: Navy

to has to l
at one po
is too cyn
thing, she
mistake t
with the r
to impress
high prin
lenge and
ever so i
movies, of
shoot.
Apart
tonal char

IT ARRIVED ACCOMPANIED BY A PORTAL TO A STRANGE NEW DIMENSION. A DIMENSION WHERE LIFE REQUIRED BALACLAVAS, ANORAKS, GAITERS, AND TROUSERS MADE OF MOLESKIN.

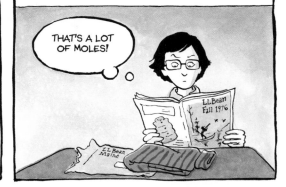

THAT'S A LOT OF MOLES!

A HARDY, UNISEX DIMENSION WHERE THE AIR SMELLED OF WOODSMOKE AND IMPENDING SNOW.

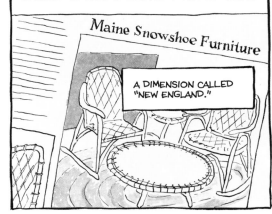

Maine Snowshoe Furniture

A DIMENSION CALLED "NEW ENGLAND."

NEW ENGLAND SEEMED AT ONCE MORE CIVILIZED AND MUCH WILDER THAN THE APPALACHIAN BACKWATER WHERE I WAS CURRENTLY STRANDED.

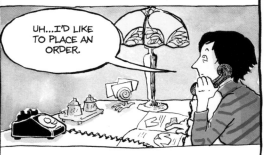

UH...I'D LIKE TO PLACE AN ORDER.

BUT UNTIL I MANAGED TO GET THERE MYSELF, I COULD APPARENTLY PURCHASE IT IN INSTALLMENTS.

AS IT HAPPENS, BUCKMINSTER FULLER WAS NOT THE SOLE INSPIRATION FOR THE *WHOLE EARTH CATALOG*. STEWART BRAND HAD MANY FRIENDS WHO HAD GONE "BACK TO THE LAND" AND WERE LIVING ON COMMUNES.

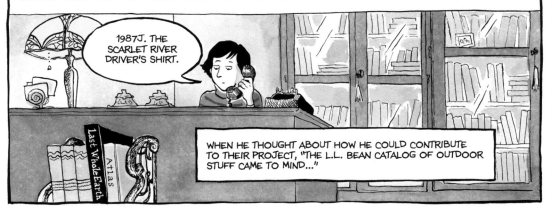

1987J. THE SCARLET RIVER DRIVER'S SHIRT.

Last Whole Earth
Atlas

WHEN HE THOUGHT ABOUT HOW HE COULD CONTRIBUTE TO THEIR PROJECT, "THE L.L. BEAN CATALOG OF OUTDOOR STUFF CAME TO MIND..."

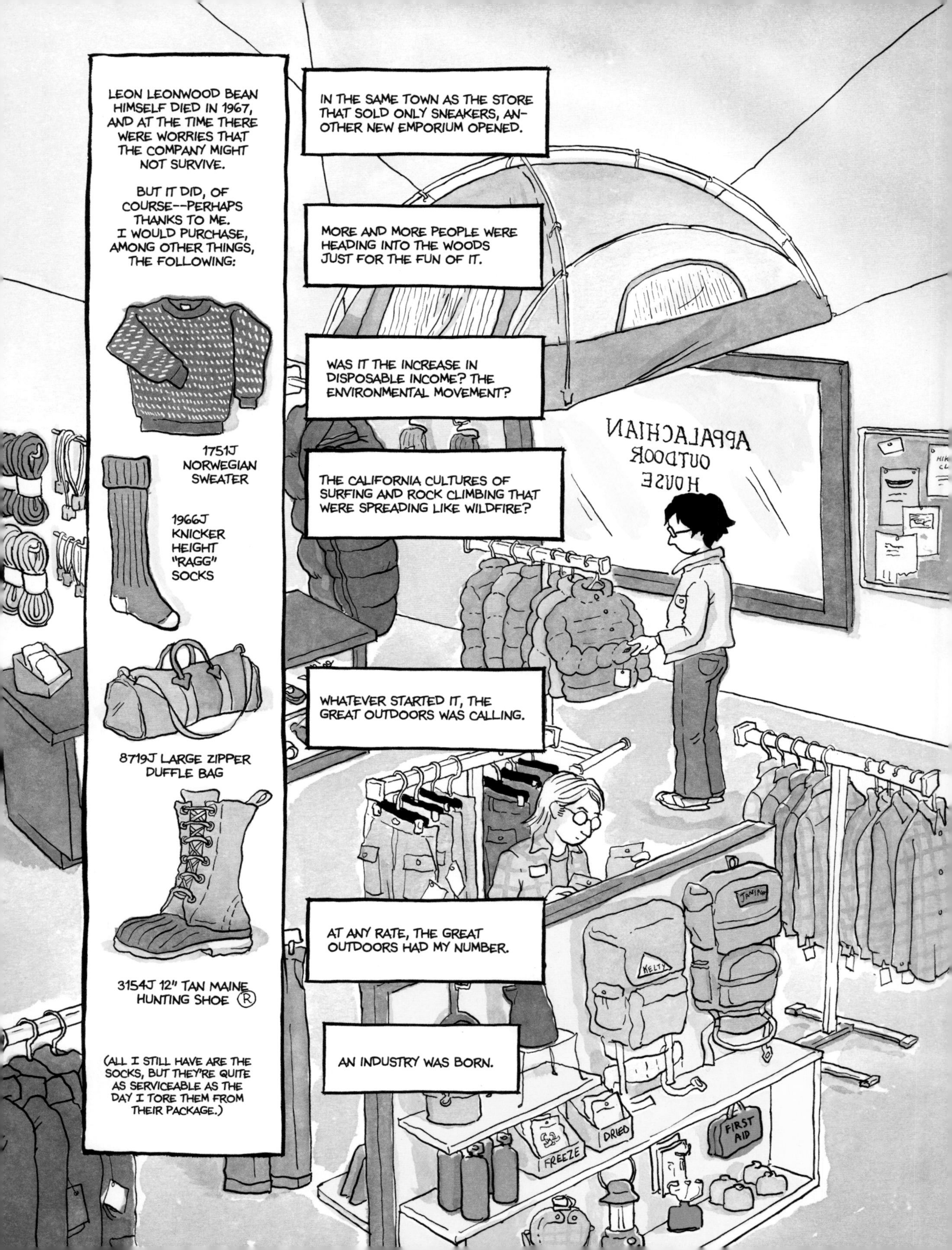

LEON LEONWOOD BEAN HIMSELF DIED IN 1967, AND AT THE TIME THERE WERE WORRIES THAT THE COMPANY MIGHT NOT SURVIVE.
BUT IT DID, OF COURSE--PERHAPS THANKS TO ME. I WOULD PURCHASE, AMONG OTHER THINGS, THE FOLLOWING:
1751J NORWEGIAN SWEATER
1966J KNICKER HEIGHT "RAGG" SOCKS
8719J LARGE ZIPPER DUFFLE BAG
3154J 12" TAN MAINE HUNTING SHOE ®
(ALL I STILL HAVE ARE THE SOCKS, BUT THEY'RE QUITE AS SERVICEABLE AS THE DAY I TORE THEM FROM THEIR PACKAGE.)
IN THE SAME TOWN AS THE STORE THAT SOLD ONLY SNEAKERS, ANOTHER NEW EMPORIUM OPENED.
MORE AND MORE PEOPLE WERE HEADING INTO THE WOODS JUST FOR THE FUN OF IT.
WAS IT THE INCREASE IN DISPOSABLE INCOME? THE ENVIRONMENTAL MOVEMENT?
APPALACHIAN OUTDOOR HOUSE
THE CALIFORNIA CULTURES OF SURFING AND ROCK CLIMBING THAT WERE SPREADING LIKE WILDFIRE?
WHATEVER STARTED IT, THE GREAT OUTDOORS WAS CALLING.
AT ANY RATE, THE GREAT OUTDOORS HAD MY NUMBER.
KELTY
JANSPORT
AN INDUSTRY WAS BORN.
FREEZE
DRIED
FIRST AID

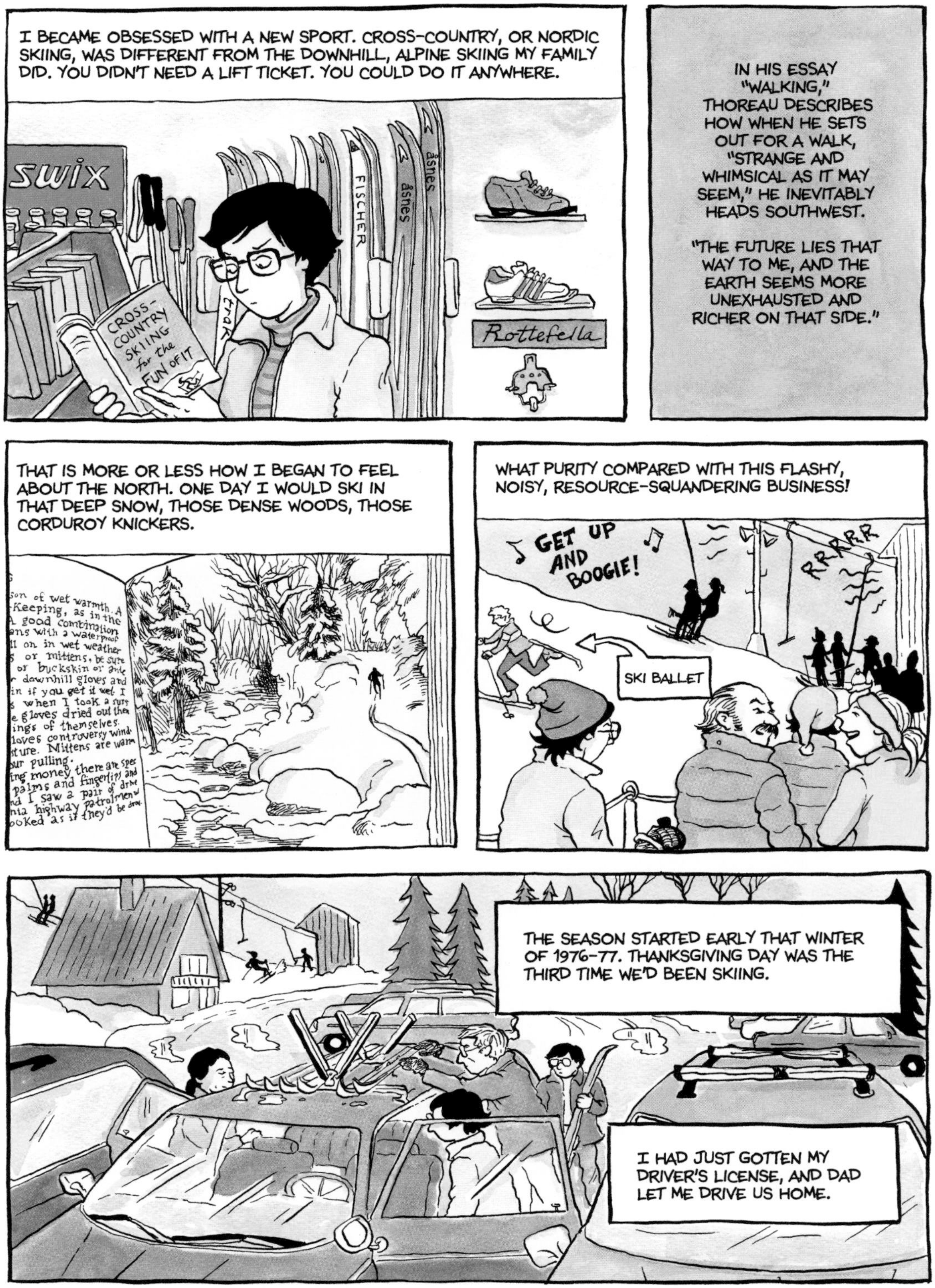
I BECAME OBSESSED WITH A NEW SPORT. CROSS-COUNTRY, OR NORDIC SKIING, WAS DIFFERENT FROM THE DOWNHILL, ALPINE SKIING MY FAMILY DID. YOU DIDN'T NEED A LIFT TICKET. YOU COULD DO IT ANYWHERE.
SWIX
FISCHER
åsnes
CROSS-COUNTRY SKIING for the FUN OF IT
Rottefella
IN HIS ESSAY "WALKING," THOREAU DESCRIBES HOW WHEN HE SETS OUT FOR A WALK, "STRANGE AND WHIMSICAL AS IT MAY SEEM," HE INEVITABLY HEADS SOUTHWEST.
"THE FUTURE LIES THAT WAY TO ME, AND THE EARTH SEEMS MORE UNEXHAUSTED AND RICHER ON THAT SIDE."
THAT IS MORE OR LESS HOW I BEGAN TO FEEL ABOUT THE NORTH. ONE DAY I WOULD SKI IN THAT DEEP SNOW, THOSE DENSE WOODS, THOSE CORDUROY KNICKERS.
WHAT PURITY COMPARED WITH THIS FLASHY, NOISY, RESOURCE-SQUANDERING BUSINESS!
GET UP AND BOOGIE!
RRRRR
SKI BALLET
THE SEASON STARTED EARLY THAT WINTER OF 1976–77. THANKSGIVING DAY WAS THE THIRD TIME WE'D BEEN SKIING.
I HAD JUST GOTTEN MY DRIVER'S LICENSE, AND DAD LET ME DRIVE US HOME.

WE HADN'T GONE FAR WHEN I LOST CONTROL ON A DOWNHILL CURVE.

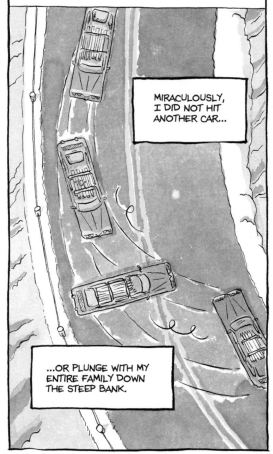

MIRACULOUSLY, I DID NOT HIT ANOTHER CAR...

...OR PLUNGE WITH MY ENTIRE FAMILY DOWN THE STEEP BANK.

AFTER WE CAME TO A STOP, FACING IN THE OPPOSITE DIRECTION, NO ONE SAID A WORD. DAD AND I EXCHANGED PLACES.

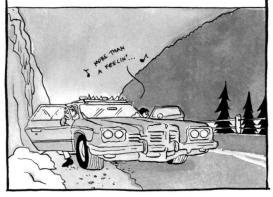

TEN MILES LATER, HE PULLED OVER, STILL WITHOUT SPEAKING. I SOMEHOW KNEW WHAT HAD TO BE DONE.

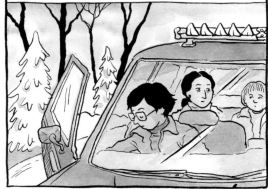

WHILE IT'S TRUE THAT I SUFFER FROM UNSEEMLY SPASMS OF SELF-DOUBT AND SELF-CRITICISM, I SIMULTANEOUSLY POSSESS A SELF-CONFIDENCE AS SOLID AS A SEVENTIES STATION WAGON...

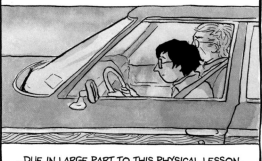

...DUE IN LARGE PART TO THIS PHYSICAL LESSON.

IT CERTAINLY ALLOWED ME TO DO WHAT CAME NEXT. IT WAS MY TENTH SEASON OF SKIING, AND WHILE I ROUTINELY PLIED THE EXPERT SLOPES WITHOUT FALLING...

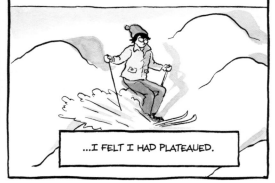

...I FELT I HAD PLATEAUED.

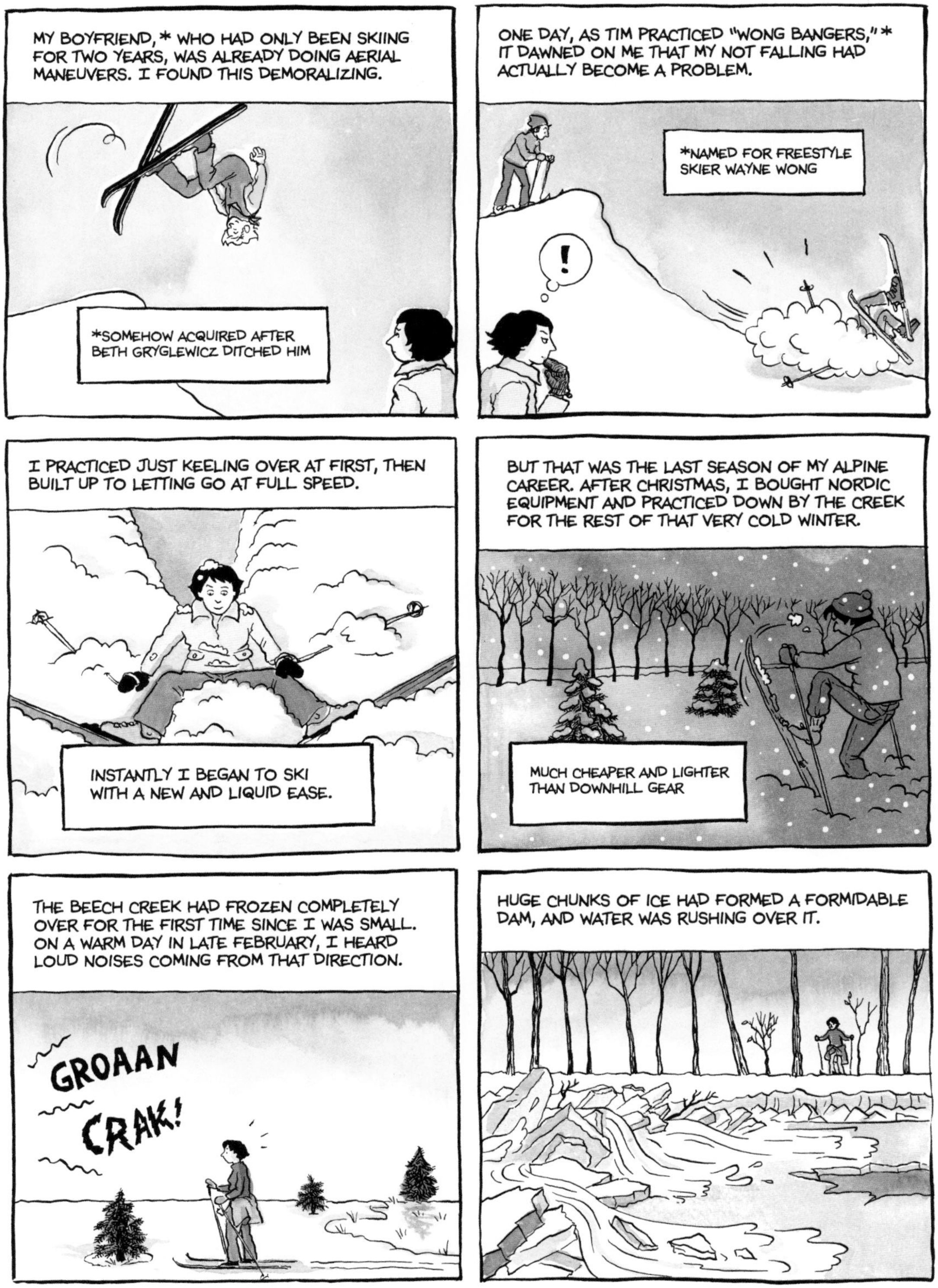
MY BOYFRIEND,* WHO HAD ONLY BEEN SKIING FOR TWO YEARS, WAS ALREADY DOING AERIAL MANEUVERS. I FOUND THIS DEMORALIZING.
*SOMEHOW ACQUIRED AFTER BETH GRYGLEWICZ DITCHED HIM
ONE DAY, AS TIM PRACTICED "WONG BANGERS,"* IT DAWNED ON ME THAT MY NOT FALLING HAD ACTUALLY BECOME A PROBLEM.
*NAMED FOR FREESTYLE SKIER WAYNE WONG
!
I PRACTICED JUST KEELING OVER AT FIRST, THEN BUILT UP TO LETTING GO AT FULL SPEED.
INSTANTLY I BEGAN TO SKI WITH A NEW AND LIQUID EASE.
BUT THAT WAS THE LAST SEASON OF MY ALPINE CAREER. AFTER CHRISTMAS, I BOUGHT NORDIC EQUIPMENT AND PRACTICED DOWN BY THE CREEK FOR THE REST OF THAT VERY COLD WINTER.
MUCH CHEAPER AND LIGHTER THAN DOWNHILL GEAR
THE BEECH CREEK HAD FROZEN COMPLETELY OVER FOR THE FIRST TIME SINCE I WAS SMALL. ON A WARM DAY IN LATE FEBRUARY, I HEARD LOUD NOISES COMING FROM THAT DIRECTION.
GROAAN
CRAK!
HUGE CHUNKS OF ICE HAD FORMED A FORMIDABLE DAM, AND WATER WAS RUSHING OVER IT.

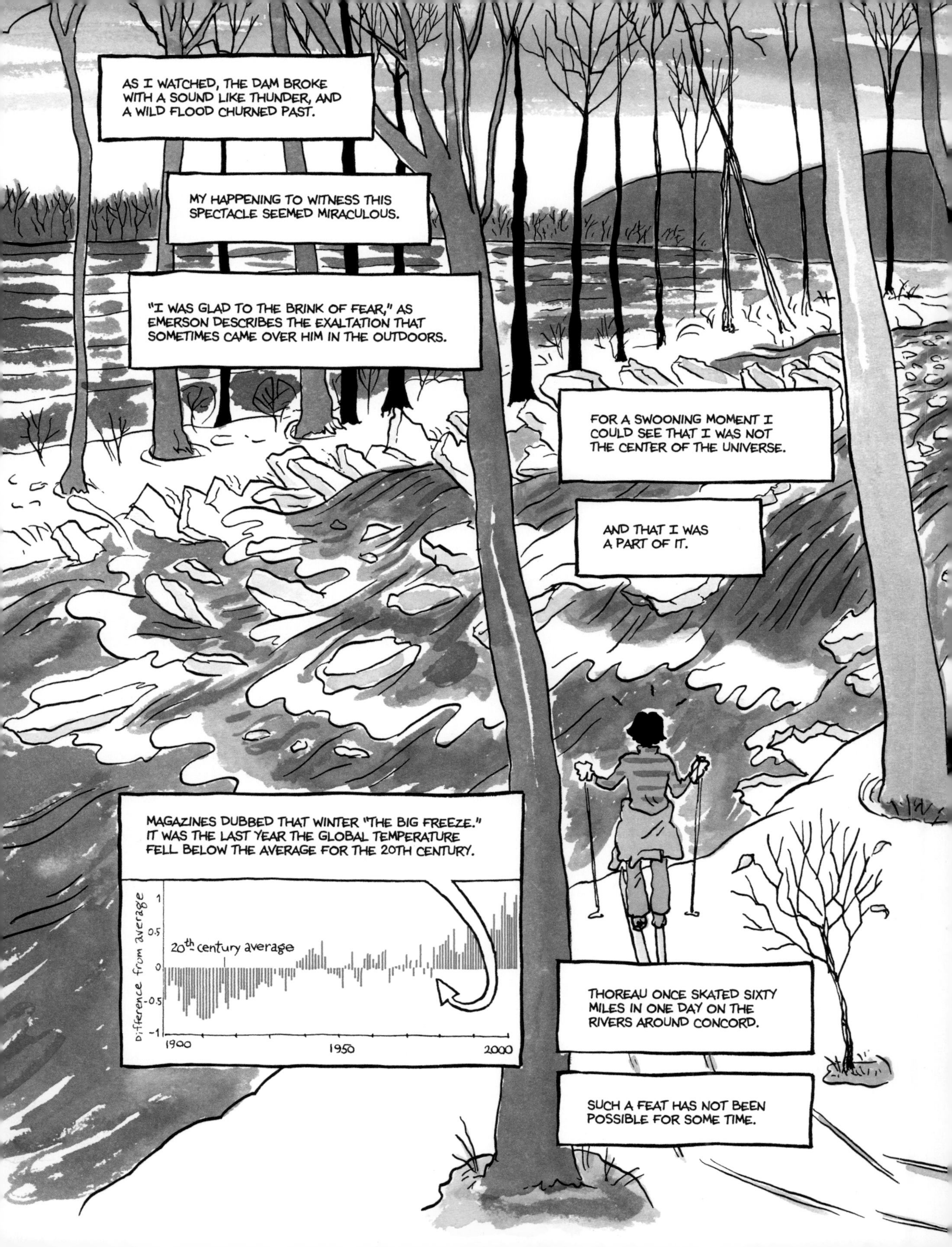
AS I WATCHED, THE DAM BROKE WITH A SOUND LIKE THUNDER, AND A WILD FLOOD CHURNED PAST.
MY HAPPENING TO WITNESS THIS SPECTACLE SEEMED MIRACULOUS.
"I WAS GLAD TO THE BRINK OF FEAR," AS EMERSON DESCRIBES THE EXALTATION THAT SOMETIMES CAME OVER HIM IN THE OUTDOORS.
FOR A SWOONING MOMENT I COULD SEE THAT I WAS NOT THE CENTER OF THE UNIVERSE.
AND THAT I WAS A PART OF IT.
MAGAZINES DUBBED THAT WINTER "THE BIG FREEZE." IT WAS THE LAST YEAR THE GLOBAL TEMPERATURE FELL BELOW THE AVERAGE FOR THE 20TH CENTURY.
difference from average
1
0.5
0
-0.5
-1
20th-century average
1900
1950
2000
THOREAU ONCE SKATED SIXTY MILES IN ONE DAY ON THE RIVERS AROUND CONCORD.
SUCH A FEAT HAS NOT BEEN POSSIBLE FOR SOME TIME.

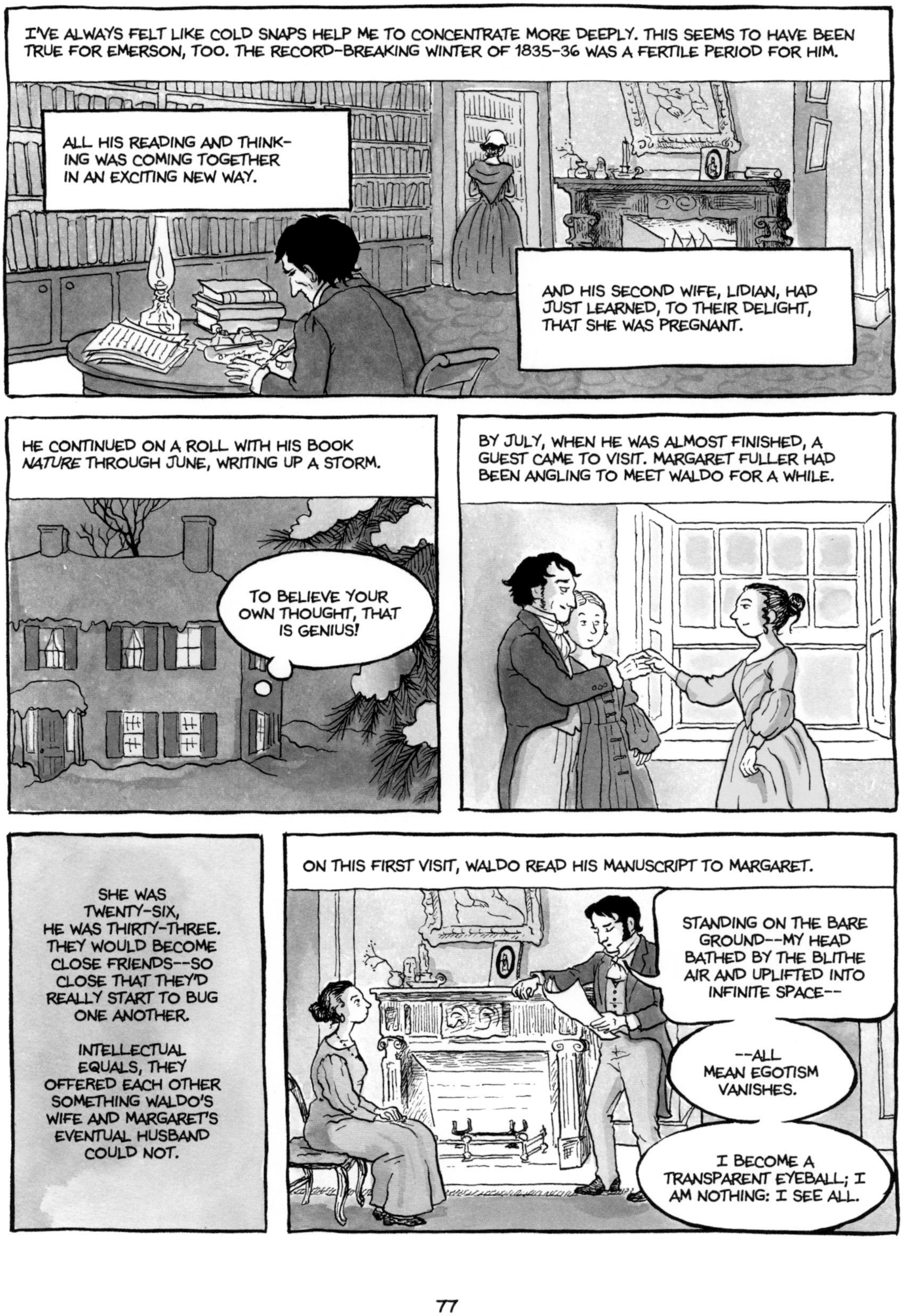
I'VE ALWAYS FELT LIKE COLD SNAPS HELP ME TO CONCENTRATE MORE DEEPLY. THIS SEEMS TO HAVE BEEN TRUE FOR EMERSON, TOO. THE RECORD-BREAKING WINTER OF 1835-36 WAS A FERTILE PERIOD FOR HIM.
ALL HIS READING AND THINKING WAS COMING TOGETHER IN AN EXCITING NEW WAY.
AND HIS SECOND WIFE, LIDIAN, HAD JUST LEARNED, TO THEIR DELIGHT, THAT SHE WAS PREGNANT.
HE CONTINUED ON A ROLL WITH HIS BOOK *NATURE* THROUGH JUNE, WRITING UP A STORM.
TO BELIEVE YOUR OWN THOUGHT, THAT IS GENIUS!
BY JULY, WHEN HE WAS ALMOST FINISHED, A GUEST CAME TO VISIT. MARGARET FULLER HAD BEEN ANGLING TO MEET WALDO FOR A WHILE.
SHE WAS TWENTY-SIX, HE WAS THIRTY-THREE. THEY WOULD BECOME CLOSE FRIENDS--SO CLOSE THAT THEY'D REALLY START TO BUG ONE ANOTHER.
INTELLECTUAL EQUALS, THEY OFFERED EACH OTHER SOMETHING WALDO'S WIFE AND MARGARET'S EVENTUAL HUSBAND COULD NOT.
ON THIS FIRST VISIT, WALDO READ HIS MANUSCRIPT TO MARGARET.
STANDING ON THE BARE GROUND--MY HEAD BATHED BY THE BLITHE AIR AND UPLIFTED INTO INFINITE SPACE--
--ALL MEAN EGOTISM VANISHES.
I BECOME A TRANSPARENT EYEBALL; I AM NOTHING: I SEE ALL.

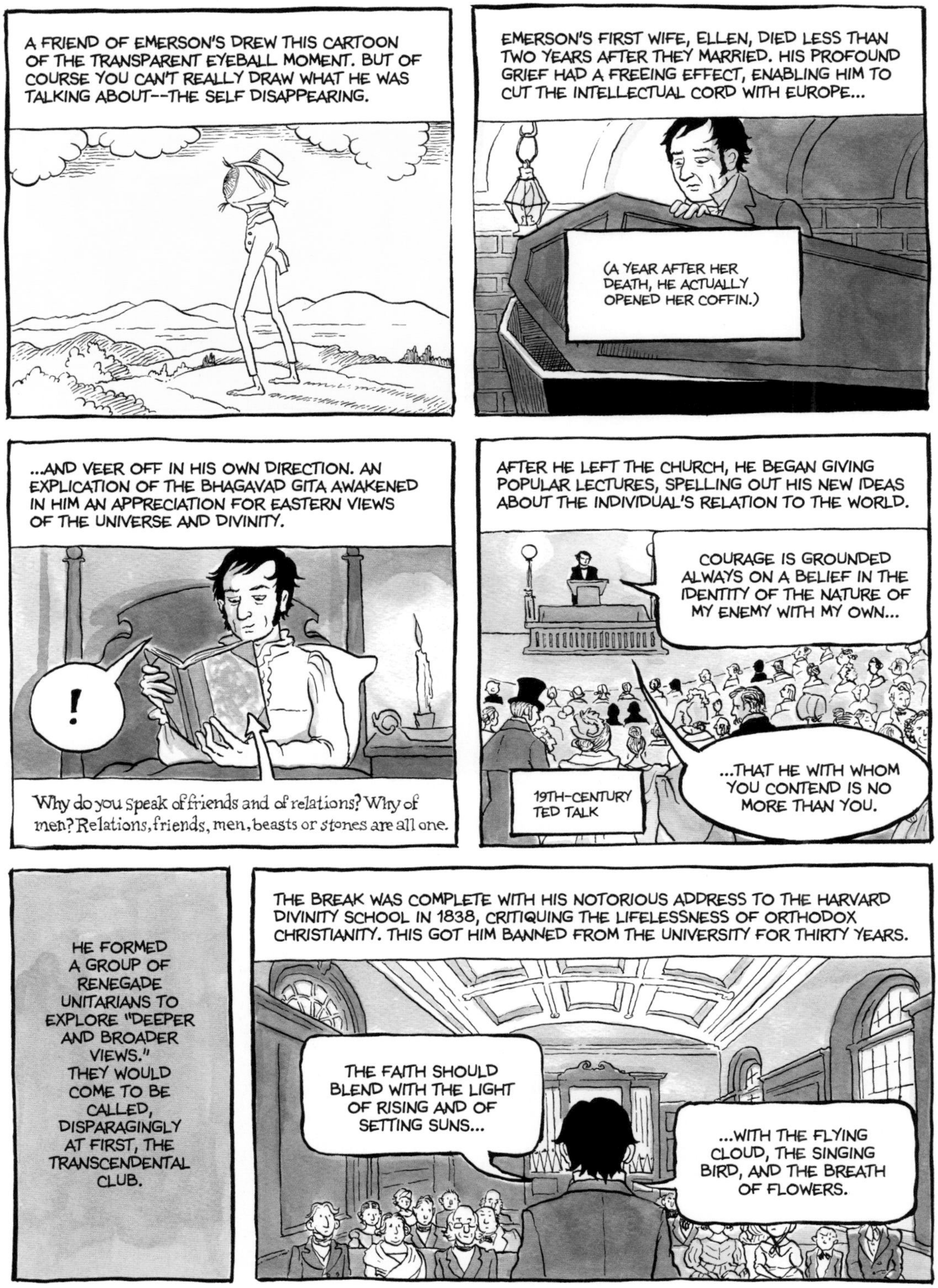
A FRIEND OF EMERSON'S DREW THIS CARTOON OF THE TRANSPARENT EYEBALL MOMENT. BUT OF COURSE YOU CAN'T REALLY DRAW WHAT HE WAS TALKING ABOUT--THE SELF DISAPPEARING.
EMERSON'S FIRST WIFE, ELLEN, DIED LESS THAN TWO YEARS AFTER THEY MARRIED. HIS PROFOUND GRIEF HAD A FREEING EFFECT, ENABLING HIM TO CUT THE INTELLECTUAL CORD WITH EUROPE...
(A YEAR AFTER HER DEATH, HE ACTUALLY OPENED HER COFFIN.)
...AND VEER OFF IN HIS OWN DIRECTION. AN EXPLICATION OF THE BHAGAVAD GITA AWAKENED IN HIM AN APPRECIATION FOR EASTERN VIEWS OF THE UNIVERSE AND DIVINITY.
!
Why do you speak of friends and of relations? Why of men? Relations, friends, men, beasts or stones are all one.
AFTER HE LEFT THE CHURCH, HE BEGAN GIVING POPULAR LECTURES, SPELLING OUT HIS NEW IDEAS ABOUT THE INDIVIDUAL'S RELATION TO THE WORLD.
COURAGE IS GROUNDED ALWAYS ON A BELIEF IN THE IDENTITY OF THE NATURE OF MY ENEMY WITH MY OWN...
19TH-CENTURY TED TALK
...THAT HE WITH WHOM YOU CONTEND IS NO MORE THAN YOU.
HE FORMED A GROUP OF RENEGADE UNITARIANS TO EXPLORE "DEEPER AND BROADER VIEWS." THEY WOULD COME TO BE CALLED, DISPARAGINGLY AT FIRST, THE TRANSCENDENTAL CLUB.
THE BREAK WAS COMPLETE WITH HIS NOTORIOUS ADDRESS TO THE HARVARD DIVINITY SCHOOL IN 1838, CRITIQUING THE LIFELESSNESS OF ORTHODOX CHRISTIANITY. THIS GOT HIM BANNED FROM THE UNIVERSITY FOR THIRTY YEARS.
THE FAITH SHOULD BLEND WITH THE LIGHT OF RISING AND OF SETTING SUNS...
...WITH THE FLYING CLOUD, THE SINGING BIRD, AND THE BREATH OF FLOWERS.

A PLAN SUDDENLY EMERGED FOR ME TO SKIP MY LAST YEAR OF HIGH SCHOOL AND HEAD STRAIGHT TO COLLEGE, IN MASSACHUSETTS. I BROKE UP WITH TIM IN A ROBOTIC WAY. I WAS OUT OF HERE.

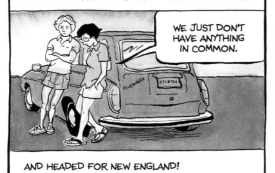

WE JUST DON'T HAVE ANYTHING IN COMMON.

AND HEADED FOR NEW ENGLAND!

I'D HAD FLICKERS OF ANXIETY THAT I MIGHT LIKE GIRLS MORE THAN BOYS, BUT I COULD BARELY NAVIGATE THE SOCIAL FRAY AS IT WAS--I COULDN'T IMAGINE ALSO BEING A HOMOSEXUAL.

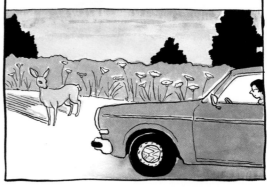

THE WORLD WAS CHANGING, THOUGH. IN FACT, THAT VERY AUGUST, IN NEW ENGLAND, ONE PERSON IN PARTICULAR WAS MAKING IT CHANGE. THE POET ADRIENNE RICH WAS UP AT HER COUNTRY HOUSE IN VERMONT.

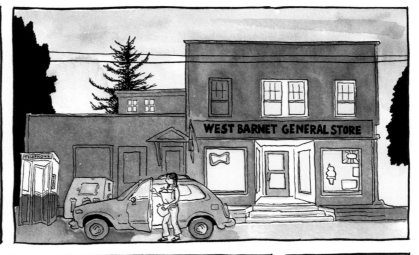

WEST BARNET GENERAL STORE

SHE AND HER HUSBAND HAD BOUGHT THE PLACE WHEN THEIR KIDS WERE SMALL.

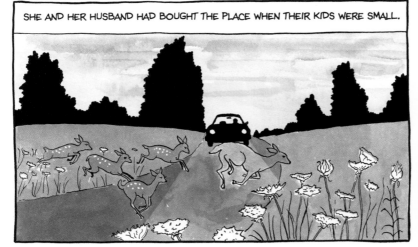

THEN THEY BOTH GOT CAUGHT UP IN THE RADICAL POLITICS OF THE LATE '60S, AND THE MARRIAGE FELL APART.

SOON AFTER THAT, HER HUSBAND CAME TO THE HOUSE ALONE AND KILLED HIMSELF.

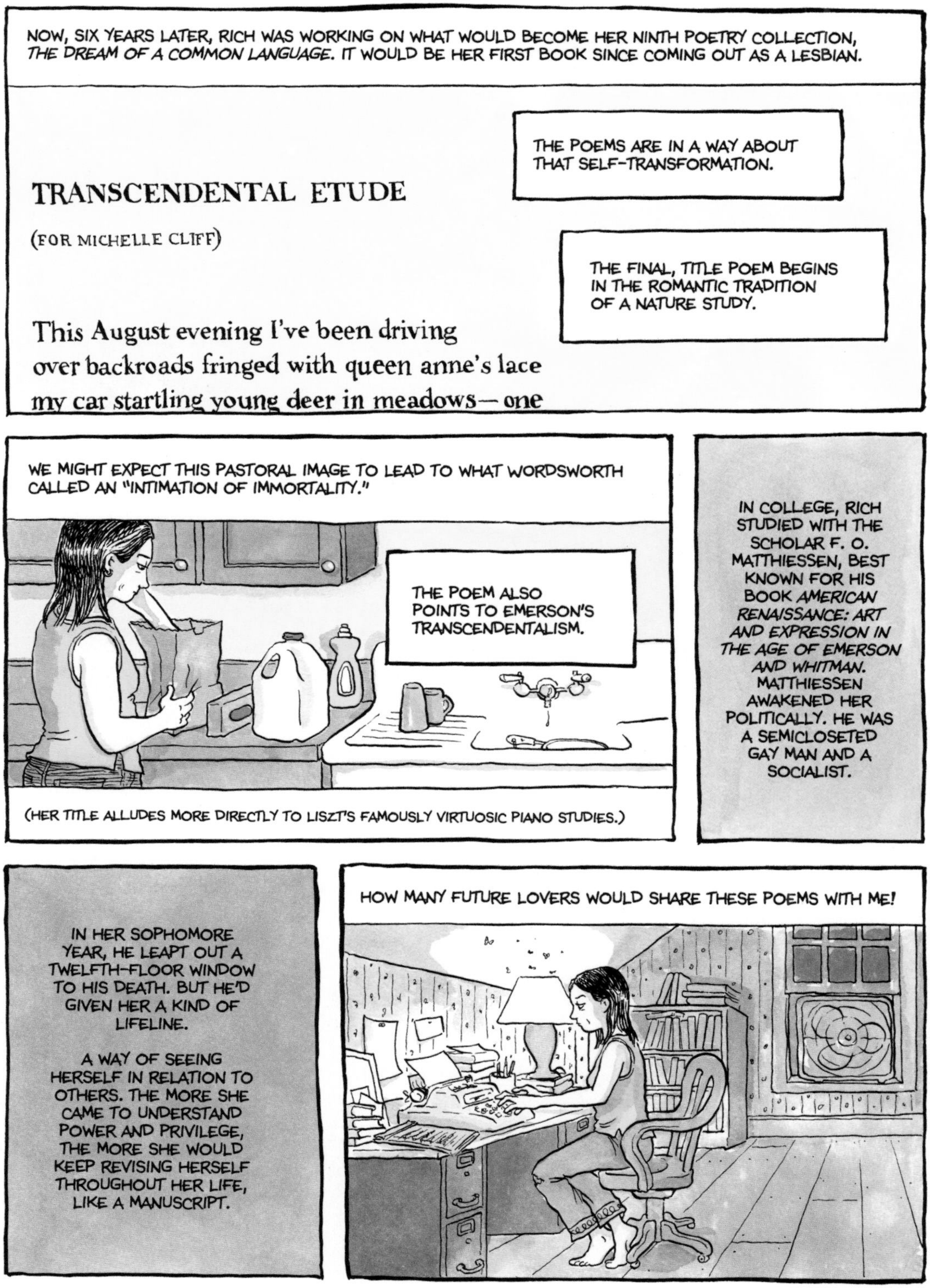
NOW, SIX YEARS LATER, RICH WAS WORKING ON WHAT WOULD BECOME HER NINTH POETRY COLLECTION, *THE DREAM OF A COMMON LANGUAGE.* IT WOULD BE HER FIRST BOOK SINCE COMING OUT AS A LESBIAN.
TRANSCENDENTAL ETUDE
(FOR MICHELLE CLIFF)
This August evening I've been driving
over backroads fringed with queen anne's lace
my car startling young deer in meadows—one
THE POEMS ARE IN A WAY ABOUT THAT SELF-TRANSFORMATION.
THE FINAL, TITLE POEM BEGINS IN THE ROMANTIC TRADITION OF A NATURE STUDY.
WE MIGHT EXPECT THIS PASTORAL IMAGE TO LEAD TO WHAT WORDSWORTH CALLED AN "INTIMATION OF IMMORTALITY."
THE POEM ALSO POINTS TO EMERSON'S TRANSCENDENTALISM.
(HER TITLE ALLUDES MORE DIRECTLY TO LISZT'S FAMOUSLY VIRTUOSIC PIANO STUDIES.)
IN COLLEGE, RICH STUDIED WITH THE SCHOLAR F. O. MATTHIESSEN, BEST KNOWN FOR HIS BOOK *AMERICAN RENAISSANCE: ART AND EXPRESSION IN THE AGE OF EMERSON AND WHITMAN.* MATTHIESSEN AWAKENED HER POLITICALLY. HE WAS A SEMICLOSETED GAY MAN AND A SOCIALIST.
IN HER SOPHOMORE YEAR, HE LEAPT OUT A TWELFTH-FLOOR WINDOW TO HIS DEATH. BUT HE'D GIVEN HER A KIND OF LIFELINE.
A WAY OF SEEING HERSELF IN RELATION TO OTHERS. THE MORE SHE CAME TO UNDERSTAND POWER AND PRIVILEGE, THE MORE SHE WOULD KEEP REVISING HERSELF THROUGHOUT HER LIFE, LIKE A MANUSCRIPT.
HOW MANY FUTURE LOVERS WOULD SHARE THESE POEMS WITH ME!

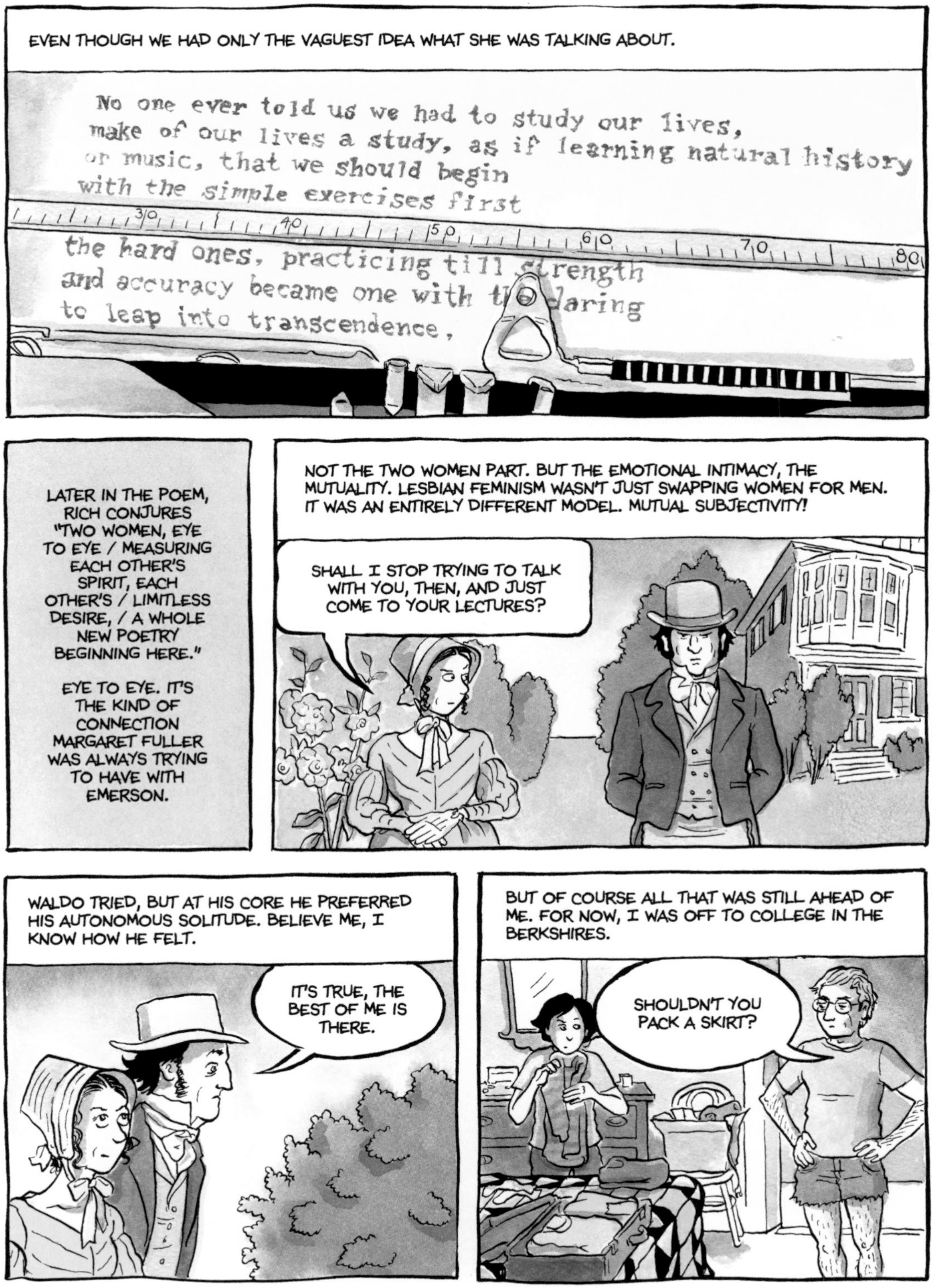
EVEN THOUGH WE HAD ONLY THE VAGUEST IDEA WHAT SHE WAS TALKING ABOUT.
No one ever told us we had to study our lives,
make of our lives a study, as if learning natural history
or music, that we should begin
with the simple exercises first
the hard ones, practicing till strength
and accuracy became one with the daring
to leap into transcendence.
LATER IN THE POEM, RICH CONJURES "TWO WOMEN, EYE TO EYE / MEASURING EACH OTHER'S SPIRIT, EACH OTHER'S / LIMITLESS DESIRE, / A WHOLE NEW POETRY BEGINNING HERE."
EYE TO EYE. IT'S THE KIND OF CONNECTION MARGARET FULLER WAS ALWAYS TRYING TO HAVE WITH EMERSON.
NOT THE TWO WOMEN PART. BUT THE EMOTIONAL INTIMACY, THE MUTUALITY. LESBIAN FEMINISM WASN'T JUST SWAPPING WOMEN FOR MEN. IT WAS AN ENTIRELY DIFFERENT MODEL. MUTUAL SUBJECTIVITY!
SHALL I STOP TRYING TO TALK WITH YOU, THEN, AND JUST COME TO YOUR LECTURES?
WALDO TRIED, BUT AT HIS CORE HE PREFERRED HIS AUTONOMOUS SOLITUDE. BELIEVE ME, I KNOW HOW HE FELT.
IT'S TRUE, THE BEST OF ME IS THERE.
BUT OF COURSE ALL THAT WAS STILL AHEAD OF ME. FOR NOW, I WAS OFF TO COLLEGE IN THE BERKSHIRES.
SHOULDN'T YOU PACK A SKIRT?

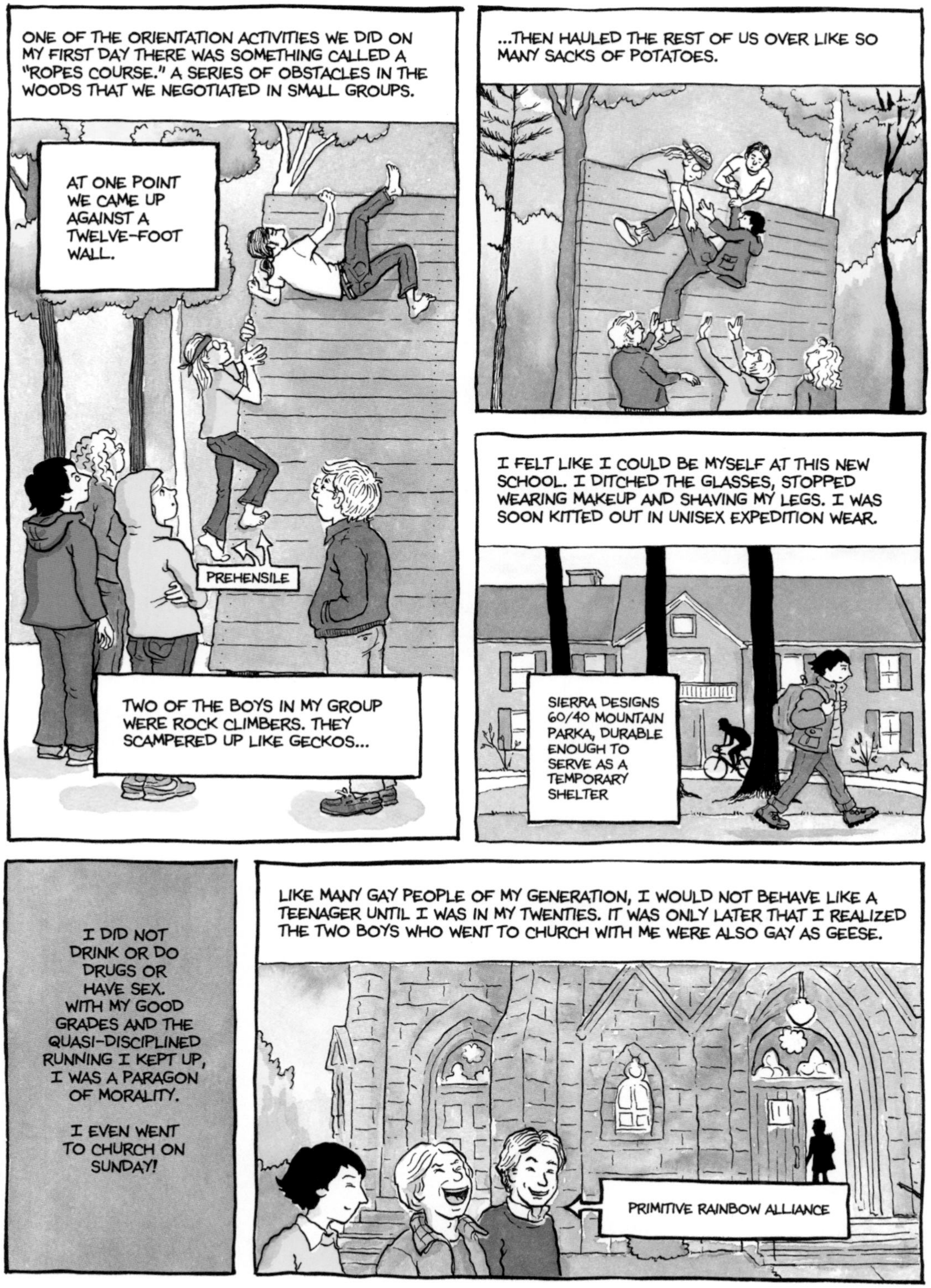
ONE OF THE ORIENTATION ACTIVITIES WE DID ON MY FIRST DAY THERE WAS SOMETHING CALLED A "ROPES COURSE." A SERIES OF OBSTACLES IN THE WOODS THAT WE NEGOTIATED IN SMALL GROUPS.
AT ONE POINT WE CAME UP AGAINST A TWELVE-FOOT WALL.
PREHENSILE
TWO OF THE BOYS IN MY GROUP WERE ROCK CLIMBERS. THEY SCAMPERED UP LIKE GECKOS...
...THEN HAULED THE REST OF US OVER LIKE SO MANY SACKS OF POTATOES.
I FELT LIKE I COULD BE MYSELF AT THIS NEW SCHOOL. I DITCHED THE GLASSES, STOPPED WEARING MAKEUP AND SHAVING MY LEGS. I WAS SOON KITTED OUT IN UNISEX EXPEDITION WEAR.
SIERRA DESIGNS 60/40 MOUNTAIN PARKA, DURABLE ENOUGH TO SERVE AS A TEMPORARY SHELTER
I DID NOT DRINK OR DO DRUGS OR HAVE SEX. WITH MY GOOD GRADES AND THE QUASI-DISCIPLINED RUNNING I KEPT UP, I WAS A PARAGON OF MORALITY.
I EVEN WENT TO CHURCH ON SUNDAY!
LIKE MANY GAY PEOPLE OF MY GENERATION, I WOULD NOT BEHAVE LIKE A TEENAGER UNTIL I WAS IN MY TWENTIES. IT WAS ONLY LATER THAT I REALIZED THE TWO BOYS WHO WENT TO CHURCH WITH ME WERE ALSO GAY AS GEESE.
PRIMITIVE RAINBOW ALLIANCE

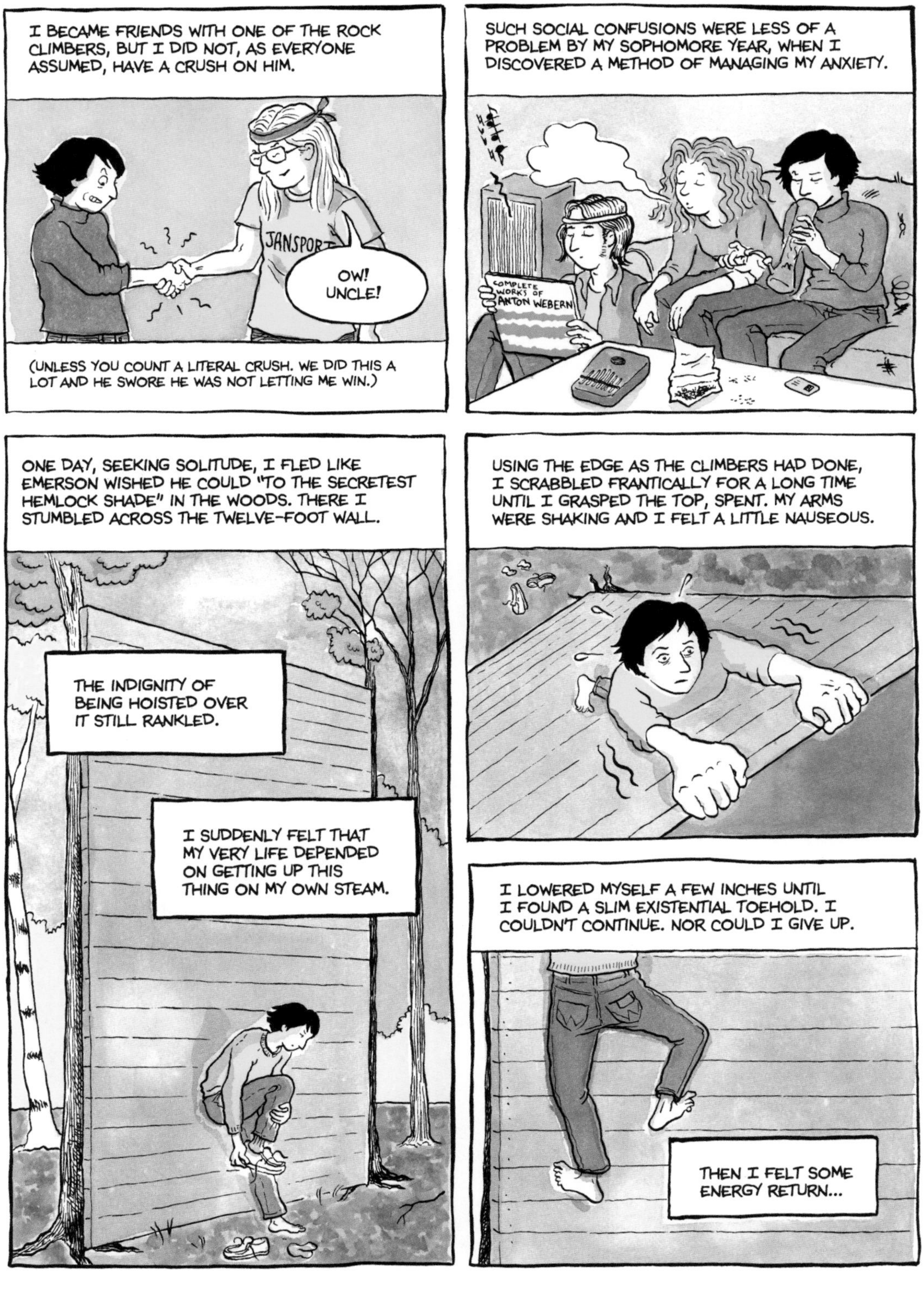
I BECAME FRIENDS WITH ONE OF THE ROCK CLIMBERS, BUT I DID NOT, AS EVERYONE ASSUMED, HAVE A CRUSH ON HIM.
OW! UNCLE!
(UNLESS YOU COUNT A LITERAL CRUSH. WE DID THIS A LOT AND HE SWORE HE WAS NOT LETTING ME WIN.)
SUCH SOCIAL CONFUSIONS WERE LESS OF A PROBLEM BY MY SOPHOMORE YEAR, WHEN I DISCOVERED A METHOD OF MANAGING MY ANXIETY.
COMPLETE WORKS OF ANTON WEBERN
ONE DAY, SEEKING SOLITUDE, I FLED LIKE EMERSON WISHED HE COULD "TO THE SECRETEST HEMLOCK SHADE" IN THE WOODS. THERE I STUMBLED ACROSS THE TWELVE-FOOT WALL.
THE INDIGNITY OF BEING HOISTED OVER IT STILL RANKLED.
I SUDDENLY FELT THAT MY VERY LIFE DEPENDED ON GETTING UP THIS THING ON MY OWN STEAM.
USING THE EDGE AS THE CLIMBERS HAD DONE, I SCRABBLED FRANTICALLY FOR A LONG TIME UNTIL I GRASPED THE TOP, SPENT. MY ARMS WERE SHAKING AND I FELT A LITTLE NAUSEOUS.
I LOWERED MYSELF A FEW INCHES UNTIL I FOUND A SLIM EXISTENTIAL TOEHOLD. I COULDN'T CONTINUE. NOR COULD I GIVE UP.
THEN I FELT SOME ENERGY RETURN...

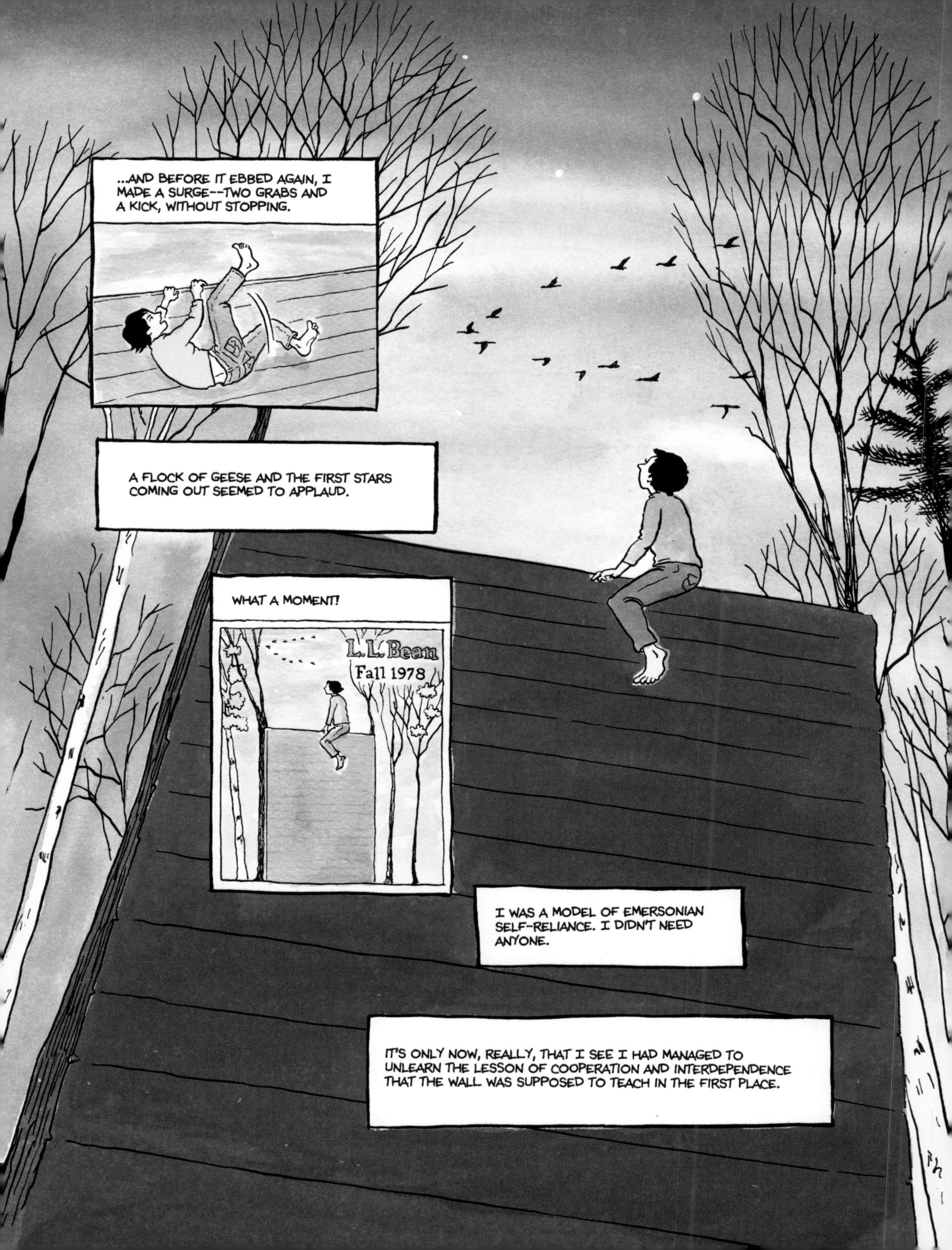
...AND BEFORE IT EBBED AGAIN, I MADE A SURGE--TWO GRABS AND A KICK, WITHOUT STOPPING.
A FLOCK OF GEESE AND THE FIRST STARS COMING OUT SEEMED TO APPLAUD.
WHAT A MOMENT!
L. L. Bean
Fall 1978
I WAS A MODEL OF EMERSONIAN SELF-RELIANCE. I DIDN'T NEED ANYONE.
IT'S ONLY NOW, REALLY, THAT I SEE I HAD MANAGED TO UNLEARN THE LESSON OF COOPERATION AND INTERDEPENDENCE THAT THE WALL WAS SUPPOSED TO TEACH IN THE FIRST PLACE.

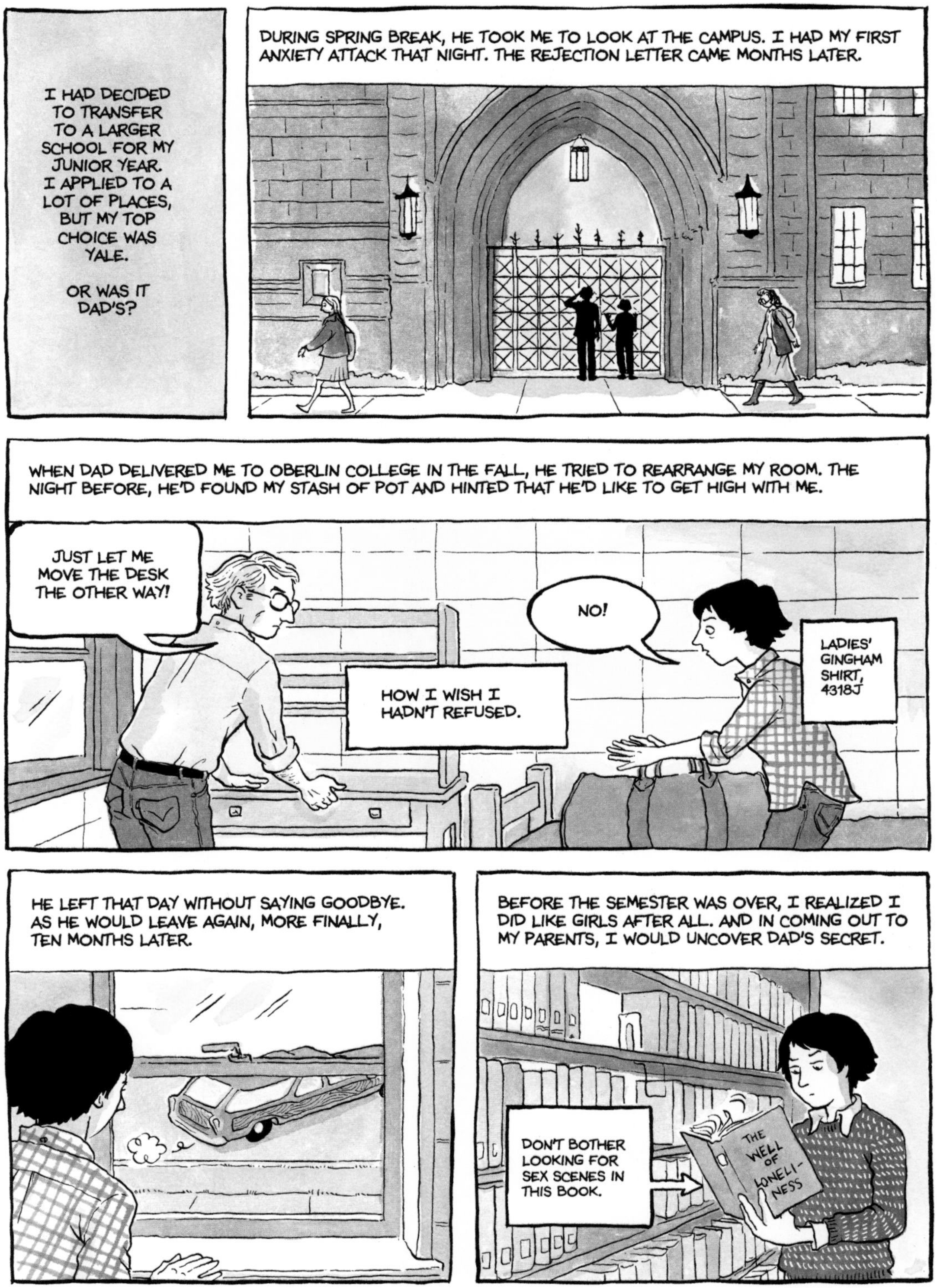
I HAD DECIDED TO TRANSFER TO A LARGER SCHOOL FOR MY JUNIOR YEAR. I APPLIED TO A LOT OF PLACES, BUT MY TOP CHOICE WAS YALE.
OR WAS IT DAD'S?
DURING SPRING BREAK, HE TOOK ME TO LOOK AT THE CAMPUS. I HAD MY FIRST ANXIETY ATTACK THAT NIGHT. THE REJECTION LETTER CAME MONTHS LATER.
WHEN DAD DELIVERED ME TO OBERLIN COLLEGE IN THE FALL, HE TRIED TO REARRANGE MY ROOM. THE NIGHT BEFORE, HE'D FOUND MY STASH OF POT AND HINTED THAT HE'D LIKE TO GET HIGH WITH ME.
JUST LET ME MOVE THE DESK THE OTHER WAY!
HOW I WISH I HADN'T REFUSED.
NO!
LADIES' GINGHAM SHIRT, 4318J
HE LEFT THAT DAY WITHOUT SAYING GOODBYE. AS HE WOULD LEAVE AGAIN, MORE FINALLY, TEN MONTHS LATER.
BEFORE THE SEMESTER WAS OVER, I REALIZED I DID LIKE GIRLS AFTER ALL. AND IN COMING OUT TO MY PARENTS, I WOULD UNCOVER DAD'S SECRET.
DON'T BOTHER LOOKING FOR SEX SCENES IN THIS BOOK.
THE WELL OF LONELINESS

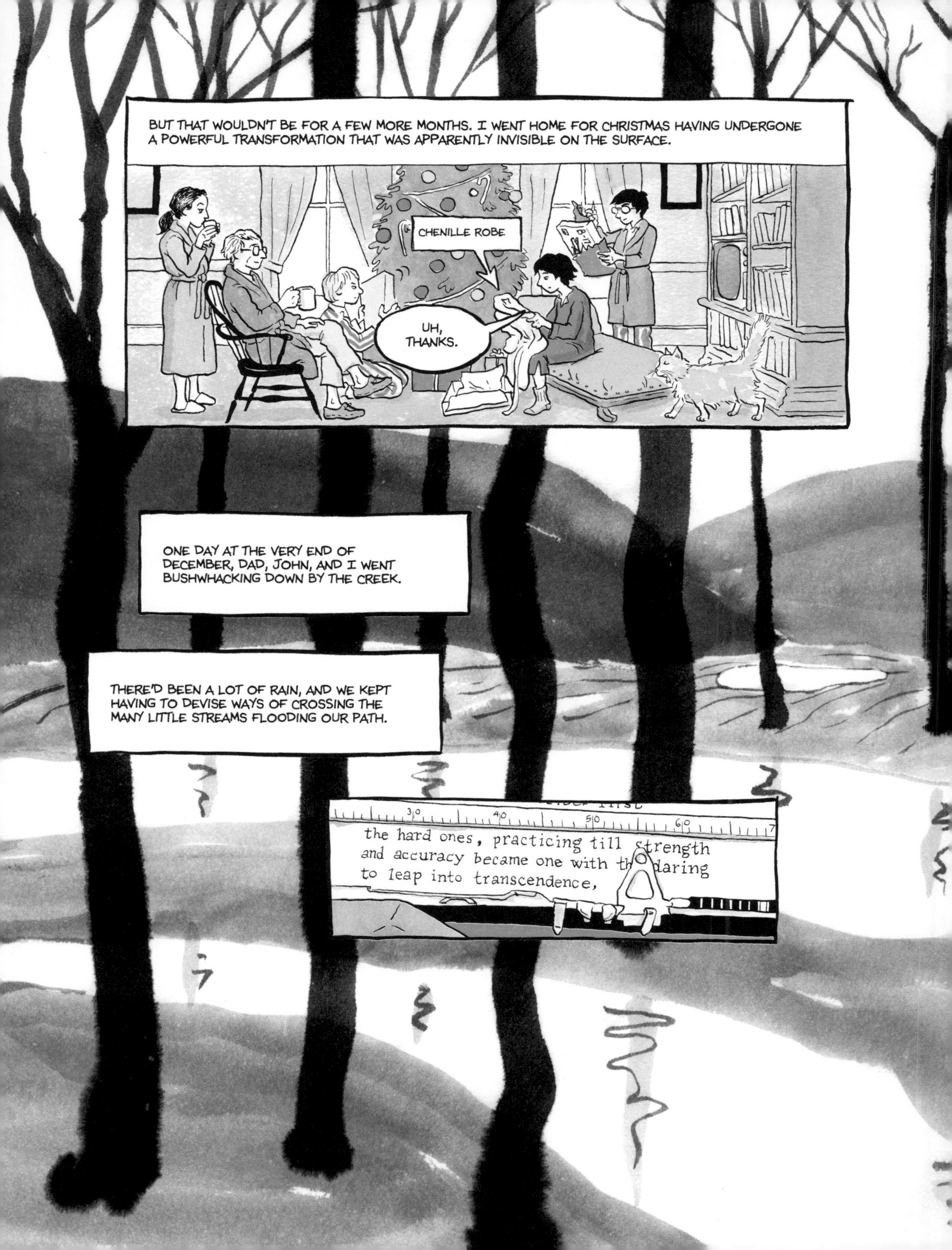

BUT THAT WOULDN'T BE FOR A FEW MORE MONTHS. I WENT HOME FOR CHRISTMAS HAVING UNDERGONE A POWERFUL TRANSFORMATION THAT WAS APPARENTLY INVISIBLE ON THE SURFACE.
CHENILLE ROBE
UH, THANKS.
ONE DAY AT THE VERY END OF DECEMBER, DAD, JOHN, AND I WENT BUSHWHACKING DOWN BY THE CREEK.
THERE'D BEEN A LOT OF RAIN, AND WE KEPT HAVING TO DEVISE WAYS OF CROSSING THE MANY LITTLE STREAMS FLOODING OUR PATH.
the hard ones, practicing till strength
and accuracy became one with th daring
to leap into transcendence,

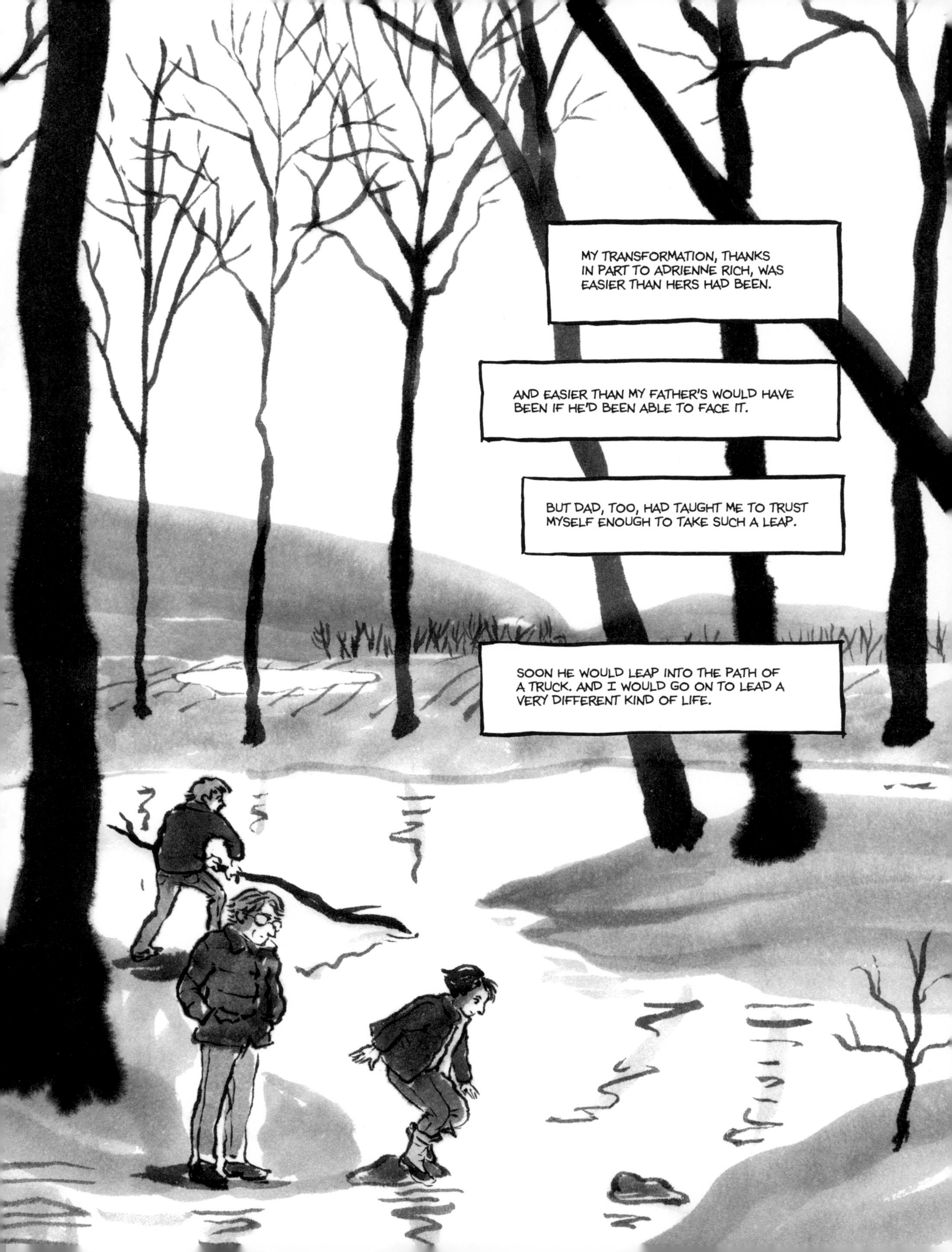
MY TRANSFORMATION, THANKS IN PART TO ADRIENNE RICH, WAS EASIER THAN HERS HAD BEEN.
AND EASIER THAN MY FATHER'S WOULD HAVE BEEN IF HE'D BEEN ABLE TO FACE IT.
BUT DAD, TOO, HAD TAUGHT ME TO TRUST MYSELF ENOUGH TO TAKE SUCH A LEAP.
SOON HE WOULD LEAP INTO THE PATH OF A TRUCK. AND I WOULD GO ON TO LEAD A VERY DIFFERENT KIND OF LIFE.

1980s

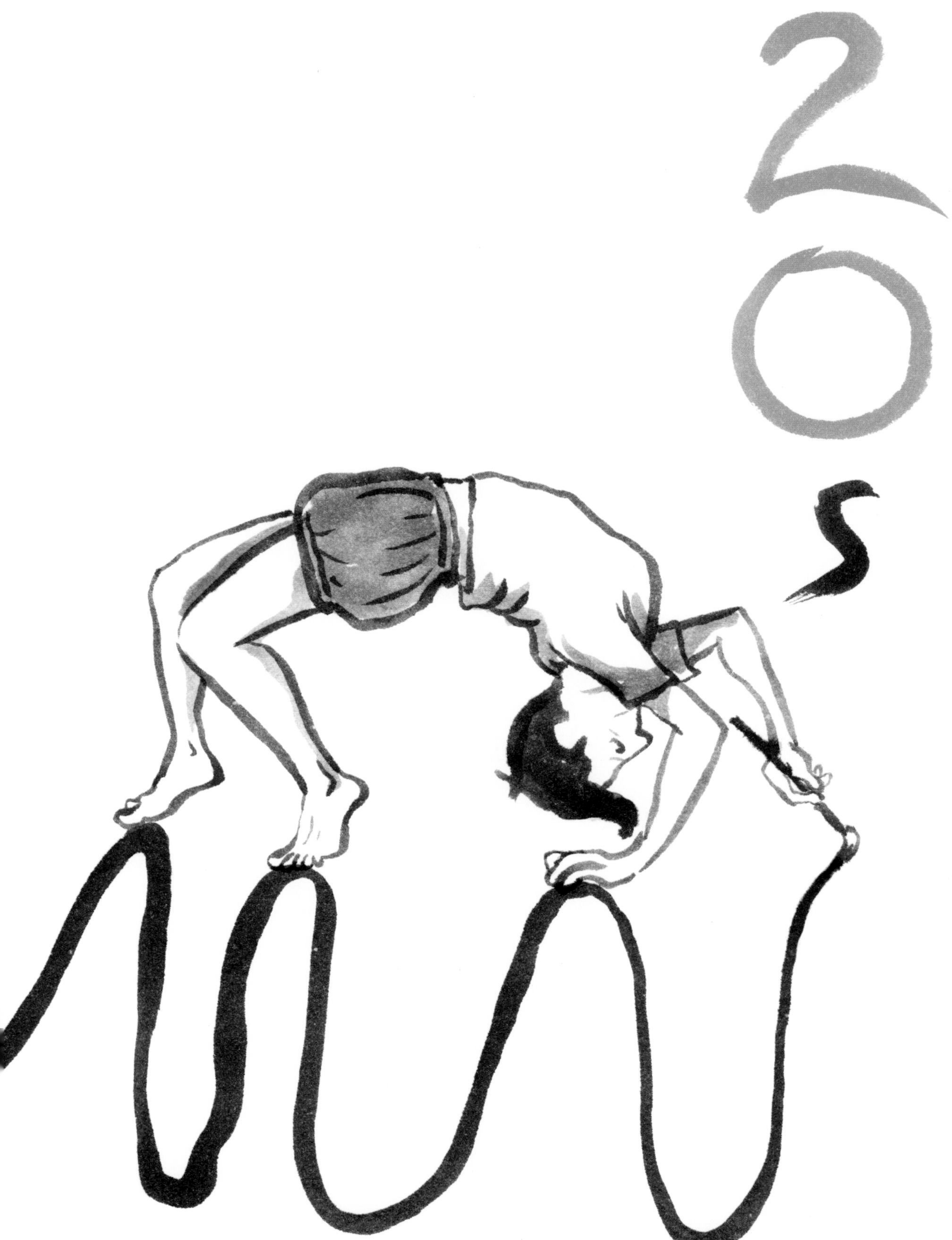
20

A MONTH AFTER DAD'S FUNERAL, AND A MONTH BEFORE MY TWENTIETH BIRTHDAY, I FOUND MYSELF HEADING WITH MY NEW GIRLFRIEND, JOAN, TO SOMETHING CALLED THE MICHIGAN WOMYN'S MUSIC FESTIVAL.

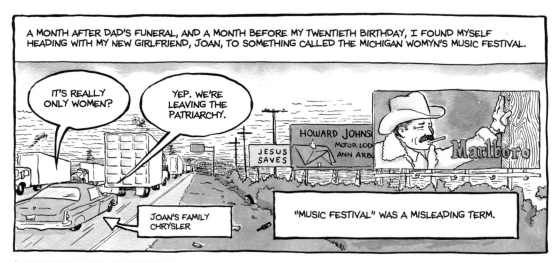

IT'S REALLY ONLY WOMEN?

YEP. WE'RE LEAVING THE PATRIARCHY.

JESUS SAVES

HOWARD JOHNS MOTOR LOD ANN ARBO

Marlboro

JOAN'S FAMILY CHRYSLER

"MUSIC FESTIVAL" WAS A MISLEADING TERM.

THERE WOULD BE MUSIC, TO BE SURE. BUT THE WEEKEND WAS A MIND-BENDING UTOPIAN EXPERIMENT, AN INSURGENCY OF WOMEN ENGAGED IN NOTHING LESS THAN DISMANTLING SAID PATRIARCHY.

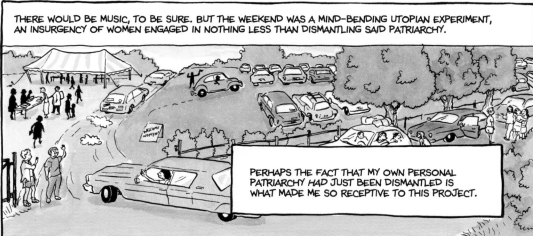

WELCOME WOMYN!

PERHAPS THE FACT THAT MY OWN PERSONAL PATRIARCHY *HAD* JUST BEEN DISMANTLED IS WHAT MADE ME SO RECEPTIVE TO THIS PROJECT.

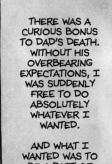

THERE WAS A CURIOUS BONUS TO DAD'S DEATH. WITHOUT HIS OVERBEARING EXPECTATIONS, I WAS SUDDENLY FREE TO DO ABSOLUTELY WHATEVER I WANTED.

AND WHAT I WANTED WAS TO BE A PART OF THIS.

IT WAS A WORLD UPSIDE DOWN! THE BOUNDARY BETWEEN SELF AND OTHER BROKE DOWN IMMEDIATELY. HIERARCHY WAS OUT. THE COLLECTIVE WAS IN!

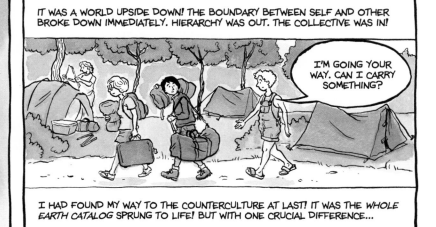

I'M GOING YOUR WAY. CAN I CARRY SOMETHING?

I HAD FOUND MY WAY TO THE COUNTERCULTURE AT LAST! IT WAS THE *WHOLE EARTH CATALOG* SPRUNG TO LIFE! BUT WITH ONE CRUCIAL DIFFERENCE...

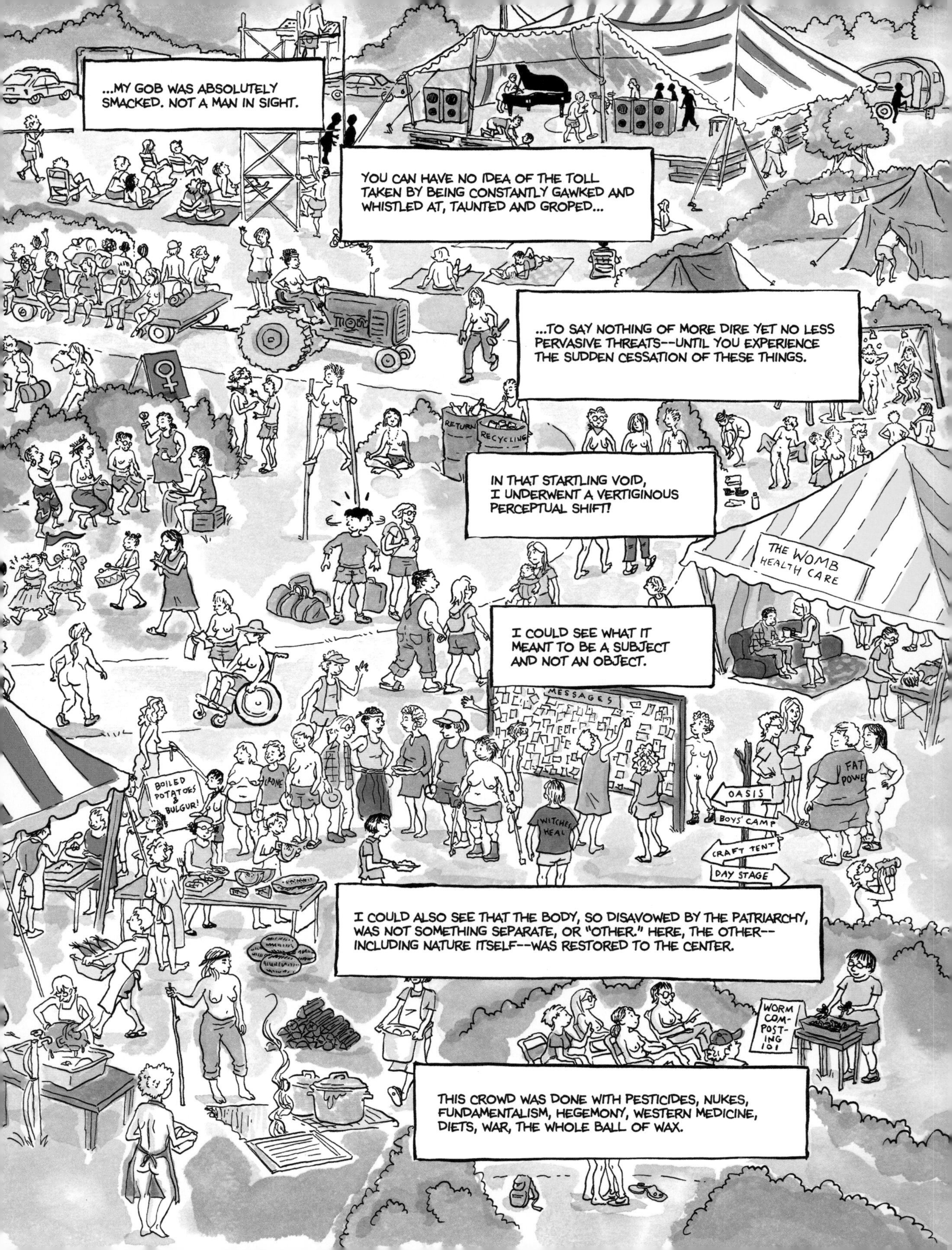
...MY GOB WAS ABSOLUTELY SMACKED. NOT A MAN IN SIGHT.
YOU CAN HAVE NO IDEA OF THE TOLL TAKEN BY BEING CONSTANTLY GAWKED AND WHISTLED AT, TAUNTED AND GROPED...
...TO SAY NOTHING OF MORE DIRE YET NO LESS PERVASIVE THREATS--UNTIL YOU EXPERIENCE THE SUDDEN CESSATION OF THESE THINGS.
RETURN
RECYCLING
IN THAT STARTLING VOID, I UNDERWENT A VERTIGINOUS PERCEPTUAL SHIFT!
THE WOMB HEALTH CARE
I COULD SEE WHAT IT MEANT TO BE A SUBJECT AND NOT AN OBJECT.
MESSAGES
BOILED POTATOES & BULGUR!
CRONE
WITCHES HEAL
FAT POWER
OASIS
BOYS' CAMP
CRAFT TENT
DAY STAGE
I COULD ALSO SEE THAT THE BODY, SO DISAVOWED BY THE PATRIARCHY, WAS NOT SOMETHING SEPARATE, OR "OTHER." HERE, THE OTHER--INCLUDING NATURE ITSELF--WAS RESTORED TO THE CENTER.
WORM COMPOSTING 101
THIS CROWD WAS DONE WITH PESTICIDES, NUKES, FUNDAMENTALISM, HEGEMONY, WESTERN MEDICINE, DIETS, WAR, THE WHOLE BALL OF WAX.

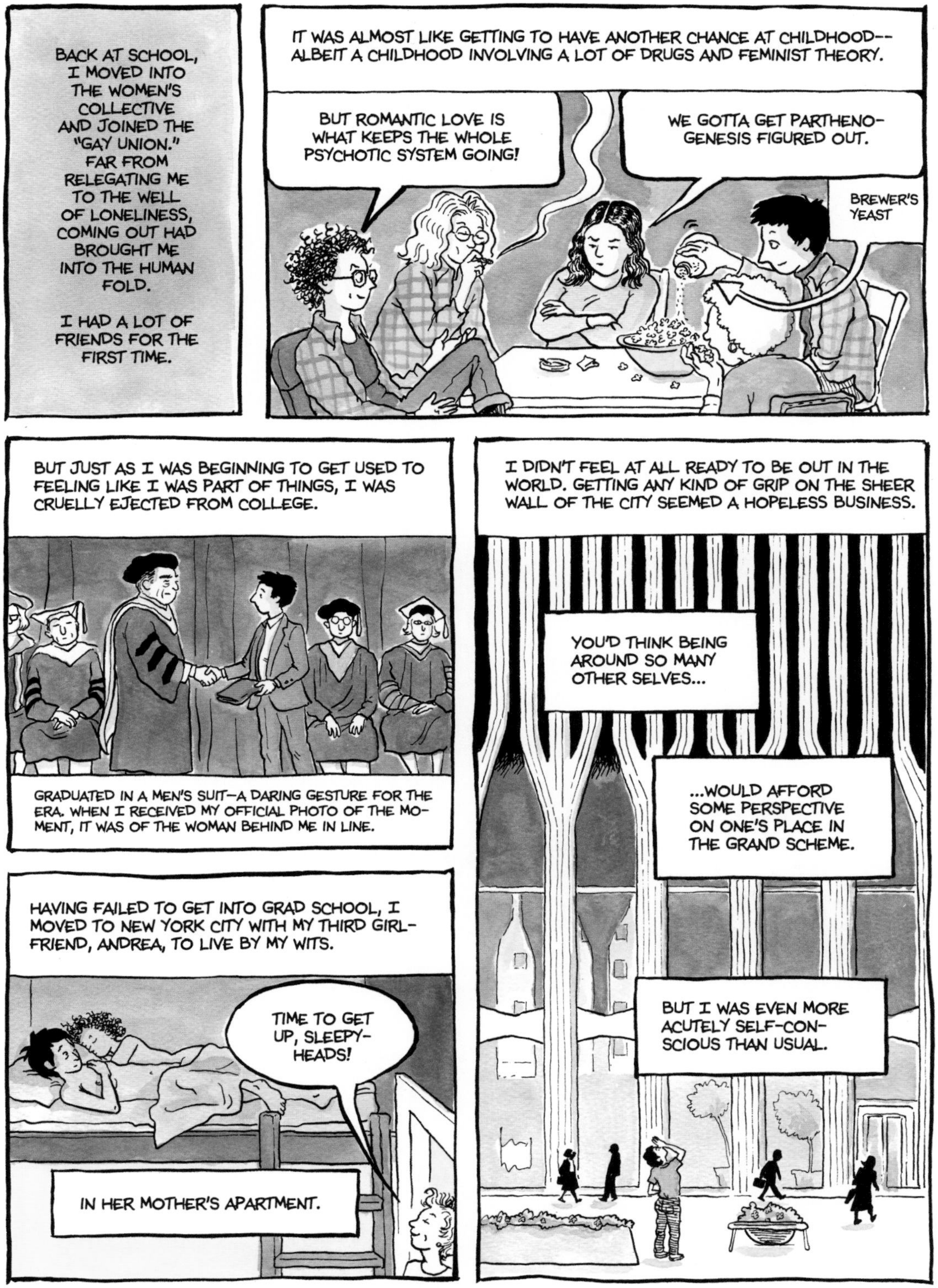
BACK AT SCHOOL, I MOVED INTO THE WOMEN'S COLLECTIVE AND JOINED THE "GAY UNION." FAR FROM RELEGATING ME TO THE WELL OF LONELINESS, COMING OUT HAD BROUGHT ME INTO THE HUMAN FOLD.
I HAD A LOT OF FRIENDS FOR THE FIRST TIME.
IT WAS ALMOST LIKE GETTING TO HAVE ANOTHER CHANCE AT CHILDHOOD--ALBEIT A CHILDHOOD INVOLVING A LOT OF DRUGS AND FEMINIST THEORY.
BUT ROMANTIC LOVE IS WHAT KEEPS THE WHOLE PSYCHOTIC SYSTEM GOING!
WE GOTTA GET PARTHENO-GENESIS FIGURED OUT.
BREWER'S YEAST
BUT JUST AS I WAS BEGINNING TO GET USED TO FEELING LIKE I WAS PART OF THINGS, I WAS CRUELLY EJECTED FROM COLLEGE.
GRADUATED IN A MEN'S SUIT—A DARING GESTURE FOR THE ERA. WHEN I RECEIVED MY OFFICIAL PHOTO OF THE MOMENT, IT WAS OF THE WOMAN BEHIND ME IN LINE.
HAVING FAILED TO GET INTO GRAD SCHOOL, I MOVED TO NEW YORK CITY WITH MY THIRD GIRLFRIEND, ANDREA, TO LIVE BY MY WITS.
TIME TO GET UP, SLEEPY-HEADS!
IN HER MOTHER'S APARTMENT.
I DIDN'T FEEL AT ALL READY TO BE OUT IN THE WORLD. GETTING ANY KIND OF GRIP ON THE SHEER WALL OF THE CITY SEEMED A HOPELESS BUSINESS.
YOU'D THINK BEING AROUND SO MANY OTHER SELVES...
...WOULD AFFORD SOME PERSPECTIVE ON ONE'S PLACE IN THE GRAND SCHEME.
BUT I WAS EVEN MORE ACUTELY SELF-CONSCIOUS THAN USUAL.

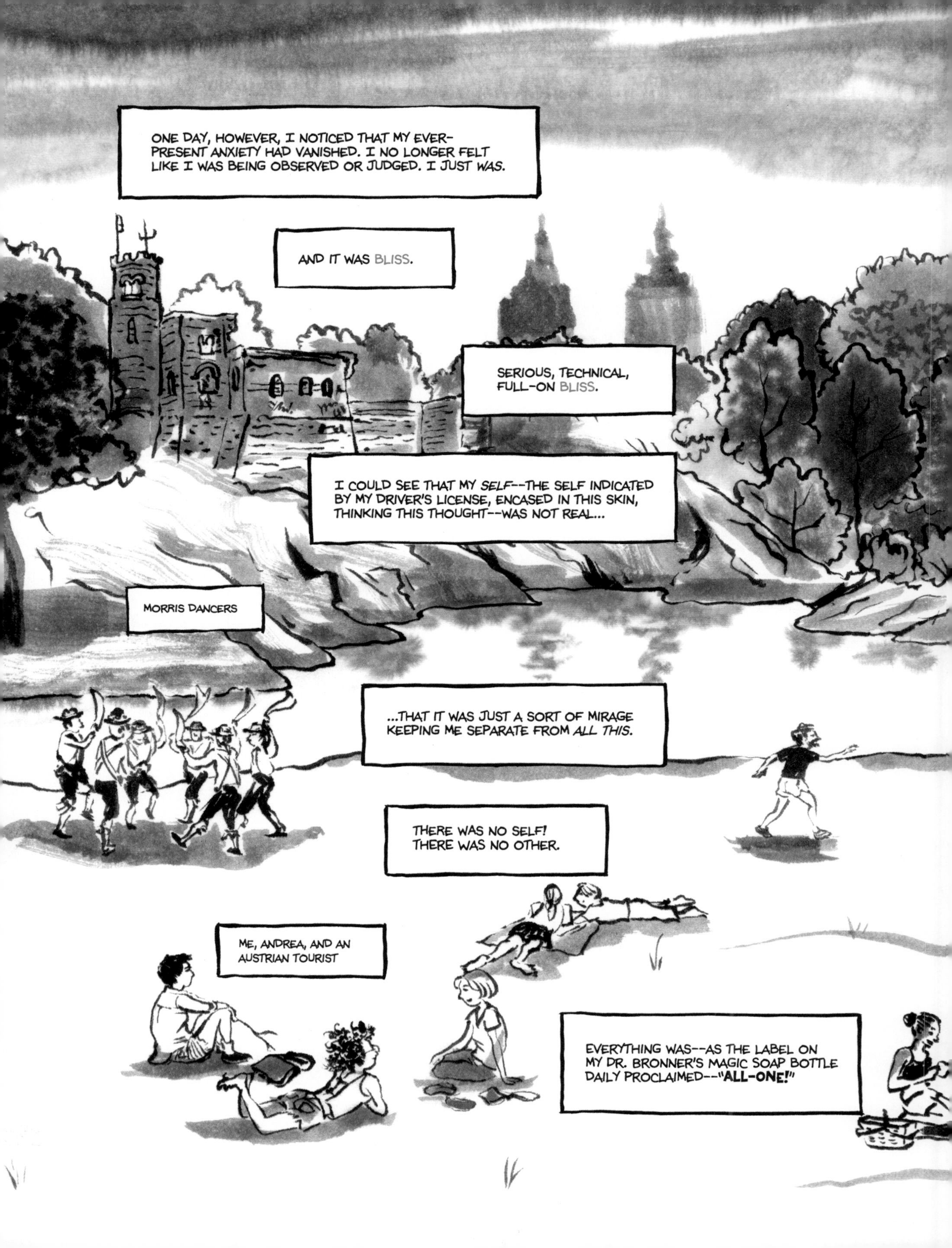
ONE DAY, HOWEVER, I NOTICED THAT MY EVER-PRESENT ANXIETY HAD VANISHED. I NO LONGER FELT LIKE I WAS BEING OBSERVED OR JUDGED. I JUST *WAS*.
AND IT WAS BLISS.
SERIOUS, TECHNICAL, FULL-ON BLISS.
I COULD SEE THAT MY *SELF*--THE SELF INDICATED BY MY DRIVER'S LICENSE, ENCASED IN THIS SKIN, THINKING THIS THOUGHT--WAS NOT REAL...
MORRIS DANCERS
...THAT IT WAS JUST A SORT OF MIRAGE KEEPING ME SEPARATE FROM *ALL THIS*.
THERE WAS NO SELF! THERE WAS NO OTHER.
ME, ANDREA, AND AN AUSTRIAN TOURIST
EVERYTHING WAS--AS THE LABEL ON MY DR. BRONNER'S MAGIC SOAP BOTTLE DAILY PROCLAIMED--"**ALL-ONE!**"

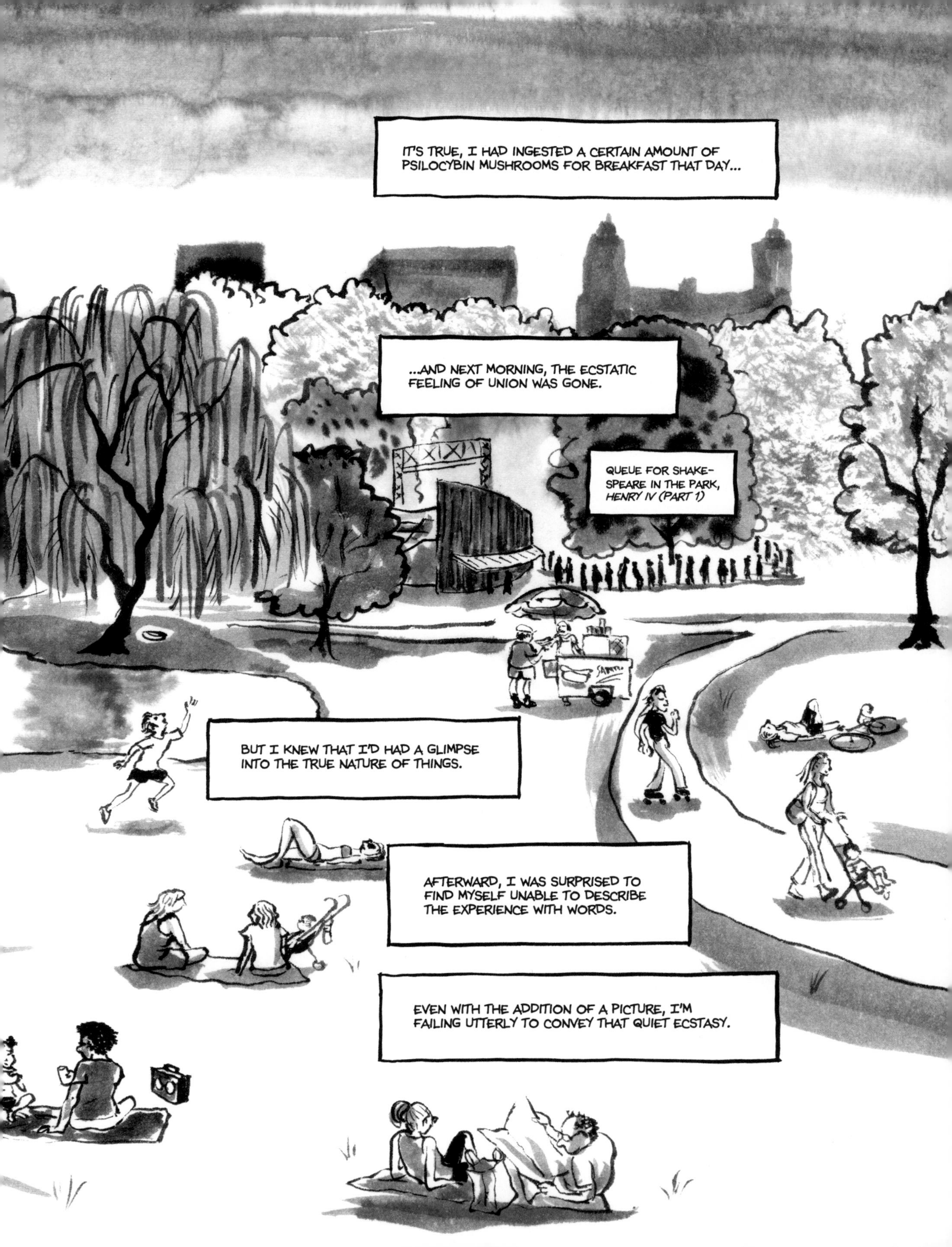
IT'S TRUE, I HAD INGESTED A CERTAIN AMOUNT OF PSILOCYBIN MUSHROOMS FOR BREAKFAST THAT DAY...
...AND NEXT MORNING, THE ECSTATIC FEELING OF UNION WAS GONE.
QUEUE FOR SHAKESPEARE IN THE PARK, *HENRY IV (PART 1)*
BUT I KNEW THAT I'D HAD A GLIMPSE INTO THE TRUE NATURE OF THINGS.
AFTERWARD, I WAS SURPRISED TO FIND MYSELF UNABLE TO DESCRIBE THE EXPERIENCE WITH WORDS.
EVEN WITH THE ADDITION OF A PICTURE, I'M FAILING UTTERLY TO CONVEY THAT QUIET ECSTASY.

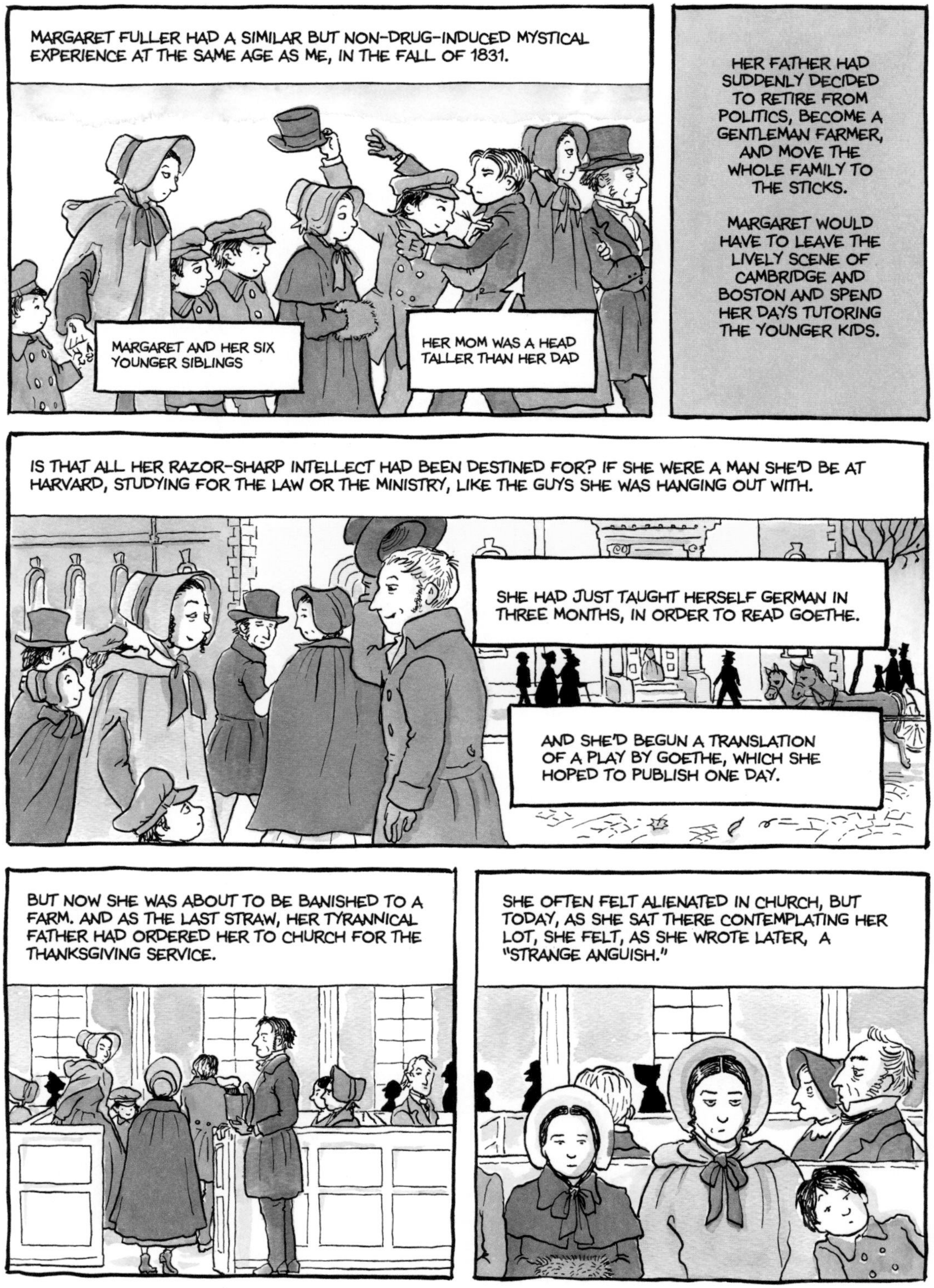
MARGARET FULLER HAD A SIMILAR BUT NON-DRUG-INDUCED MYSTICAL EXPERIENCE AT THE SAME AGE AS ME, IN THE FALL OF 1831.
MARGARET AND HER SIX YOUNGER SIBLINGS
HER MOM WAS A HEAD TALLER THAN HER DAD
HER FATHER HAD SUDDENLY DECIDED TO RETIRE FROM POLITICS, BECOME A GENTLEMAN FARMER, AND MOVE THE WHOLE FAMILY TO THE STICKS.
MARGARET WOULD HAVE TO LEAVE THE LIVELY SCENE OF CAMBRIDGE AND BOSTON AND SPEND HER DAYS TUTORING THE YOUNGER KIDS.
IS THAT ALL HER RAZOR-SHARP INTELLECT HAD BEEN DESTINED FOR? IF SHE WERE A MAN SHE'D BE AT HARVARD, STUDYING FOR THE LAW OR THE MINISTRY, LIKE THE GUYS SHE WAS HANGING OUT WITH.
SHE HAD JUST TAUGHT HERSELF GERMAN IN THREE MONTHS, IN ORDER TO READ GOETHE.
AND SHE'D BEGUN A TRANSLATION OF A PLAY BY GOETHE, WHICH SHE HOPED TO PUBLISH ONE DAY.
BUT NOW SHE WAS ABOUT TO BE BANISHED TO A FARM. AND AS THE LAST STRAW, HER TYRANNICAL FATHER HAD ORDERED HER TO CHURCH FOR THE THANKSGIVING SERVICE.
SHE OFTEN FELT ALIENATED IN CHURCH, BUT TODAY, AS SHE SAT THERE CONTEMPLATING HER LOT, SHE FELT, AS SHE WROTE LATER, A "STRANGE ANGUISH."

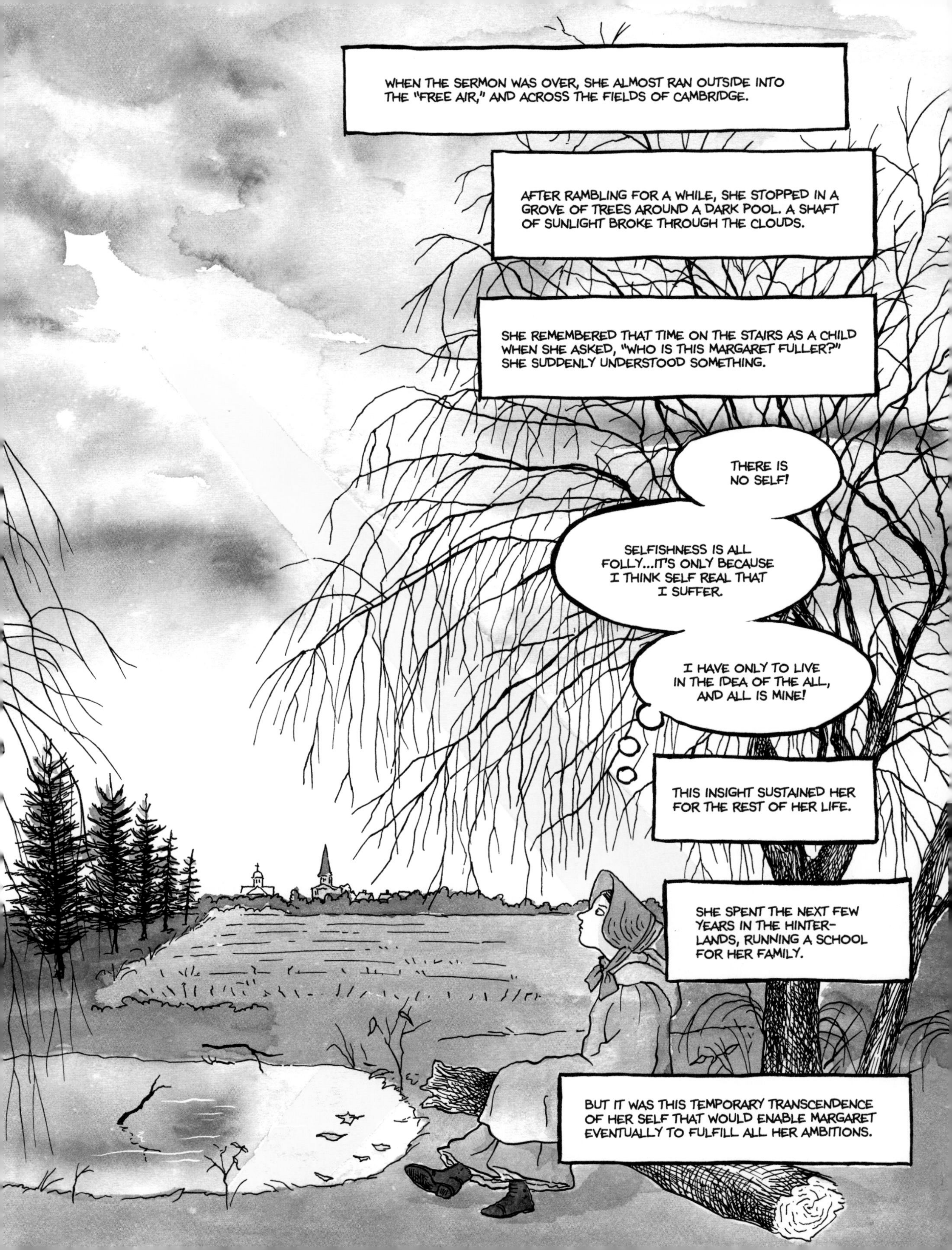
WHEN THE SERMON WAS OVER, SHE ALMOST RAN OUTSIDE INTO THE "FREE AIR," AND ACROSS THE FIELDS OF CAMBRIDGE.
AFTER RAMBLING FOR A WHILE, SHE STOPPED IN A GROVE OF TREES AROUND A DARK POOL. A SHAFT OF SUNLIGHT BROKE THROUGH THE CLOUDS.
SHE REMEMBERED THAT TIME ON THE STAIRS AS A CHILD WHEN SHE ASKED, "WHO IS THIS MARGARET FULLER?" SHE SUDDENLY UNDERSTOOD SOMETHING.
THERE IS NO SELF!
SELFISHNESS IS ALL FOLLY...IT'S ONLY BECAUSE I THINK SELF REAL THAT I SUFFER.
I HAVE ONLY TO LIVE IN THE IDEA OF THE ALL, AND ALL IS MINE!
THIS INSIGHT SUSTAINED HER FOR THE REST OF HER LIFE.
SHE SPENT THE NEXT FEW YEARS IN THE HINTER-LANDS, RUNNING A SCHOOL FOR HER FAMILY.
BUT IT WAS THIS TEMPORARY TRANSCENDENCE OF HER SELF THAT WOULD ENABLE MARGARET EVENTUALLY TO FULFILL ALL HER AMBITIONS.

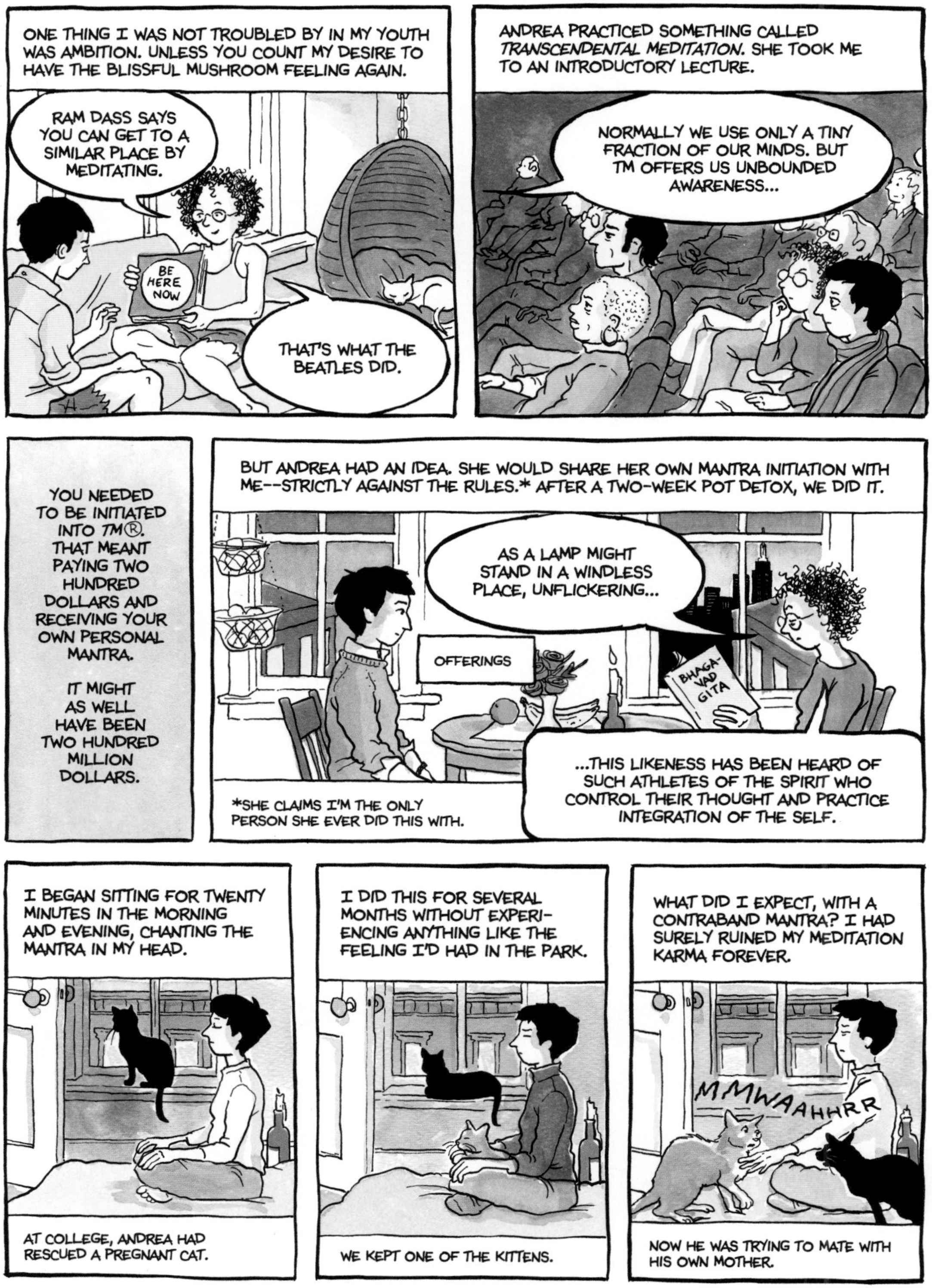
ONE THING I WAS NOT TROUBLED BY IN MY YOUTH WAS AMBITION. UNLESS YOU COUNT MY DESIRE TO HAVE THE BLISSFUL MUSHROOM FEELING AGAIN.
RAM DASS SAYS YOU CAN GET TO A SIMILAR PLACE BY MEDITATING.
BE HERE NOW
THAT'S WHAT THE BEATLES DID.
ANDREA PRACTICED SOMETHING CALLED *TRANSCENDENTAL MEDITATION.* SHE TOOK ME TO AN INTRODUCTORY LECTURE.
NORMALLY WE USE ONLY A TINY FRACTION OF OUR MINDS. BUT TM OFFERS US UNBOUNDED AWARENESS...
YOU NEEDED TO BE INITIATED INTO *TM*®. THAT MEANT PAYING TWO HUNDRED DOLLARS AND RECEIVING YOUR OWN PERSONAL MANTRA.
IT MIGHT AS WELL HAVE BEEN TWO HUNDRED MILLION DOLLARS.
BUT ANDREA HAD AN IDEA. SHE WOULD SHARE HER OWN MANTRA INITIATION WITH ME--STRICTLY AGAINST THE RULES.* AFTER A TWO-WEEK POT DETOX, WE DID IT.
AS A LAMP MIGHT STAND IN A WINDLESS PLACE, UNFLICKERING...
OFFERINGS
BHAGAVAD GITA
...THIS LIKENESS HAS BEEN HEARD OF SUCH ATHLETES OF THE SPIRIT WHO CONTROL THEIR THOUGHT AND PRACTICE INTEGRATION OF THE SELF.
*SHE CLAIMS I'M THE ONLY PERSON SHE EVER DID THIS WITH.
I BEGAN SITTING FOR TWENTY MINUTES IN THE MORNING AND EVENING, CHANTING THE MANTRA IN MY HEAD.
AT COLLEGE, ANDREA HAD RESCUED A PREGNANT CAT.
I DID THIS FOR SEVERAL MONTHS WITHOUT EXPERIENCING ANYTHING LIKE THE FEELING I'D HAD IN THE PARK.
WE KEPT ONE OF THE KITTENS.
WHAT DID I EXPECT, WITH A CONTRABAND MANTRA? I HAD SURELY RUINED MY MEDITATION KARMA FOREVER.
MMWAAHHRR
NOW HE WAS TRYING TO MATE WITH HIS OWN MOTHER.

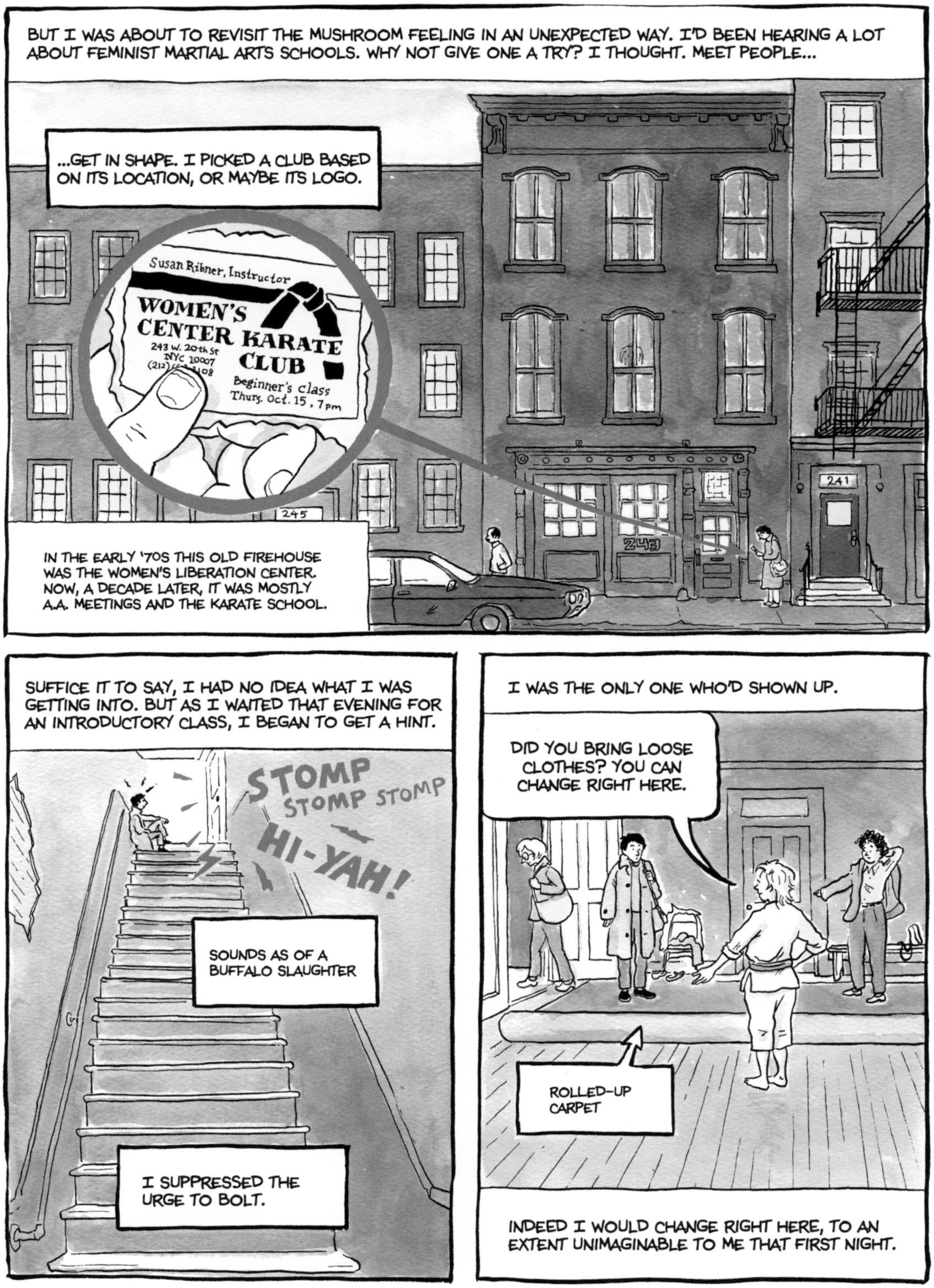

BUT I WAS ABOUT TO REVISIT THE MUSHROOM FEELING IN AN UNEXPECTED WAY. I'D BEEN HEARING A LOT ABOUT FEMINIST MARTIAL ARTS SCHOOLS. WHY NOT GIVE ONE A TRY? I THOUGHT. MEET PEOPLE...
...GET IN SHAPE. I PICKED A CLUB BASED ON ITS LOCATION, OR MAYBE ITS LOGO.
Susan Ribner, Instructor
WOMEN'S CENTER KARATE CLUB
243 W. 20th St
NYC 10007
Beginner's class
Thurs. Oct. 15, 7pm
245
243
241
IN THE EARLY '70S THIS OLD FIREHOUSE WAS THE WOMEN'S LIBERATION CENTER. NOW, A DECADE LATER, IT WAS MOSTLY A.A. MEETINGS AND THE KARATE SCHOOL.
SUFFICE IT TO SAY, I HAD NO IDEA WHAT I WAS GETTING INTO. BUT AS I WAITED THAT EVENING FOR AN INTRODUCTORY CLASS, I BEGAN TO GET A HINT.
STOMP STOMP STOMP
HI-YAH!
SOUNDS AS OF A BUFFALO SLAUGHTER
I SUPPRESSED THE URGE TO BOLT.
I WAS THE ONLY ONE WHO'D SHOWN UP.
DID YOU BRING LOOSE CLOTHES? YOU CAN CHANGE RIGHT HERE.
ROLLED-UP CARPET
INDEED I WOULD CHANGE RIGHT HERE, TO AN EXTENT UNIMAGINABLE TO ME THAT FIRST NIGHT.

I LEARNED HOW TO MAKE A PROPER FIST. NEXT DAY, I LEARNED TO KICK.

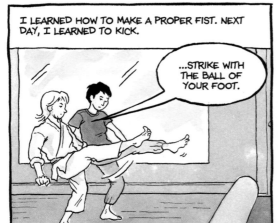

...STRIKE WITH THE BALL OF YOUR FOOT.

THE DAY AFTER THAT, RACKED WITH PAIN, I BOUGHT A UNIFORM AT A MIDTOWN WAREHOUSE.

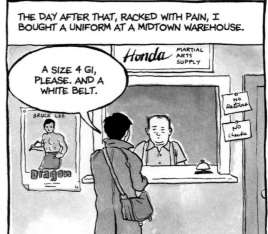

A SIZE 4 GI, PLEASE. AND A WHITE BELT.

Honda MARTIAL ARTS SUPPLY

NO Returns

NO Checks

BRUCE LEE
Dragon

I HAD A BIT OF A LEG UP, AS IT TURNED OUT. A LOW, SOLID STANCE IS KEY IN KARATE, AND THANKS TO ALL THE SKIING AND RUNNING, I HAD THE QUADRICEPS OF A SOVIET SPEED SKATER.

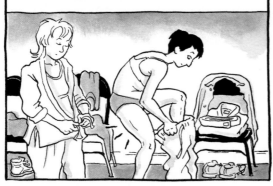

I WOULDN'T MEET SUSAN, THE SENSEI AND FOUNDER OF THE SCHOOL, UNTIL MY THIRD CLASS. SHE WAS A SECOND-DEGREE BLACK BELT.

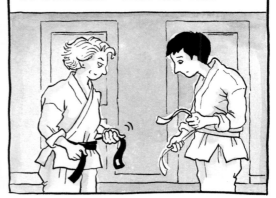

THERE WERE FOUR CLASSES A WEEK, AND I STARTED GOING TO ALL OF THEM. SOON I WAS LEARNING MY FIRST *KATA*--A CHOREOGRAPHED SEQUENCE OF ATTACKS AND DEFENSES AGAINST IMAGINARY OPPONENTS.

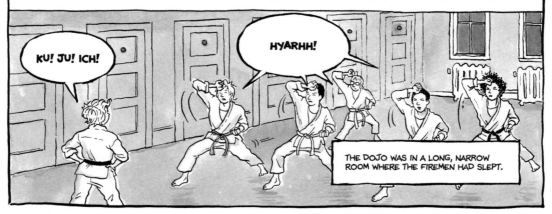

KU! JU! ICH!

HYARHH!

THE DOJO WAS IN A LONG, NARROW ROOM WHERE THE FIREMEN HAD SLEPT.

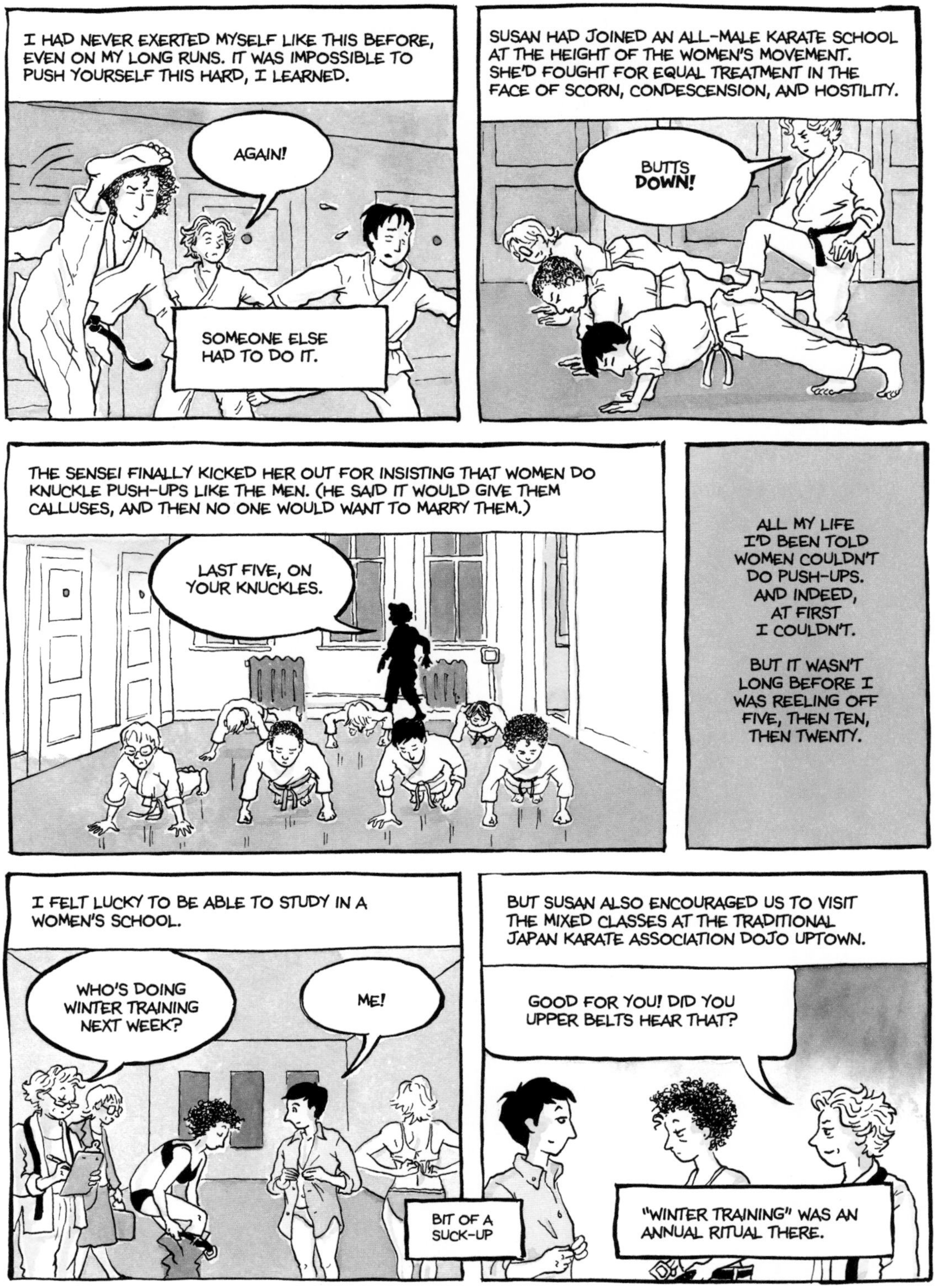
I HAD NEVER EXERTED MYSELF LIKE THIS BEFORE, EVEN ON MY LONG RUNS. IT WAS IMPOSSIBLE TO PUSH YOURSELF THIS HARD, I LEARNED.
AGAIN!
SOMEONE ELSE HAD TO DO IT.
SUSAN HAD JOINED AN ALL-MALE KARATE SCHOOL AT THE HEIGHT OF THE WOMEN'S MOVEMENT. SHE'D FOUGHT FOR EQUAL TREATMENT IN THE FACE OF SCORN, CONDESCENSION, AND HOSTILITY.
BUTTS DOWN!
THE SENSEI FINALLY KICKED HER OUT FOR INSISTING THAT WOMEN DO KNUCKLE PUSH-UPS LIKE THE MEN. (HE SAID IT WOULD GIVE THEM CALLUSES, AND THEN NO ONE WOULD WANT TO MARRY THEM.)
LAST FIVE, ON YOUR KNUCKLES.
ALL MY LIFE I'D BEEN TOLD WOMEN COULDN'T DO PUSH-UPS. AND INDEED, AT FIRST I COULDN'T.
BUT IT WASN'T LONG BEFORE I WAS REELING OFF FIVE, THEN TEN, THEN TWENTY.
I FELT LUCKY TO BE ABLE TO STUDY IN A WOMEN'S SCHOOL.
WHO'S DOING WINTER TRAINING NEXT WEEK?
ME!
BIT OF A SUCK-UP
BUT SUSAN ALSO ENCOURAGED US TO VISIT THE MIXED CLASSES AT THE TRADITIONAL JAPAN KARATE ASSOCIATION DOJO UPTOWN.
GOOD FOR YOU! DID YOU UPPER BELTS HEAR THAT?
"WINTER TRAINING" WAS AN ANNUAL RITUAL THERE.

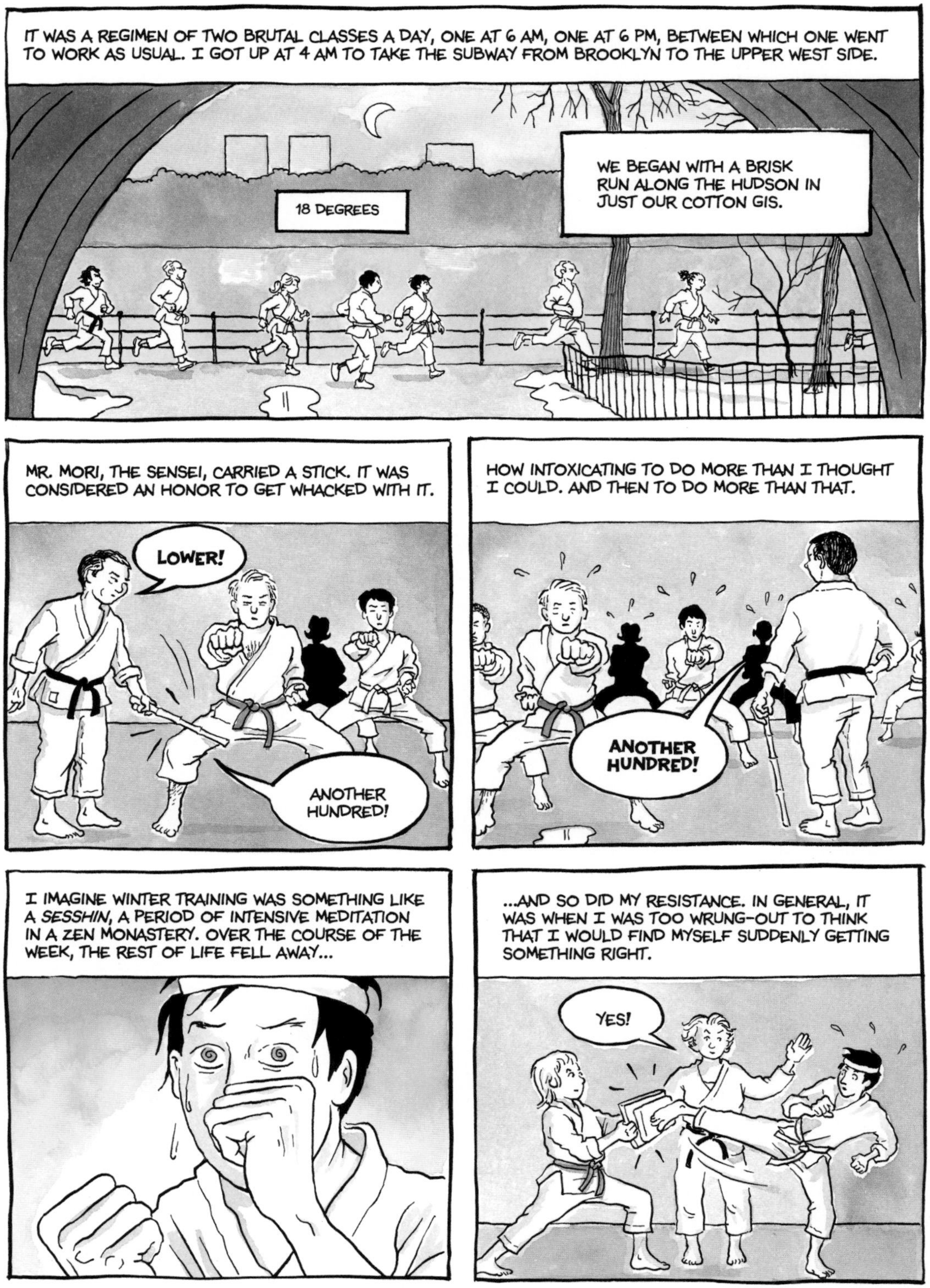
IT WAS A REGIMEN OF TWO BRUTAL CLASSES A DAY, ONE AT 6 AM, ONE AT 6 PM, BETWEEN WHICH ONE WENT TO WORK AS USUAL. I GOT UP AT 4 AM TO TAKE THE SUBWAY FROM BROOKLYN TO THE UPPER WEST SIDE.
18 DEGREES
WE BEGAN WITH A BRISK RUN ALONG THE HUDSON IN JUST OUR COTTON GIS.
MR. MORI, THE SENSEI, CARRIED A STICK. IT WAS CONSIDERED AN HONOR TO GET WHACKED WITH IT.
LOWER!
ANOTHER HUNDRED!
HOW INTOXICATING TO DO MORE THAN I THOUGHT I COULD. AND THEN TO DO MORE THAN THAT.
ANOTHER HUNDRED!
I IMAGINE WINTER TRAINING WAS SOMETHING LIKE A *SESSHIN*, A PERIOD OF INTENSIVE MEDITATION IN A ZEN MONASTERY. OVER THE COURSE OF THE WEEK, THE REST OF LIFE FELL AWAY...
...AND SO DID MY RESISTANCE. IN GENERAL, IT WAS WHEN I WAS TOO WRUNG-OUT TO THINK THAT I WOULD FIND MYSELF SUDDENLY GETTING SOMETHING RIGHT.
YES!

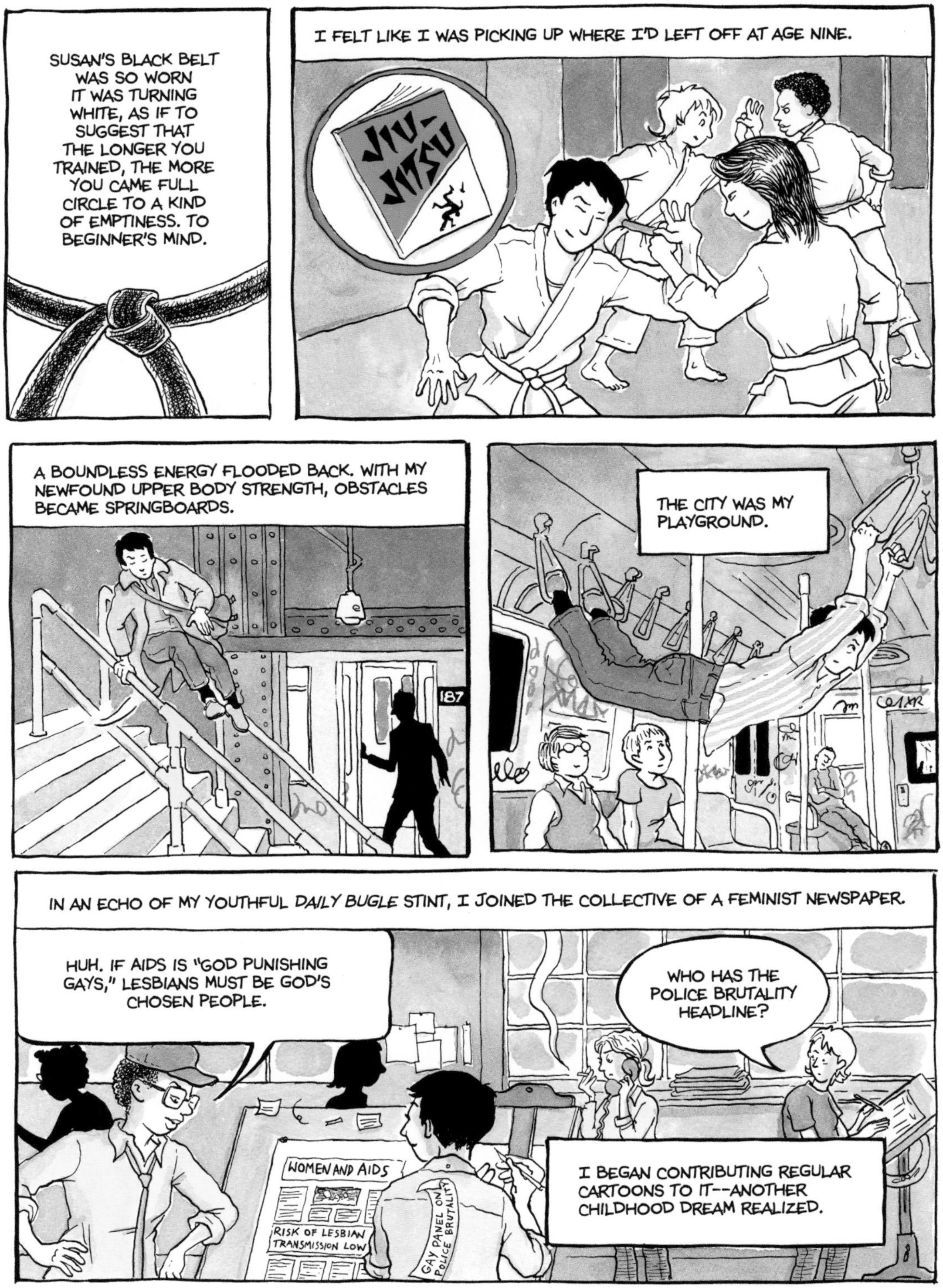
SUSAN'S BLACK BELT WAS SO WORN IT WAS TURNING WHITE, AS IF TO SUGGEST THAT THE LONGER YOU TRAINED, THE MORE YOU CAME FULL CIRCLE TO A KIND OF EMPTINESS. TO BEGINNER'S MIND.
I FELT LIKE I WAS PICKING UP WHERE I'D LEFT OFF AT AGE NINE.
JIU-JITSU
A BOUNDLESS ENERGY FLOODED BACK. WITH MY NEWFOUND UPPER BODY STRENGTH, OBSTACLES BECAME SPRINGBOARDS.
187
THE CITY WAS MY PLAYGROUND.
IN AN ECHO OF MY YOUTHFUL *DAILY BUGLE* STINT, I JOINED THE COLLECTIVE OF A FEMINIST NEWSPAPER.
HUH. IF AIDS IS "GOD PUNISHING GAYS," LESBIANS MUST BE GOD'S CHOSEN PEOPLE.
WHO HAS THE POLICE BRUTALITY HEADLINE?
WOMEN AND AIDS
RISK OF LESBIAN TRANSMISSION LOW
GAY PANEL ON POLICE BRUTALITY
I BEGAN CONTRIBUTING REGULAR CARTOONS TO IT--ANOTHER CHILDHOOD DREAM REALIZED.

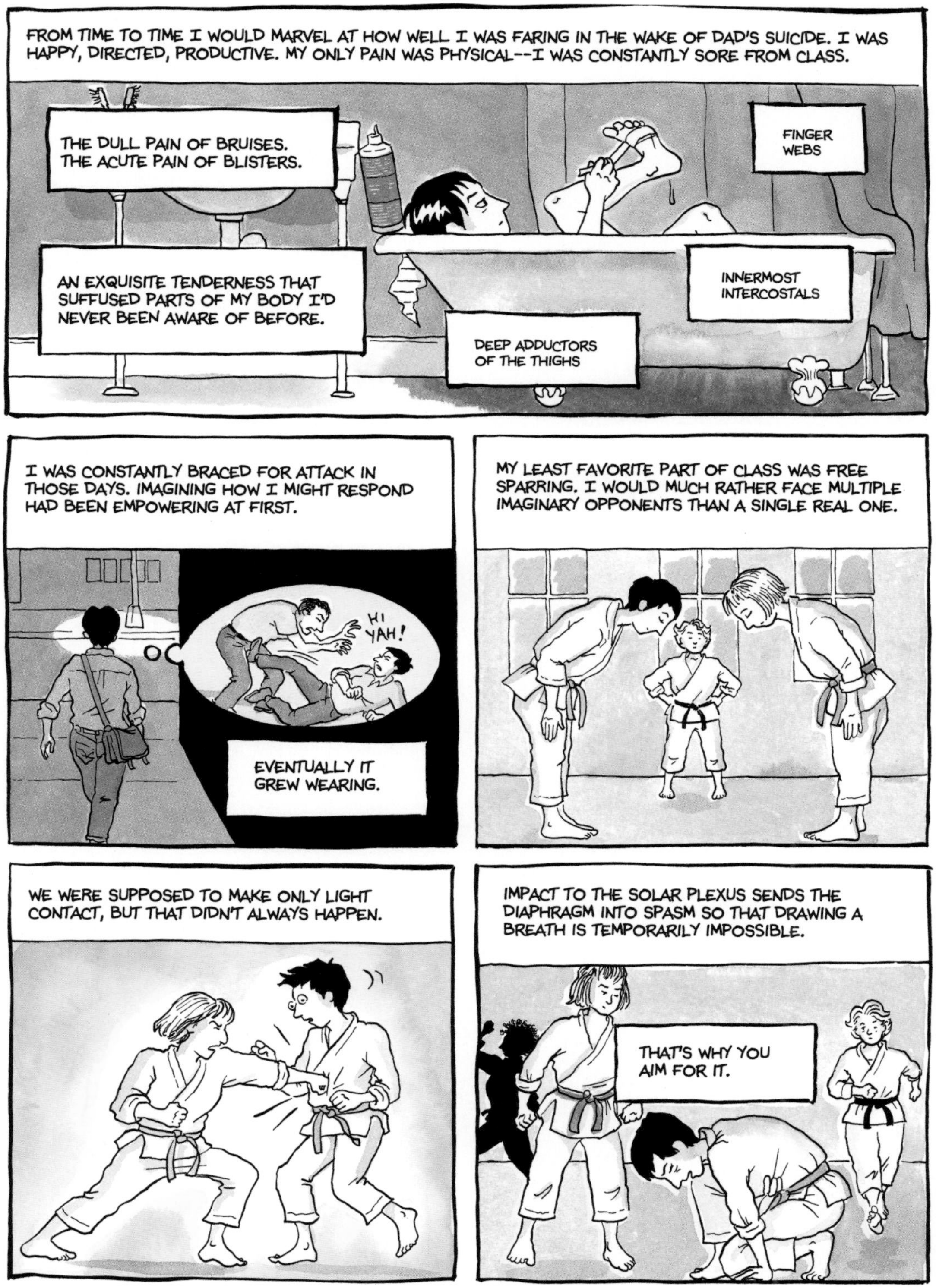
FROM TIME TO TIME I WOULD MARVEL AT HOW WELL I WAS FARING IN THE WAKE OF DAD'S SUICIDE. I WAS HAPPY, DIRECTED, PRODUCTIVE. MY ONLY PAIN WAS PHYSICAL--I WAS CONSTANTLY SORE FROM CLASS.
THE DULL PAIN OF BRUISES. THE ACUTE PAIN OF BLISTERS.
AN EXQUISITE TENDERNESS THAT SUFFUSED PARTS OF MY BODY I'D NEVER BEEN AWARE OF BEFORE.
DEEP ADDUCTORS OF THE THIGHS
INNERMOST INTERCOSTALS
FINGER WEBS
I WAS CONSTANTLY BRACED FOR ATTACK IN THOSE DAYS. IMAGINING HOW I MIGHT RESPOND HAD BEEN EMPOWERING AT FIRST.
HI YAH!
EVENTUALLY IT GREW WEARING.
MY LEAST FAVORITE PART OF CLASS WAS FREE SPARRING. I WOULD MUCH RATHER FACE MULTIPLE IMAGINARY OPPONENTS THAN A SINGLE REAL ONE.
WE WERE SUPPOSED TO MAKE ONLY LIGHT CONTACT, BUT THAT DIDN'T ALWAYS HAPPEN.
IMPACT TO THE SOLAR PLEXUS SENDS THE DIAPHRAGM INTO SPASM SO THAT DRAWING A BREATH IS TEMPORARILY IMPOSSIBLE.
THAT'S WHY YOU AIM FOR IT.

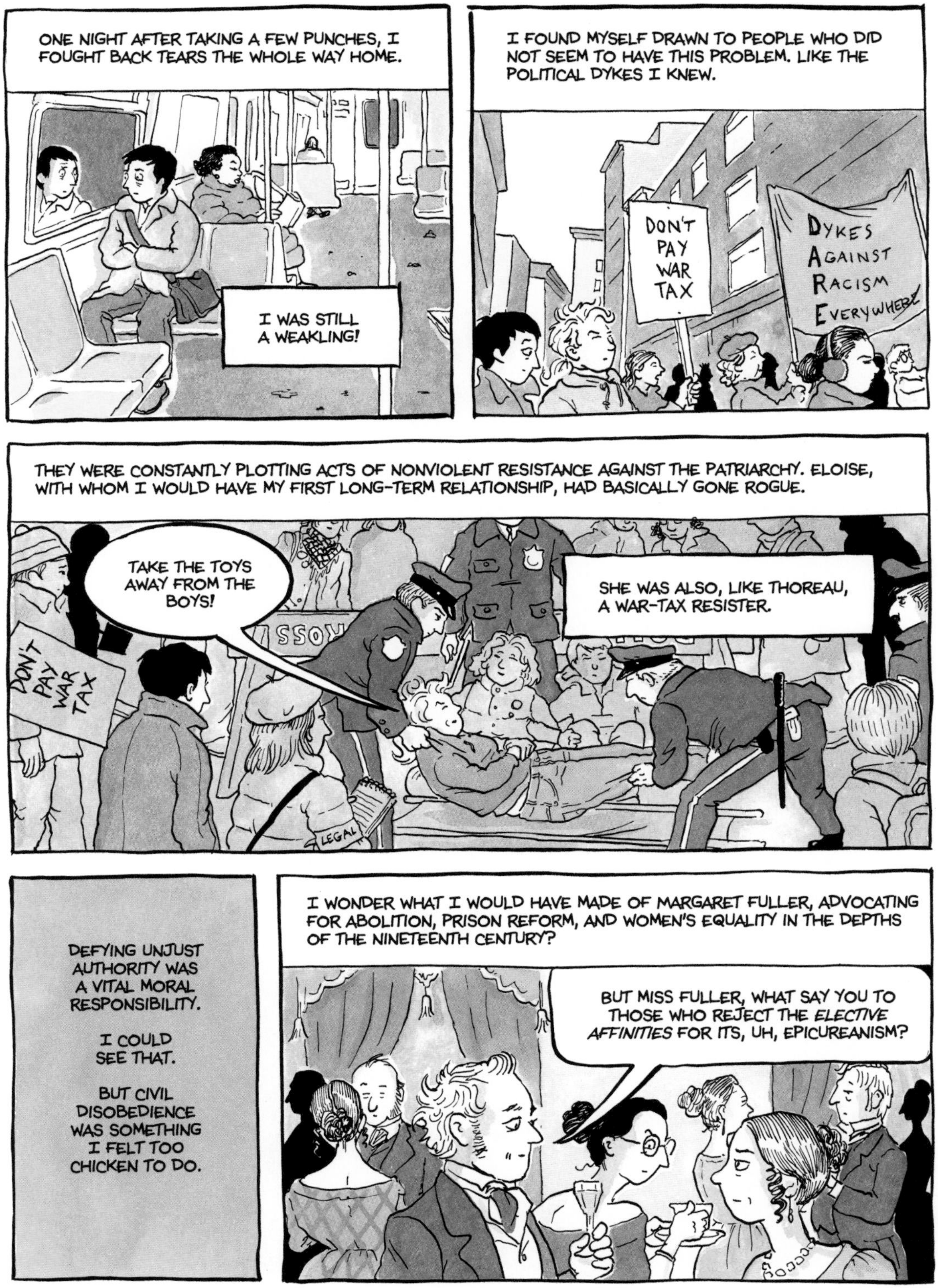
ONE NIGHT AFTER TAKING A FEW PUNCHES, I FOUGHT BACK TEARS THE WHOLE WAY HOME.
I WAS STILL A WEAKLING!
I FOUND MYSELF DRAWN TO PEOPLE WHO DID NOT SEEM TO HAVE THIS PROBLEM. LIKE THE POLITICAL DYKES I KNEW.
DON'T PAY WAR TAX
DYKES AGAINST RACISM EVERYWHERE
THEY WERE CONSTANTLY PLOTTING ACTS OF NONVIOLENT RESISTANCE AGAINST THE PATRIARCHY. ELOISE, WITH WHOM I WOULD HAVE MY FIRST LONG-TERM RELATIONSHIP, HAD BASICALLY GONE ROGUE.
TAKE THE TOYS AWAY FROM THE BOYS!
SHE WAS ALSO, LIKE THOREAU, A WAR-TAX RESISTER.
DON'T PAY WAR TAX
LEGAL
DEFYING UNJUST AUTHORITY WAS A VITAL MORAL RESPONSIBILITY.
I COULD SEE THAT.
BUT CIVIL DISOBEDIENCE WAS SOMETHING I FELT TOO CHICKEN TO DO.
I WONDER WHAT I WOULD HAVE MADE OF MARGARET FULLER, ADVOCATING FOR ABOLITION, PRISON REFORM, AND WOMEN'S EQUALITY IN THE DEPTHS OF THE NINETEENTH CENTURY?
BUT MISS FULLER, WHAT SAY YOU TO THOSE WHO REJECT THE *ELECTIVE AFFINITIES* FOR ITS, UH, EPICUREANISM?

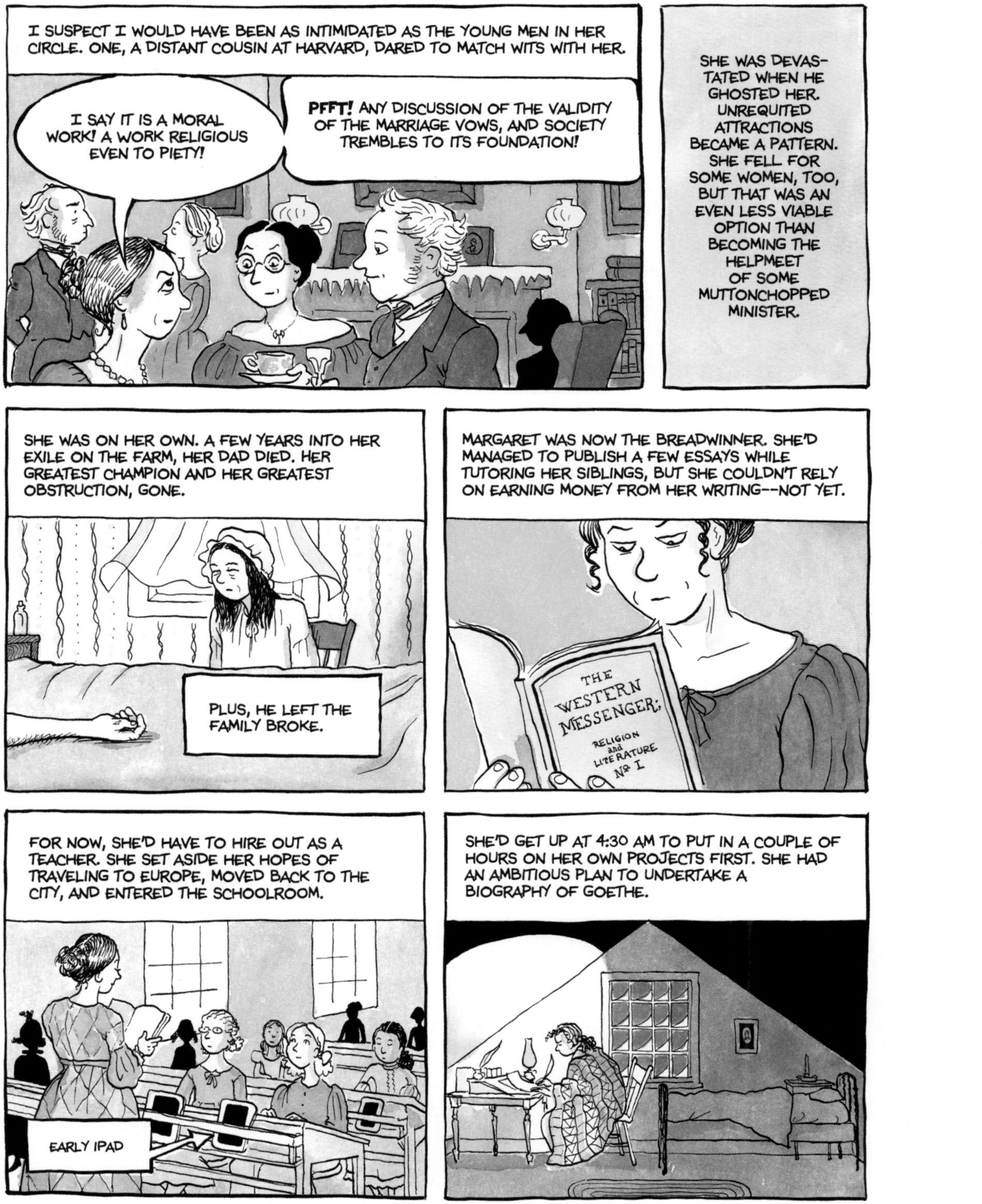
I SUSPECT I WOULD HAVE BEEN AS INTIMIDATED AS THE YOUNG MEN IN HER CIRCLE. ONE, A DISTANT COUSIN AT HARVARD, DARED TO MATCH WITS WITH HER.
I SAY IT IS A MORAL WORK! A WORK RELIGIOUS EVEN TO PIETY!
PFFT! ANY DISCUSSION OF THE VALIDITY OF THE MARRIAGE VOWS, AND SOCIETY TREMBLES TO ITS FOUNDATION!
SHE WAS DEVASTATED WHEN HE GHOSTED HER. UNREQUITED ATTRACTIONS BECAME A PATTERN. SHE FELL FOR SOME WOMEN, TOO, BUT THAT WAS AN EVEN LESS VIABLE OPTION THAN BECOMING THE HELPMEET OF SOME MUTTONCHOPPED MINISTER.
SHE WAS ON HER OWN. A FEW YEARS INTO HER EXILE ON THE FARM, HER DAD DIED. HER GREATEST CHAMPION AND HER GREATEST OBSTRUCTION, GONE.
PLUS, HE LEFT THE FAMILY BROKE.
MARGARET WAS NOW THE BREADWINNER. SHE'D MANAGED TO PUBLISH A FEW ESSAYS WHILE TUTORING HER SIBLINGS, BUT SHE COULDN'T RELY ON EARNING MONEY FROM HER WRITING--NOT YET.
THE WESTERN MESSENGER; RELIGION and LITERATURE No I
FOR NOW, SHE'D HAVE TO HIRE OUT AS A TEACHER. SHE SET ASIDE HER HOPES OF TRAVELING TO EUROPE, MOVED BACK TO THE CITY, AND ENTERED THE SCHOOLROOM.
EARLY IPAD
SHE'D GET UP AT 4:30 AM TO PUT IN A COUPLE OF HOURS ON HER OWN PROJECTS FIRST. SHE HAD AN AMBITIOUS PLAN TO UNDERTAKE A BIOGRAPHY OF GOETHE.

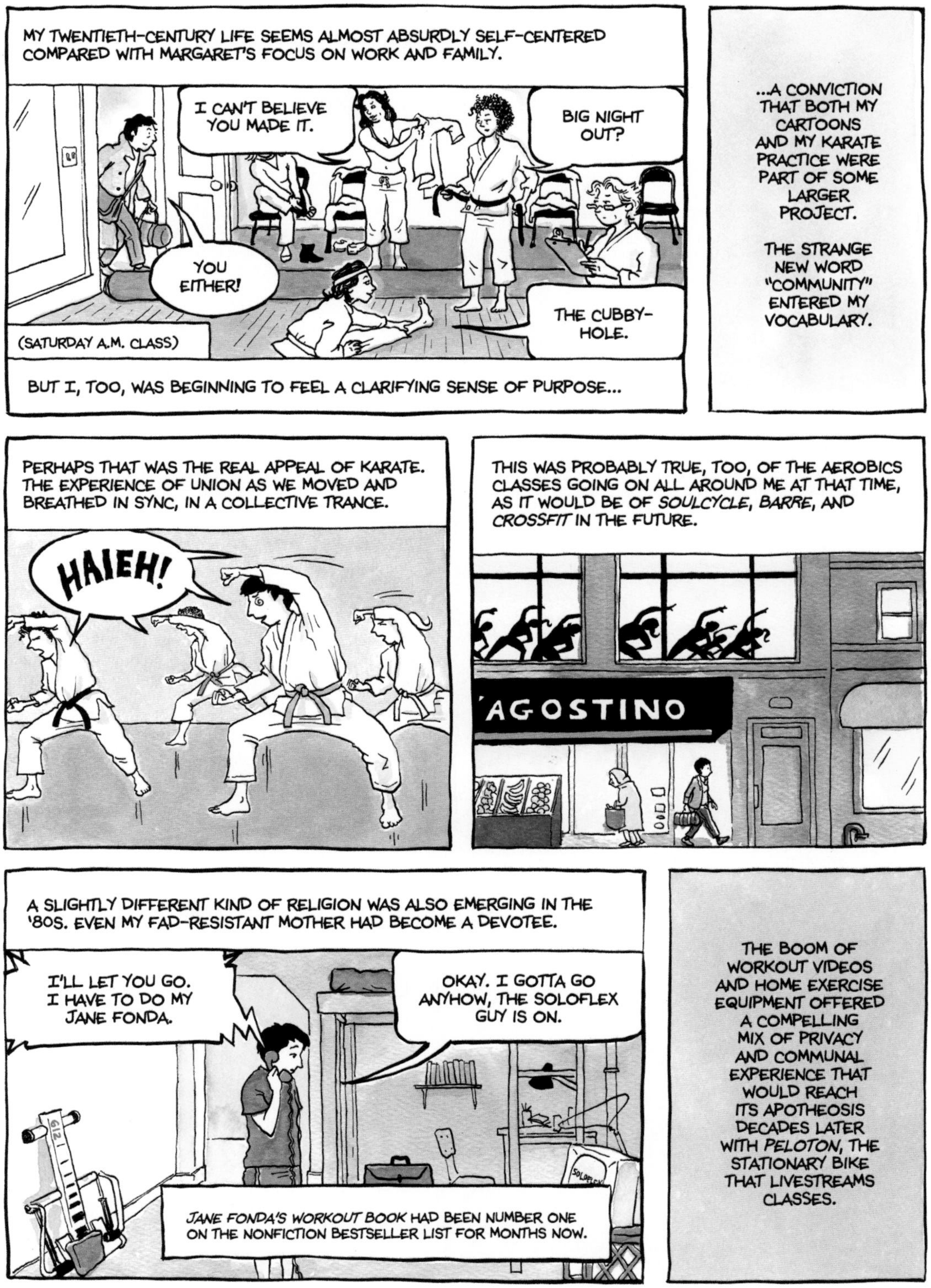
MY TWENTIETH-CENTURY LIFE SEEMS ALMOST ABSURDLY SELF-CENTERED COMPARED WITH MARGARET'S FOCUS ON WORK AND FAMILY.
I CAN'T BELIEVE YOU MADE IT.
YOU EITHER!
BIG NIGHT OUT?
THE CUBBY-HOLE.
(SATURDAY A.M. CLASS)
BUT I, TOO, WAS BEGINNING TO FEEL A CLARIFYING SENSE OF PURPOSE...
...A CONVICTION THAT BOTH MY CARTOONS AND MY KARATE PRACTICE WERE PART OF SOME LARGER PROJECT.
THE STRANGE NEW WORD "COMMUNITY" ENTERED MY VOCABULARY.
PERHAPS THAT WAS THE REAL APPEAL OF KARATE. THE EXPERIENCE OF UNION AS WE MOVED AND BREATHED IN SYNC, IN A COLLECTIVE TRANCE.
HAIEH!
THIS WAS PROBABLY TRUE, TOO, OF THE AEROBICS CLASSES GOING ON ALL AROUND ME AT THAT TIME, AS IT WOULD BE OF *SOULCYCLE*, *BARRE*, AND *CROSSFIT* IN THE FUTURE.
'AGOSTINO
A SLIGHTLY DIFFERENT KIND OF RELIGION WAS ALSO EMERGING IN THE '80S. EVEN MY FAD-RESISTANT MOTHER HAD BECOME A DEVOTEE.
I'LL LET YOU GO. I HAVE TO DO MY JANE FONDA.
OKAY. I GOTTA GO ANYHOW, THE SOLOFLEX GUY IS ON.
JANE FONDA'S WORKOUT BOOK HAD BEEN NUMBER ONE ON THE NONFICTION BESTSELLER LIST FOR MONTHS NOW.
THE BOOM OF WORKOUT VIDEOS AND HOME EXERCISE EQUIPMENT OFFERED A COMPELLING MIX OF PRIVACY AND COMMUNAL EXPERIENCE THAT WOULD REACH ITS APOTHEOSIS DECADES LATER WITH *PELOTON*, THE STATIONARY BIKE THAT LIVESTREAMS CLASSES.

SOLOFLEX, THE HOME GYM! EVEN THE NAME CONNOTED RUGGED INDIVIDUALISM, SELF-SUFFICIENCY, A DASH OF AUTOEROTICISM. I COULDN'T AFFORD A HOME GYM, BUT I DID GET A ROWING MACHINE.
ONE OF THE FIRST INFOMERCIALS
SOLOFLEX
THIS GUY WAS SO PRETTY, EVEN LESBIANS WERE TRANSFIXED.
IMAGINE THE LANDFILL SPACE THESE THINGS ARE OCCUPYING.
I ALSO BEGAN LIFTING WEIGHTS TO HELP PREVENT KARATE INJURIES.
I WAS TRAINING MORE INTENSELY THAN EVER IN PREPARATION FOR MY BLACK BELT EXAM.
BAMBOO-SHAPED WELT FROM MR. MORI'S STICK
I WOULD GET TO THE DOJO WELL BEFORE CLASS TO GET IN AN EXTRA WORKOUT.
RALPH MACCHIO! CAN I GET YOUR AUTOGRAPH?
(THE KARATE KID HAD JUST COME OUT.)
I'D BEGUN EXPERIENCING PERIODIC EPISODES OF EXERCISE-INDUCED RAPID HEARTBEAT. BUT IF I STOPPED FOR A MINUTE, THEY'D SUBSIDE AND I COULD RESUME WITH NO TROUBLE.
IN GENERAL, BETWEEN THE RUNNING, THE ROWING, THE WEIGHTS, AND THE KARATE, I WAS FILLED WITH A TERRIBLE VIGOR!
I SAW NO CONFLICT BETWEEN THIS SPARTAN REGIMEN AND MY SUBSTANCE USE. I WOULD HYDRATE AFTER CLASS WITH A TALLBOY OF BUD.
ONE WAY
DRINK Coca-Cola
CIGARS
LUNCH
WALK
PARK
THERE WAS NO CONSTANT, NAMBY-PAMBY SUCKLING ON WATER BOTTLES IN THOSE DAYS.
CATS

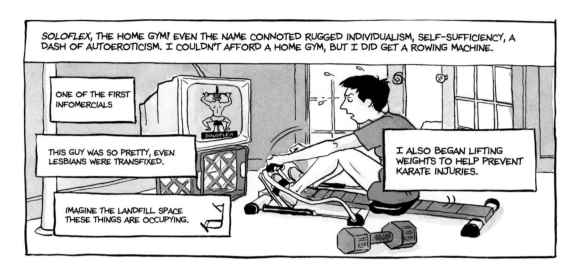

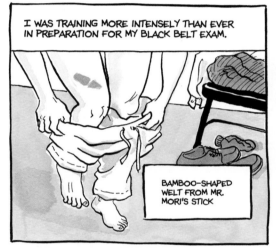

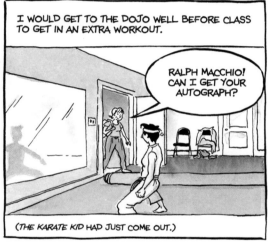

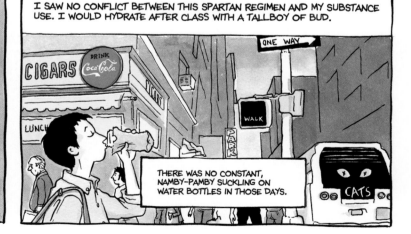

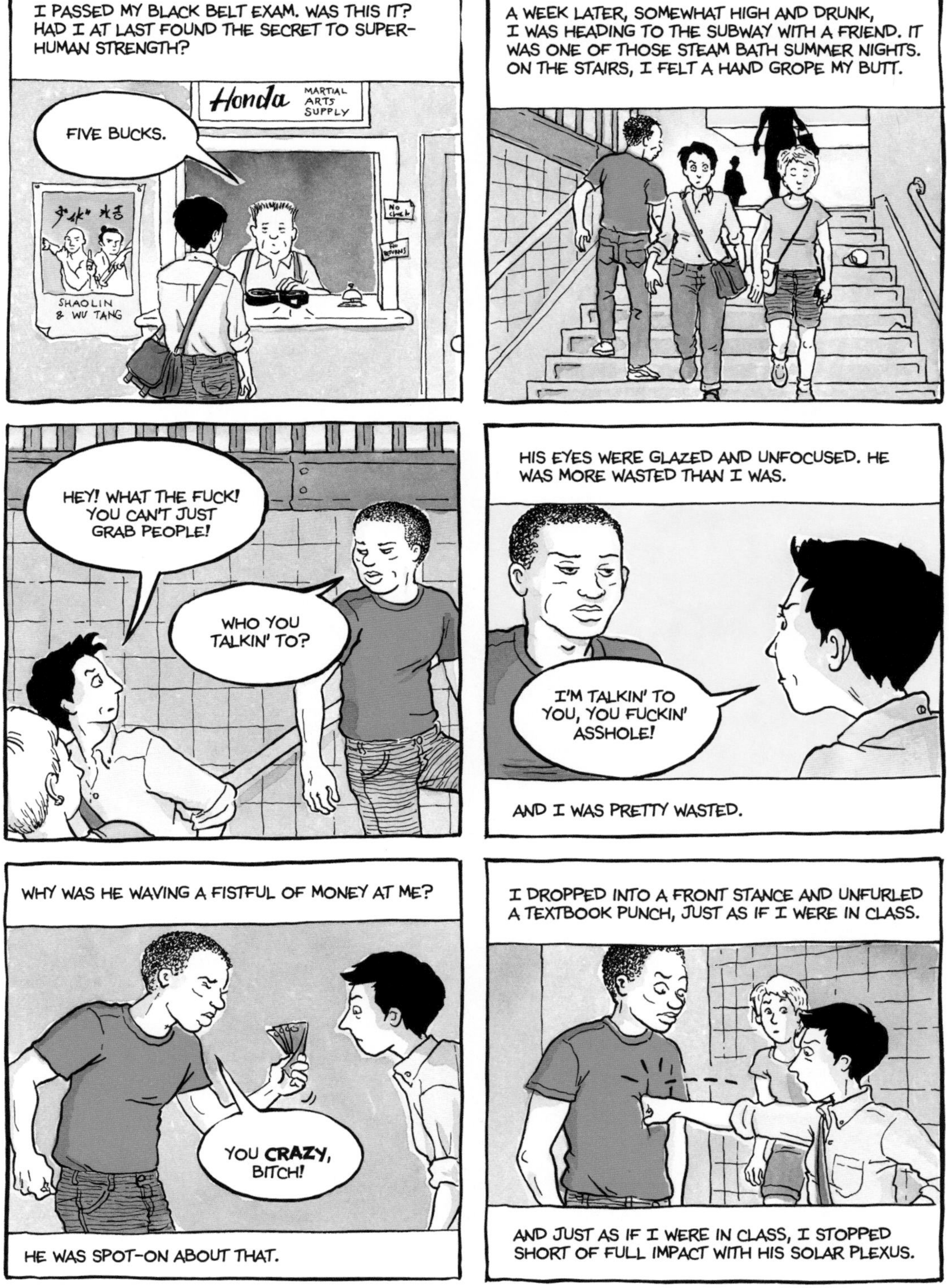
I PASSED MY BLACK BELT EXAM. WAS THIS IT? HAD I AT LAST FOUND THE SECRET TO SUPER-HUMAN STRENGTH?
Honda MARTIAL ARTS SUPPLY
SHAOLIN & WU TANG
FIVE BUCKS.
A WEEK LATER, SOMEWHAT HIGH AND DRUNK, I WAS HEADING TO THE SUBWAY WITH A FRIEND. IT WAS ONE OF THOSE STEAM BATH SUMMER NIGHTS. ON THE STAIRS, I FELT A HAND GROPE MY BUTT.
HEY! WHAT THE FUCK! YOU CAN'T JUST GRAB PEOPLE!
WHO YOU TALKIN' TO?
HIS EYES WERE GLAZED AND UNFOCUSED. HE WAS MORE WASTED THAN I WAS.
I'M TALKIN' TO YOU, YOU FUCKIN' ASSHOLE!
AND I WAS PRETTY WASTED.
WHY WAS HE WAVING A FISTFUL OF MONEY AT ME?
YOU **CRAZY**, BITCH!
HE WAS SPOT-ON ABOUT THAT.
I DROPPED INTO A FRONT STANCE AND UNFURLED A TEXTBOOK PUNCH, JUST AS IF I WERE IN CLASS.
AND JUST AS IF I WERE IN CLASS, I STOPPED SHORT OF FULL IMPACT WITH HIS SOLAR PLEXUS.

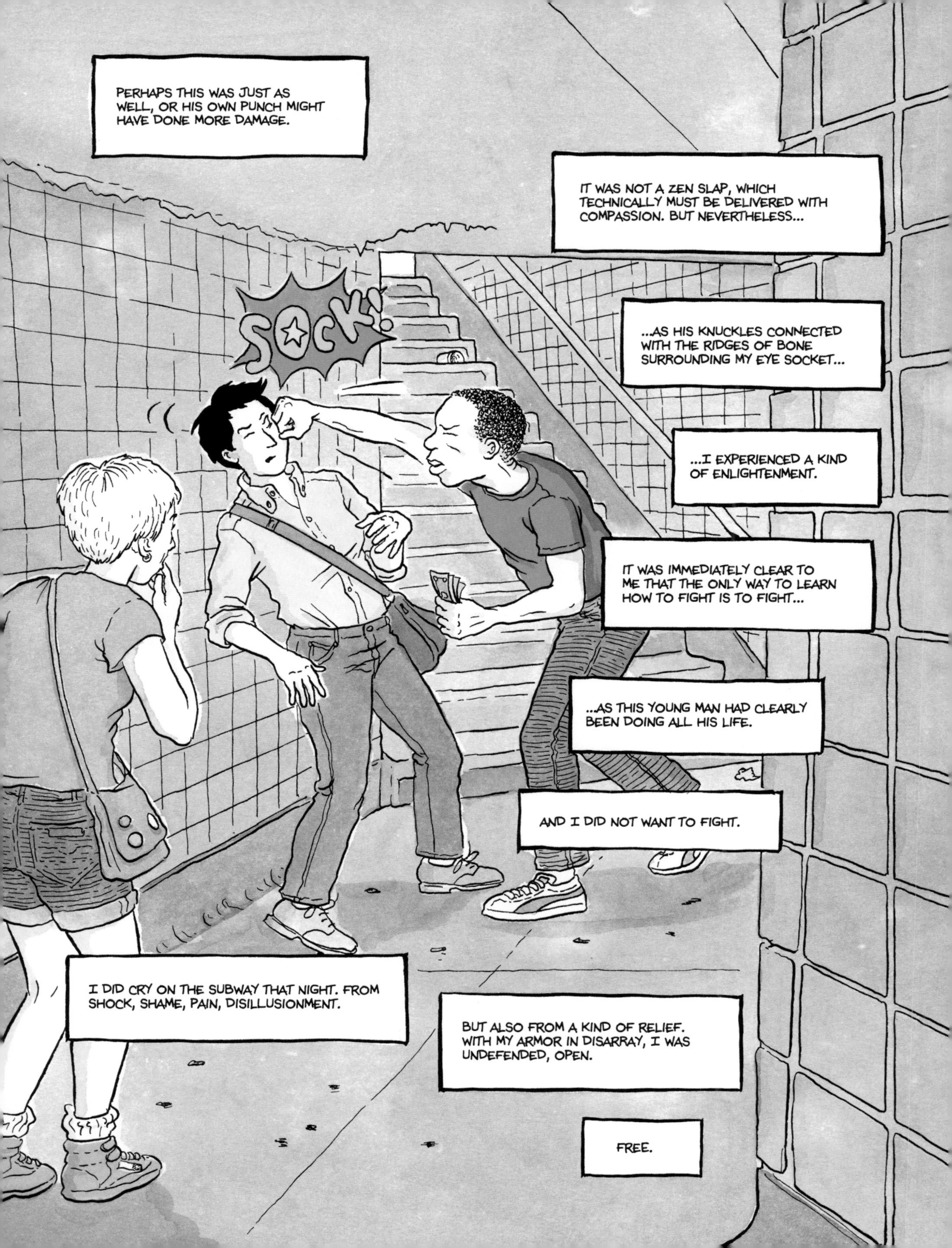
PERHAPS THIS WAS JUST AS WELL, OR HIS OWN PUNCH MIGHT HAVE DONE MORE DAMAGE.
IT WAS NOT A ZEN SLAP, WHICH TECHNICALLY MUST BE DELIVERED WITH COMPASSION. BUT NEVERTHELESS...
SOCK!
...AS HIS KNUCKLES CONNECTED WITH THE RIDGES OF BONE SURROUNDING MY EYE SOCKET...
...I EXPERIENCED A KIND OF ENLIGHTENMENT.
IT WAS IMMEDIATELY CLEAR TO ME THAT THE ONLY WAY TO LEARN HOW TO FIGHT IS TO FIGHT...
...AS THIS YOUNG MAN HAD CLEARLY BEEN DOING ALL HIS LIFE.
AND I DID NOT WANT TO FIGHT.
I DID CRY ON THE SUBWAY THAT NIGHT. FROM SHOCK, SHAME, PAIN, DISILLUSIONMENT.
BUT ALSO FROM A KIND OF RELIEF. WITH MY ARMOR IN DISARRAY, I WAS UNDEFENDED, OPEN.
FREE.

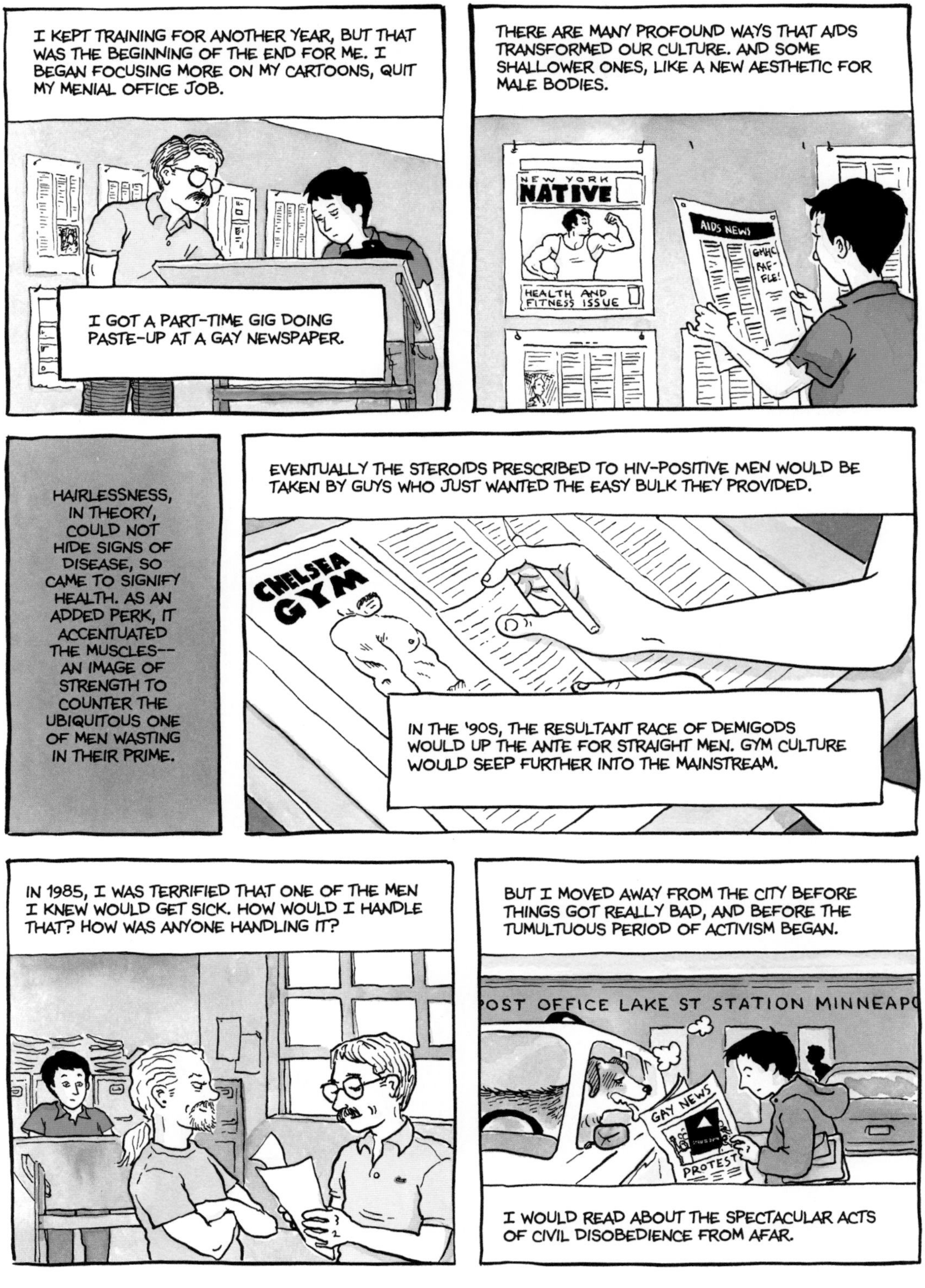
I KEPT TRAINING FOR ANOTHER YEAR, BUT THAT WAS THE BEGINNING OF THE END FOR ME. I BEGAN FOCUSING MORE ON MY CARTOONS, QUIT MY MENIAL OFFICE JOB.
I GOT A PART-TIME GIG DOING PASTE-UP AT A GAY NEWSPAPER.
THERE ARE MANY PROFOUND WAYS THAT AIDS TRANSFORMED OUR CULTURE. AND SOME SHALLOWER ONES, LIKE A NEW AESTHETIC FOR MALE BODIES.
NEW YORK NATIVE
HEALTH AND FITNESS ISSUE
AIDS NEWS
GMHC RAF-FLE!
HAIRLESSNESS, IN THEORY, COULD NOT HIDE SIGNS OF DISEASE, SO CAME TO SIGNIFY HEALTH. AS AN ADDED PERK, IT ACCENTUATED THE MUSCLES-- AN IMAGE OF STRENGTH TO COUNTER THE UBIQUITOUS ONE OF MEN WASTING IN THEIR PRIME.
EVENTUALLY THE STEROIDS PRESCRIBED TO HIV-POSITIVE MEN WOULD BE TAKEN BY GUYS WHO JUST WANTED THE EASY BULK THEY PROVIDED.
CHELSEA GYM
IN THE '90S, THE RESULTANT RACE OF DEMIGODS WOULD UP THE ANTE FOR STRAIGHT MEN. GYM CULTURE WOULD SEEP FURTHER INTO THE MAINSTREAM.
IN 1985, I WAS TERRIFIED THAT ONE OF THE MEN I KNEW WOULD GET SICK. HOW WOULD I HANDLE THAT? HOW WAS ANYONE HANDLING IT?
BUT I MOVED AWAY FROM THE CITY BEFORE THINGS GOT REALLY BAD, AND BEFORE THE TUMULTUOUS PERIOD OF ACTIVISM BEGAN.
POST OFFICE LAKE ST STATION MINNEAPO
GAY NEWS
PROTEST
I WOULD READ ABOUT THE SPECTACULAR ACTS OF CIVIL DISOBEDIENCE FROM AFAR.

I FOLLOWED ELOISE TO WESTERN MASSACHUSETTS FOR A YEAR, THEN WE BOTH MOVED TO MINNESOTA. IN THE REAR OF OUR HOUSE LIVED A WOMAN WHO WAS IN SOME SORT OF HALFWAY PROGRAM FOR RECOVERING DRUG ADDICTS.

THIS WAS MY FIRST ENCOUNTER WITH THE GENIUS LOCI OF THE TWIN CITIES...

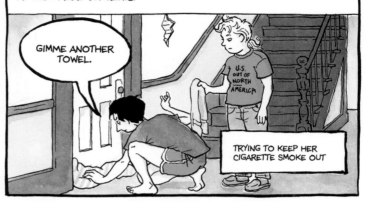

...THE RECOVERY MOVEMENT. ALCOHOLICS AND ABUSERS OF SUBSTANCES OF ALL KINDS FLOCKED HERE TO BE REHABILITATED AT THE HAZELDEN CLINIC.

GIMME ANOTHER TOWEL.

TRYING TO KEEP HER CIGARETTE SMOKE OUT

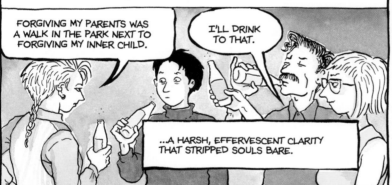

THE NEW FRIENDS I WAS MAKING WERE ALL "SOBER." AT PARTIES THERE WAS NO LUBRICATING BEER OR WINE. JUST ENDLESS BOTTLES OF SOMETHING CALLED "LACROIX WATER," WHICH HAD THE OPPOSITE EFFECT...

FORGIVING MY PARENTS WAS A WALK IN THE PARK NEXT TO FORGIVING MY INNER CHILD.

I'LL DRINK TO THAT.

...A HARSH, EFFERVESCENT CLARITY THAT STRIPPED SOULS BARE.

I WAS GLAD I HAD NOTHING TO RECOVER FROM. I WAS HAPPY WITH ELOISE. MY FIRST BOOK OF CARTOONS HAD JUST BEEN PUBLISHED.

BUT THEN, NOT LONG AFTER THAT SIGNAL EVENT...

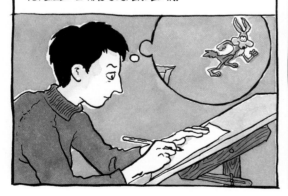

...I STARTED HAVING TROUBLE PRODUCING MY COMIC STRIP EVERY TWO WEEKS OUT OF THIN AIR. INDEED, THIN AIR WAS WHAT I SUDDENLY REALIZED I WAS SUSPENDED IN.

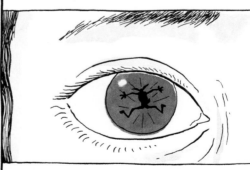

THE TRICK IN THAT CASE, OF COURSE, IS NOT TO LOOK DOWN. BUT IT WAS TOO LATE. YOU CAN'T UNSEE THE ABYSS.

I MUSCLED THROUGH THE FIRST ANXIETY ATTACK.

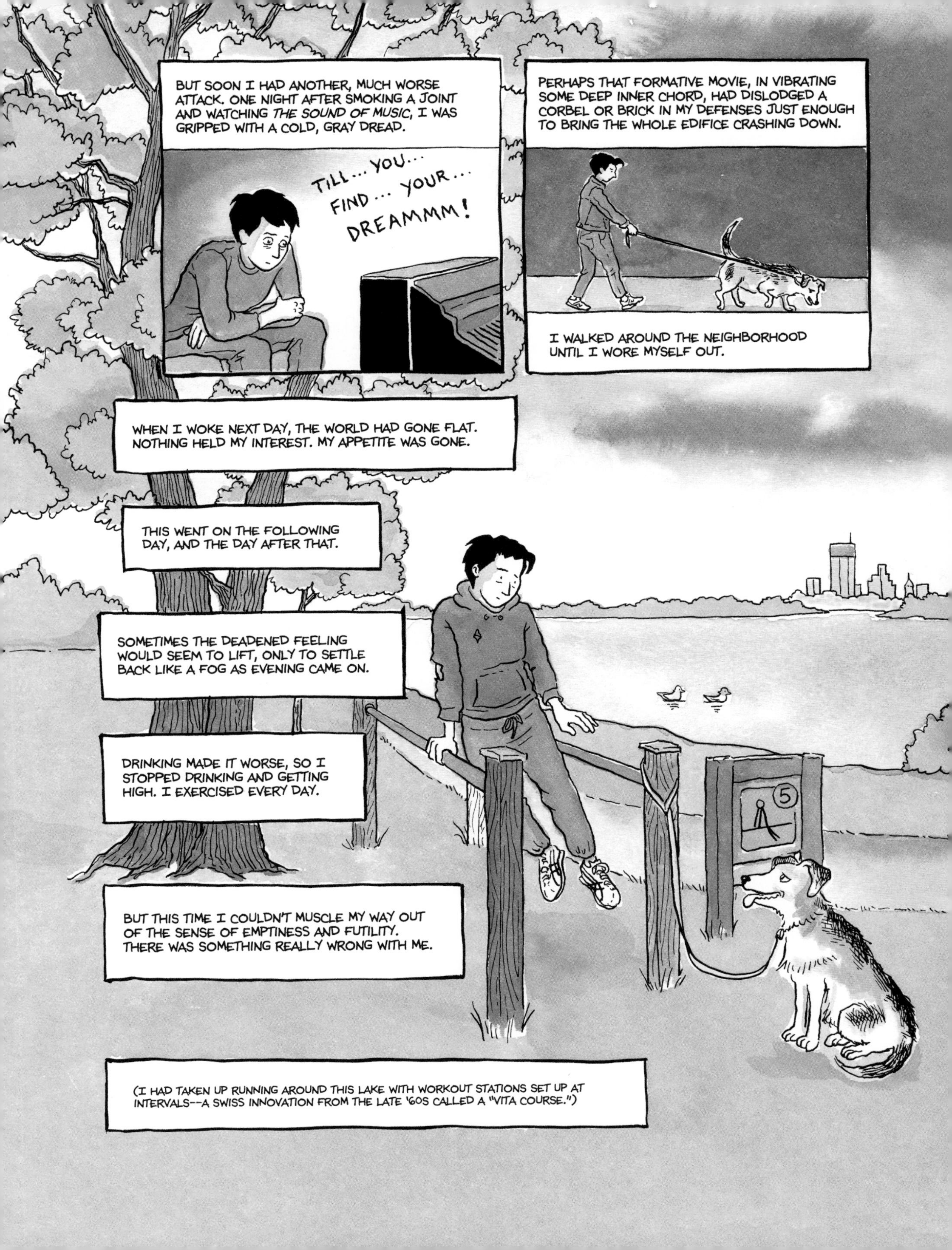
BUT SOON I HAD ANOTHER, MUCH WORSE ATTACK. ONE NIGHT AFTER SMOKING A JOINT AND WATCHING *THE SOUND OF MUSIC*, I WAS GRIPPED WITH A COLD, GRAY DREAD.
TILL... YOU... FIND... YOUR... DREAMMM!
PERHAPS THAT FORMATIVE MOVIE, IN VIBRATING SOME DEEP INNER CHORD, HAD DISLODGED A CORBEL OR BRICK IN MY DEFENSES JUST ENOUGH TO BRING THE WHOLE EDIFICE CRASHING DOWN.
I WALKED AROUND THE NEIGHBORHOOD UNTIL I WORE MYSELF OUT.
WHEN I WOKE NEXT DAY, THE WORLD HAD GONE FLAT. NOTHING HELD MY INTEREST. MY APPETITE WAS GONE.
THIS WENT ON THE FOLLOWING DAY, AND THE DAY AFTER THAT.
SOMETIMES THE DEADENED FEELING WOULD SEEM TO LIFT, ONLY TO SETTLE BACK LIKE A FOG AS EVENING CAME ON.
DRINKING MADE IT WORSE, SO I STOPPED DRINKING AND GETTING HIGH. I EXERCISED EVERY DAY.
BUT THIS TIME I COULDN'T MUSCLE MY WAY OUT OF THE SENSE OF EMPTINESS AND FUTILITY. THERE WAS SOMETHING REALLY WRONG WITH ME.
5
(I HAD TAKEN UP RUNNING AROUND THIS LAKE WITH WORKOUT STATIONS SET UP AT INTERVALS--A SWISS INNOVATION FROM THE LATE '60S CALLED A "VITA COURSE.")

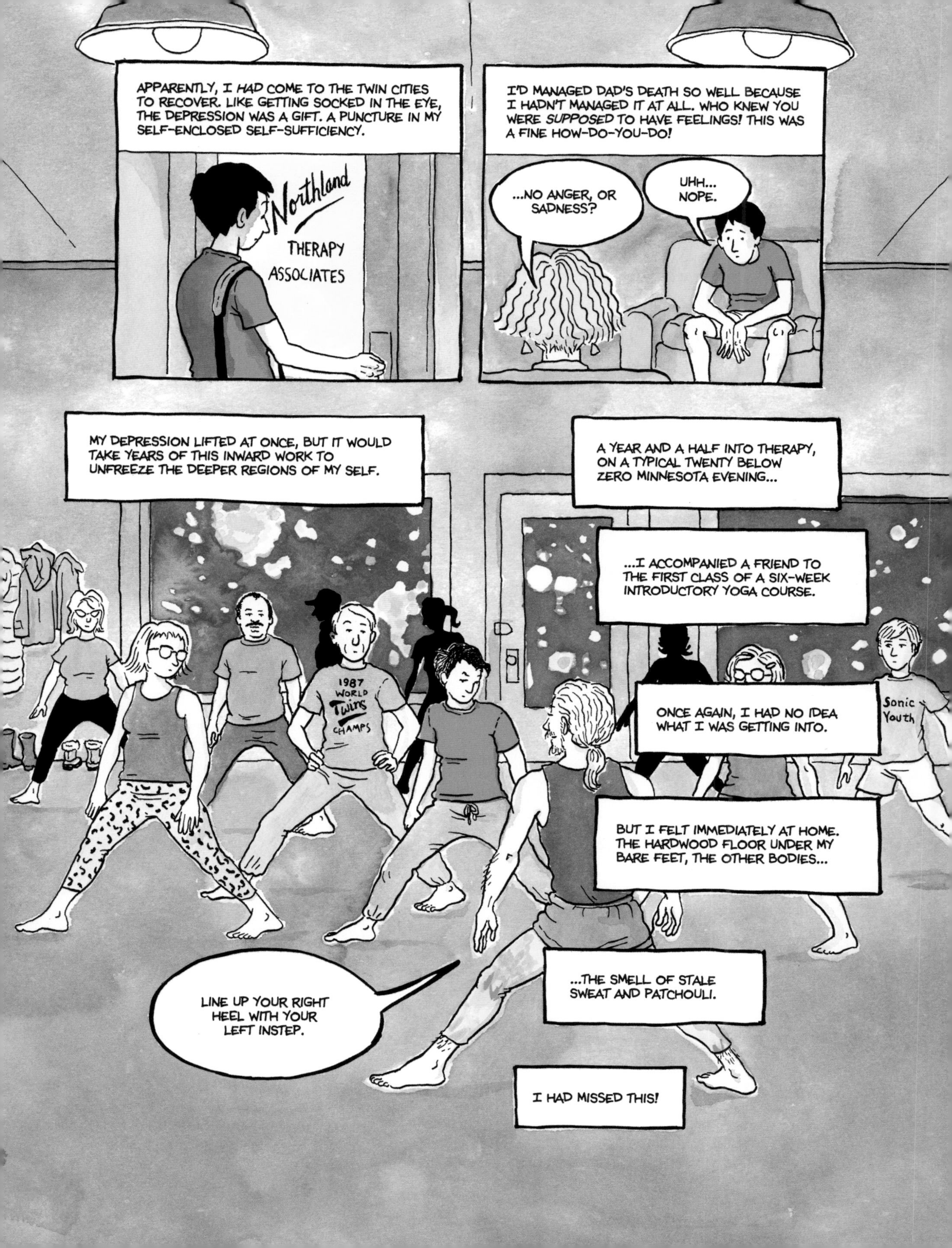
APPARENTLY, I *HAD* COME TO THE TWIN CITIES TO RECOVER. LIKE GETTING SOCKED IN THE EYE, THE DEPRESSION WAS A GIFT. A PUNCTURE IN MY SELF-ENCLOSED SELF-SUFFICIENCY.
Northland
THERAPY
ASSOCIATES
I'D MANAGED DAD'S DEATH SO WELL BECAUSE I HADN'T MANAGED IT AT ALL. WHO KNEW YOU WERE *SUPPOSED* TO HAVE FEELINGS! THIS WAS A FINE HOW-DO-YOU-DO!
...NO ANGER, OR SADNESS?
UHH... NOPE.
MY DEPRESSION LIFTED AT ONCE, BUT IT WOULD TAKE YEARS OF THIS INWARD WORK TO UNFREEZE THE DEEPER REGIONS OF MY SELF.
A YEAR AND A HALF INTO THERAPY, ON A TYPICAL TWENTY BELOW ZERO MINNESOTA EVENING...
...I ACCOMPANIED A FRIEND TO THE FIRST CLASS OF A SIX-WEEK INTRODUCTORY YOGA COURSE.
1987 WORLD Twins CHAMPS
Sonic Youth
ONCE AGAIN, I HAD NO IDEA WHAT I WAS GETTING INTO.
BUT I FELT IMMEDIATELY AT HOME. THE HARDWOOD FLOOR UNDER MY BARE FEET, THE OTHER BODIES...
LINE UP YOUR RIGHT HEEL WITH YOUR LEFT INSTEP.
...THE SMELL OF STALE SWEAT AND PATCHOULI.
I HAD MISSED THIS!

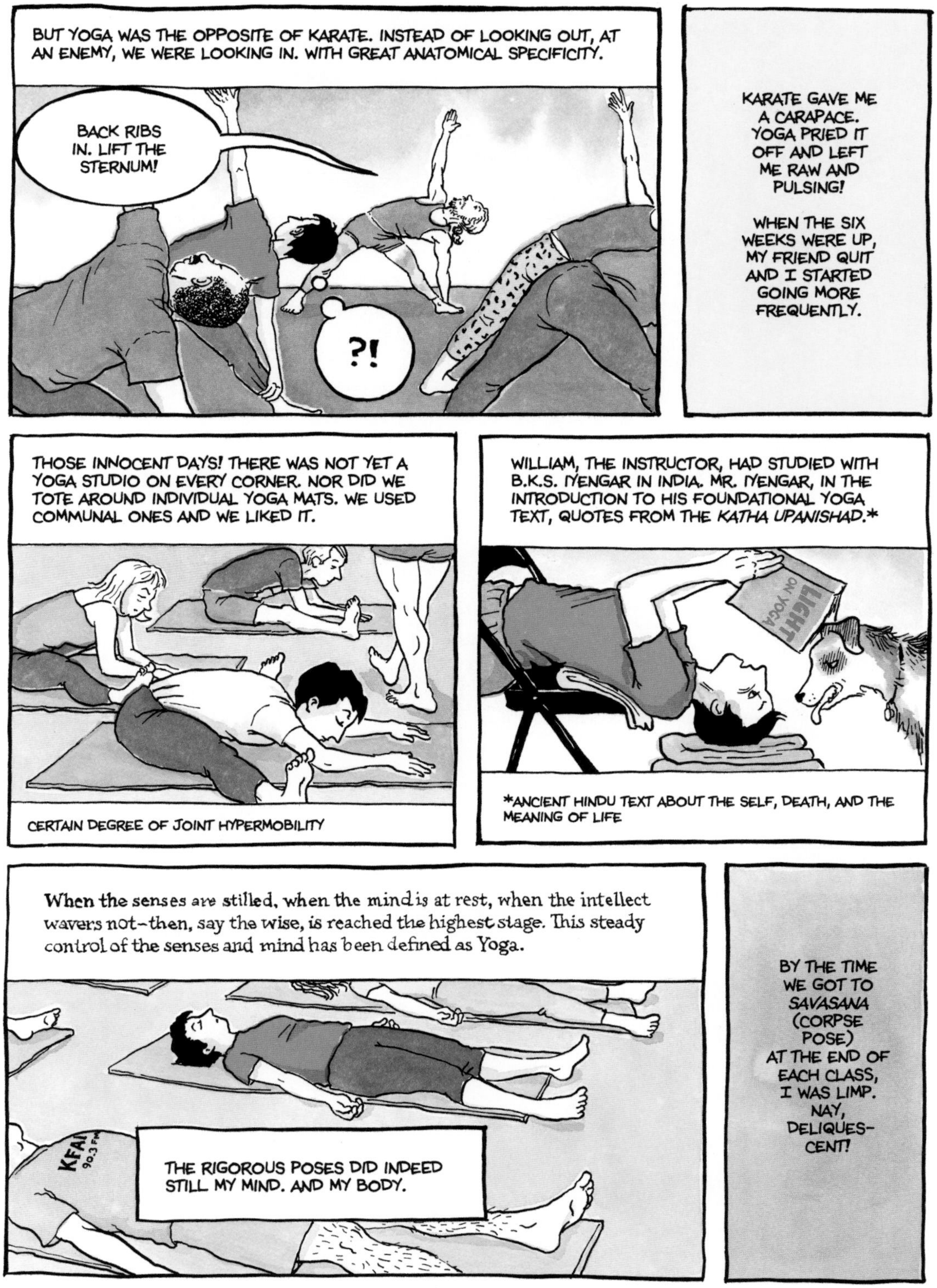
BUT YOGA WAS THE OPPOSITE OF KARATE. INSTEAD OF LOOKING OUT, AT AN ENEMY, WE WERE LOOKING IN. WITH GREAT ANATOMICAL SPECIFICITY.
BACK RIBS IN. LIFT THE STERNUM!
?!
KARATE GAVE ME A CARAPACE. YOGA PRIED IT OFF AND LEFT ME RAW AND PULSING!
WHEN THE SIX WEEKS WERE UP, MY FRIEND QUIT AND I STARTED GOING MORE FREQUENTLY.
THOSE INNOCENT DAYS! THERE WAS NOT YET A YOGA STUDIO ON EVERY CORNER. NOR DID WE TOTE AROUND INDIVIDUAL YOGA MATS. WE USED COMMUNAL ONES AND WE LIKED IT.
CERTAIN DEGREE OF JOINT HYPERMOBILITY
WILLIAM, THE INSTRUCTOR, HAD STUDIED WITH B.K.S. IYENGAR IN INDIA. MR. IYENGAR, IN THE INTRODUCTION TO HIS FOUNDATIONAL YOGA TEXT, QUOTES FROM THE *KATHA UPANISHAD*.*
LIGHT ON YOGA
*ANCIENT HINDU TEXT ABOUT THE SELF, DEATH, AND THE MEANING OF LIFE
When the senses are stilled, when the mind is at rest, when the intellect wavers not—then, say the wise, is reached the highest stage. This steady control of the senses and mind has been defined as Yoga.
KFAI 90.3 FM
THE RIGOROUS POSES DID INDEED STILL MY MIND. AND MY BODY.
BY THE TIME WE GOT TO *SAVASANA* (CORPSE POSE) AT THE END OF EACH CLASS, I WAS LIMP. NAY, DELIQUES-CENT!

WHAT A WORKOUT! INVERSIONS, TWISTS, ARM BALANCES, BACKBENDS! BUT THE POSES WERE NOT ENDS IN THEMSELVES. YOGA WAS NOT REALLY ABOUT FITNESS.

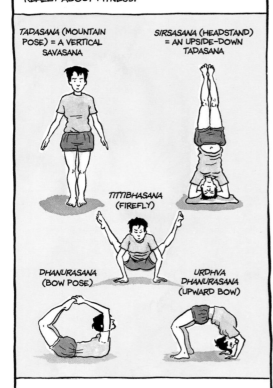

TADASANA (MOUNTAIN POSE) = A VERTICAL SAVASANA

SIRSASANA (HEADSTAND) = AN UPSIDE-DOWN TADASANA

TITTIBHASANA (FIREFLY)

DHANURASANA (BOW POSE)

URDHVA DHANURASANA (UPWARD BOW)

IN FACT, I STOPPED RUNNING AND GOING TO THE GYM, BECAUSE THOSE THINGS TIGHTENED THE BODY, AND YOGA WAS ALL ABOUT BEING SOFT.

I WAS LEARNING THE SKILL OF PRESENCE. BY SIMPLY BEING WITH MY SENSATIONS, I COULD FEEL THEM NOT AS "PAIN" BUT AS A FLUX OF TINGLINGS, PULSES, AND VIBRATIONS.

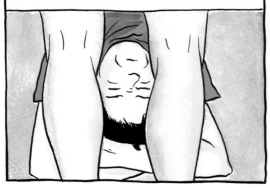

YET I FELT ALIVE AND AWARE IN EVERY CELL AS ALL MY MECHANISMS BECAME MORE FINELY TUNED.

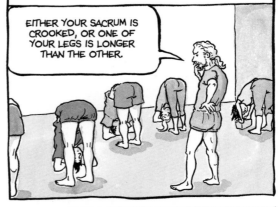

EITHER YOUR SACRUM IS CROOKED, OR ONE OF YOUR LEGS IS LONGER THAN THE OTHER.

THERE WAS INDEED SOMETHING SLIGHTLY ASKEW IN MY PELVIS--PERHAPS FROM THE TIME I SLAMMED INTO THE TREE WHILE SKIING, JUST BEFORE THE GROWTH SPURT OF PUBERTY.

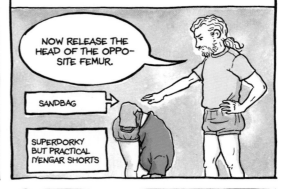

NOW RELEASE THE HEAD OF THE OPPO-SITE FEMUR.

SANDBAG

SUPERDORKY BUT PRACTICAL IYENGAR SHORTS

THIS WAY OF TURNING DISCOMFORT INTO AN OBJECT OF INTEREST WAS NOT UNLIKE WRITING. AS MY YOGA PRACTICE DEEPENED, MY CARTOONS GREW LESS SUPERFICIAL, MORE LIKE REAL LIFE.

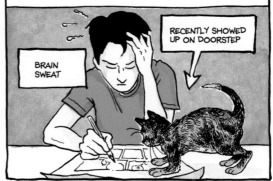

BRAIN SWEAT

RECENTLY SHOWED UP ON DOORSTEP

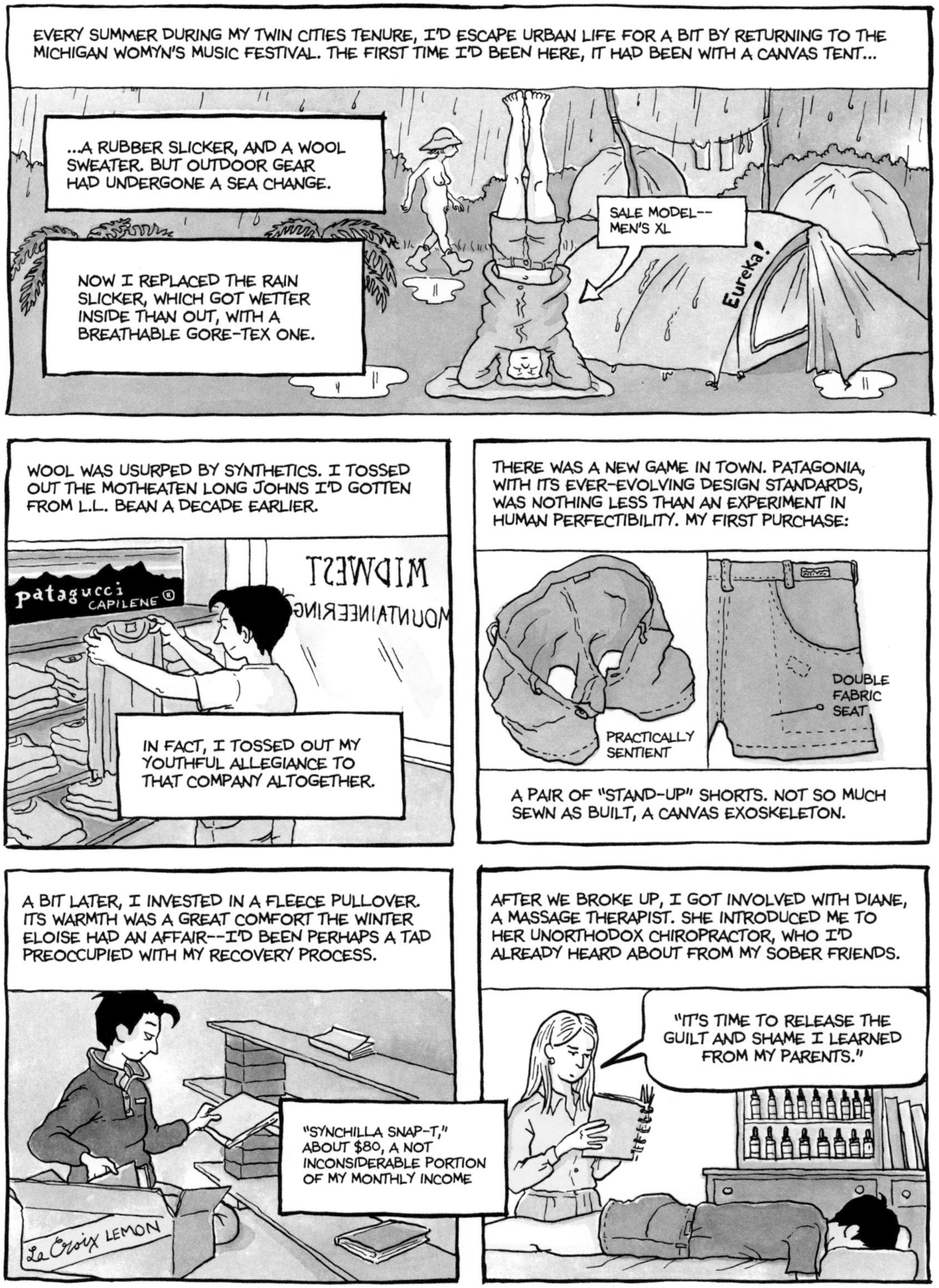
EVERY SUMMER DURING MY TWIN CITIES TENURE, I'D ESCAPE URBAN LIFE FOR A BIT BY RETURNING TO THE MICHIGAN WOMYN'S MUSIC FESTIVAL. THE FIRST TIME I'D BEEN HERE, IT HAD BEEN WITH A CANVAS TENT...
...A RUBBER SLICKER, AND A WOOL SWEATER. BUT OUTDOOR GEAR HAD UNDERGONE A SEA CHANGE.
NOW I REPLACED THE RAIN SLICKER, WHICH GOT WETTER INSIDE THAN OUT, WITH A BREATHABLE GORE-TEX ONE.
SALE MODEL-- MEN'S XL
Eureka!
WOOL WAS USURPED BY SYNTHETICS. I TOSSED OUT THE MOTHEATEN LONG JOHNS I'D GOTTEN FROM L.L. BEAN A DECADE EARLIER.
patagucci CAPILENE®
MIDWEST MOUNTAINEERING
IN FACT, I TOSSED OUT MY YOUTHFUL ALLEGIANCE TO THAT COMPANY ALTOGETHER.
THERE WAS A NEW GAME IN TOWN. PATAGONIA, WITH ITS EVER-EVOLVING DESIGN STANDARDS, WAS NOTHING LESS THAN AN EXPERIMENT IN HUMAN PERFECTIBILITY. MY FIRST PURCHASE:
PRACTICALLY SENTIENT
DOUBLE FABRIC SEAT
A PAIR OF "STAND-UP" SHORTS. NOT SO MUCH SEWN AS BUILT, A CANVAS EXOSKELETON.
A BIT LATER, I INVESTED IN A FLEECE PULLOVER. ITS WARMTH WAS A GREAT COMFORT THE WINTER ELOISE HAD AN AFFAIR--I'D BEEN PERHAPS A TAD PREOCCUPIED WITH MY RECOVERY PROCESS.
"SYNCHILLA SNAP-T," ABOUT $80, A NOT INCONSIDERABLE PORTION OF MY MONTHLY INCOME
La Croix LEMON
AFTER WE BROKE UP, I GOT INVOLVED WITH DIANE, A MASSAGE THERAPIST. SHE INTRODUCED ME TO HER UNORTHODOX CHIROPRACTOR, WHO I'D ALREADY HEARD ABOUT FROM MY SOBER FRIENDS.
"IT'S TIME TO RELEASE THE GUILT AND SHAME I LEARNED FROM MY PARENTS."

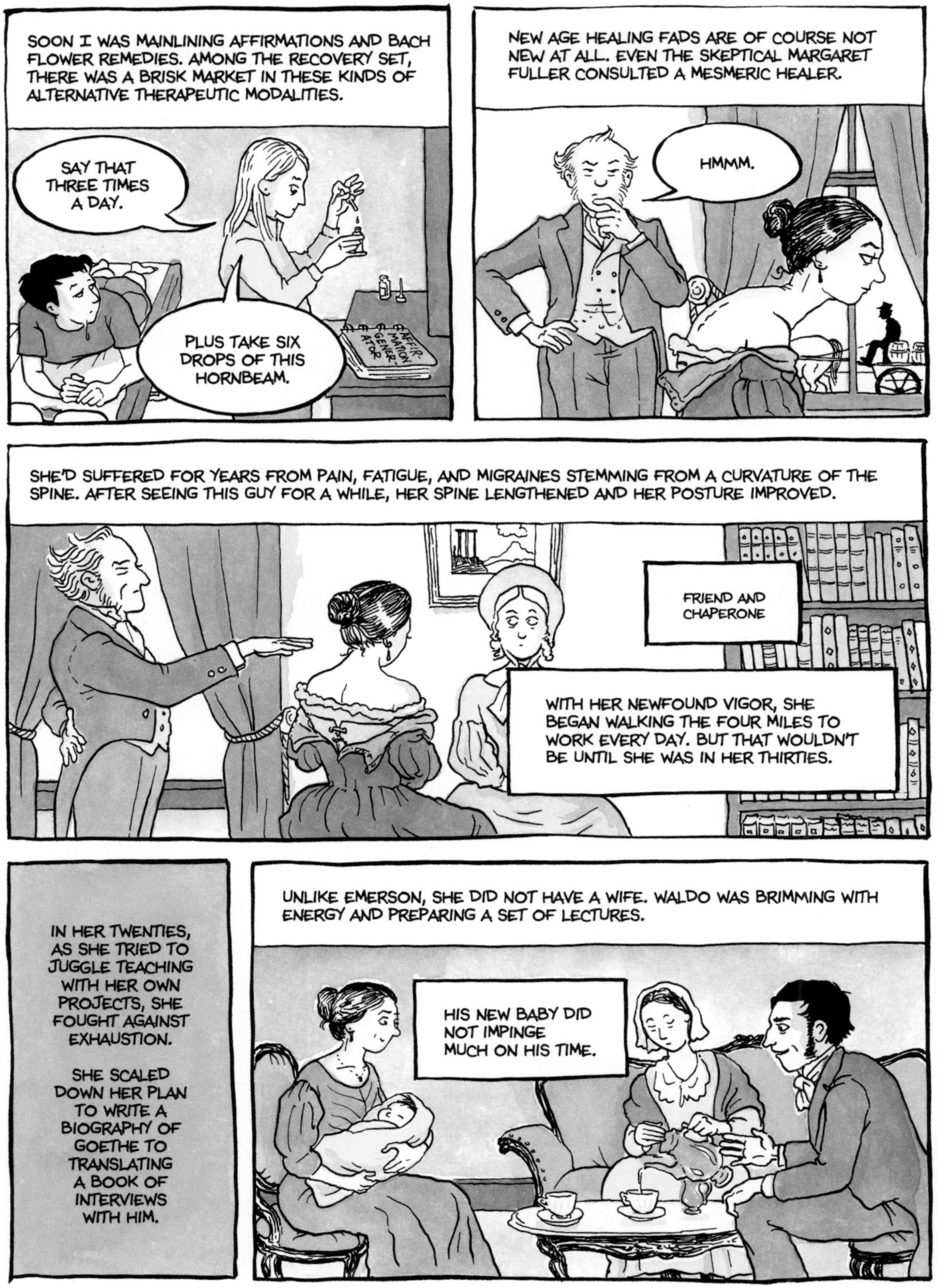
SOON I WAS MAINLINING AFFIRMATIONS AND BACH FLOWER REMEDIES. AMONG THE RECOVERY SET, THERE WAS A BRISK MARKET IN THESE KINDS OF ALTERNATIVE THERAPEUTIC MODALITIES.
SAY THAT THREE TIMES A DAY.
PLUS TAKE SIX DROPS OF THIS HORNBEAM.
AFFIR-MATION GENER-ATOR
NEW AGE HEALING FADS ARE OF COURSE NOT NEW AT ALL. EVEN THE SKEPTICAL MARGARET FULLER CONSULTED A MESMERIC HEALER.
HMMM.
SHE'D SUFFERED FOR YEARS FROM PAIN, FATIGUE, AND MIGRAINES STEMMING FROM A CURVATURE OF THE SPINE. AFTER SEEING THIS GUY FOR A WHILE, HER SPINE LENGTHENED AND HER POSTURE IMPROVED.
FRIEND AND CHAPERONE
WITH HER NEWFOUND VIGOR, SHE BEGAN WALKING THE FOUR MILES TO WORK EVERY DAY. BUT THAT WOULDN'T BE UNTIL SHE WAS IN HER THIRTIES.
IN HER TWENTIES, AS SHE TRIED TO JUGGLE TEACHING WITH HER OWN PROJECTS, SHE FOUGHT AGAINST EXHAUSTION.
SHE SCALED DOWN HER PLAN TO WRITE A BIOGRAPHY OF GOETHE TO TRANSLATING A BOOK OF INTERVIEWS WITH HIM.
UNLIKE EMERSON, SHE DID NOT HAVE A WIFE. WALDO WAS BRIMMING WITH ENERGY AND PREPARING A SET OF LECTURES.
HIS NEW BABY DID NOT IMPINGE MUCH ON HIS TIME.

ON HER SUMMER BREAK IN 1837, MARGARET HEARD WALDO GIVE HIS "AMERICAN SCHOLAR" SPEECH AND NEXT DAY WAS INVITED TO HANG WITH HIM AND THE MEMBERS OF THE TRANSCENDENTAL CLUB.

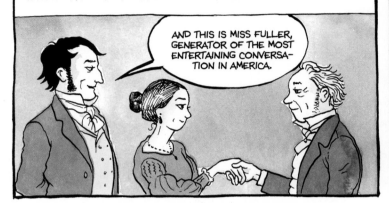

AND THIS IS MISS FULLER, GENERATOR OF THE MOST ENTERTAINING CONVERSATION IN AMERICA.

ALTHOUGH MARGARET WAS HITTING HER STRIDE AS A TEACHER AND ENJOYED INSPIRING HER STUDENTS, SHE WAS WELL AWARE THAT HER REAL GIFT WAS FOR EXTEMPORANEOUS SPEAKING.

BUT A WOMAN COULDN'T JUST TRAVEL AROUND GIVING PUBLIC TALKS, LIKE WALDO DID.

SHE FINALLY QUIT TEACHING WHEN HER HEALTH GAVE OUT. BUT SHE KEPT SLOGGING ON HER TRANSLATION PROJECT, FINISHING ON HER TWENTY-NINTH BIRTHDAY. HER FIRST BOOK.

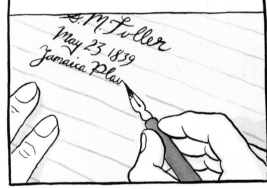

S. M. Fuller
May 23 1839
Jamaica Plain

SHE GOT AN IDEA THAT SUMMER FOR A WAY TO USE HER SPEAKING SKILLS TO MAKE A BUCK. SHE COULDN'T LECTURE, BUT SHE COULD LEAD A CLASS FOR ADULT WOMEN ON THE "GREAT QUESTIONS."

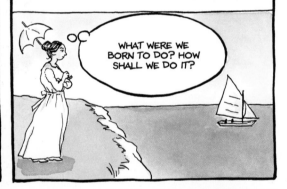

WHAT WERE WE BORN TO DO? HOW SHALL WE DO IT?

NOW THAT SHE WAS CLEAR ON HER OWN PURPOSE, SHE WOULD HELP OTHER WOMEN FIGURE OUT THEIRS. IN NOVEMBER, SHE HELD THE FIRST OF HER "CONVERSATIONS," WITH CLASSICAL MYTHOLOGY* AS THE FOCUS.

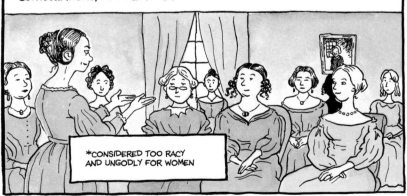

*CONSIDERED TOO RACY AND UNGODLY FOR WOMEN

THE SAME WEEK, SHE BECAME EDITOR OF THE DIAL, THE NEW TRANSCENDENTALIST JOURNAL.

SHE HAD LAUNCHED HERSELF.

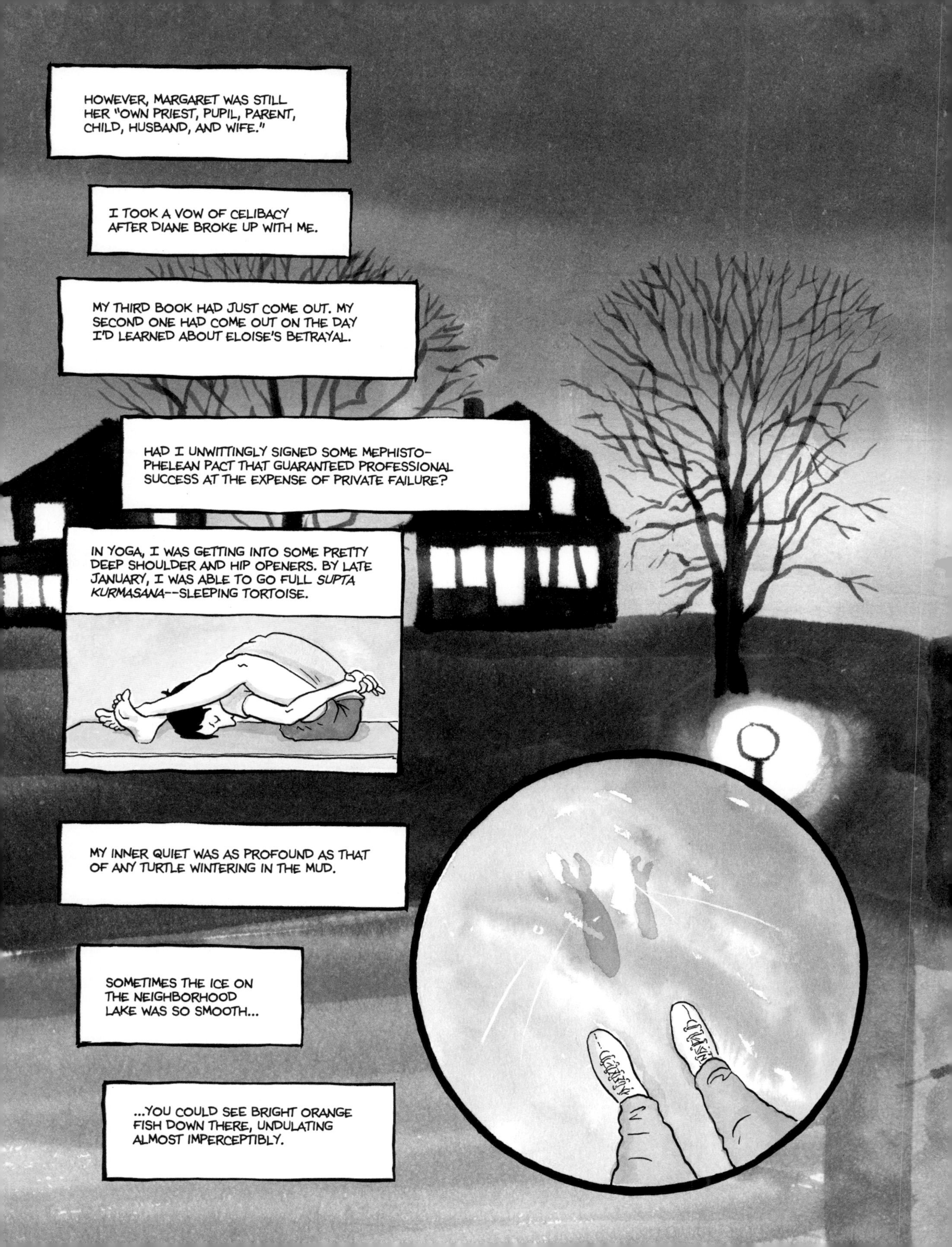

HOWEVER, MARGARET WAS STILL HER "OWN PRIEST, PUPIL, PARENT, CHILD, HUSBAND, AND WIFE."

I TOOK A VOW OF CELIBACY AFTER DIANE BROKE UP WITH ME.

MY THIRD BOOK HAD JUST COME OUT. MY SECOND ONE HAD COME OUT ON THE DAY I'D LEARNED ABOUT ELOISE'S BETRAYAL.

HAD I UNWITTINGLY SIGNED SOME MEPHISTO-PHELEAN PACT THAT GUARANTEED PROFESSIONAL SUCCESS AT THE EXPENSE OF PRIVATE FAILURE?

IN YOGA, I WAS GETTING INTO SOME PRETTY DEEP SHOULDER AND HIP OPENERS. BY LATE JANUARY, I WAS ABLE TO GO FULL *SUPTA KURMASANA*--SLEEPING TORTOISE.

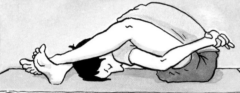

MY INNER QUIET WAS AS PROFOUND AS THAT OF ANY TURTLE WINTERING IN THE MUD.

SOMETIMES THE ICE ON THE NEIGHBORHOOD LAKE WAS SO SMOOTH...

...YOU COULD SEE BRIGHT ORANGE FISH DOWN THERE, UNDULATING ALMOST IMPERCEPTIBLY.

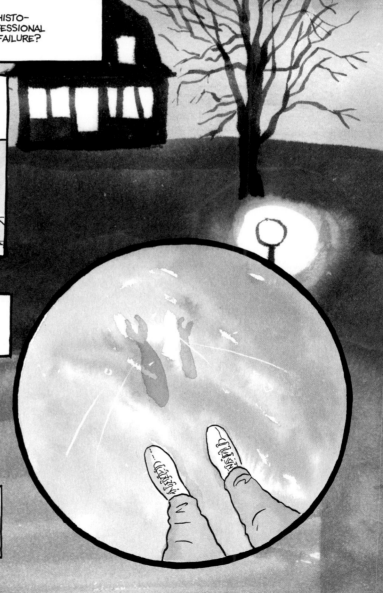

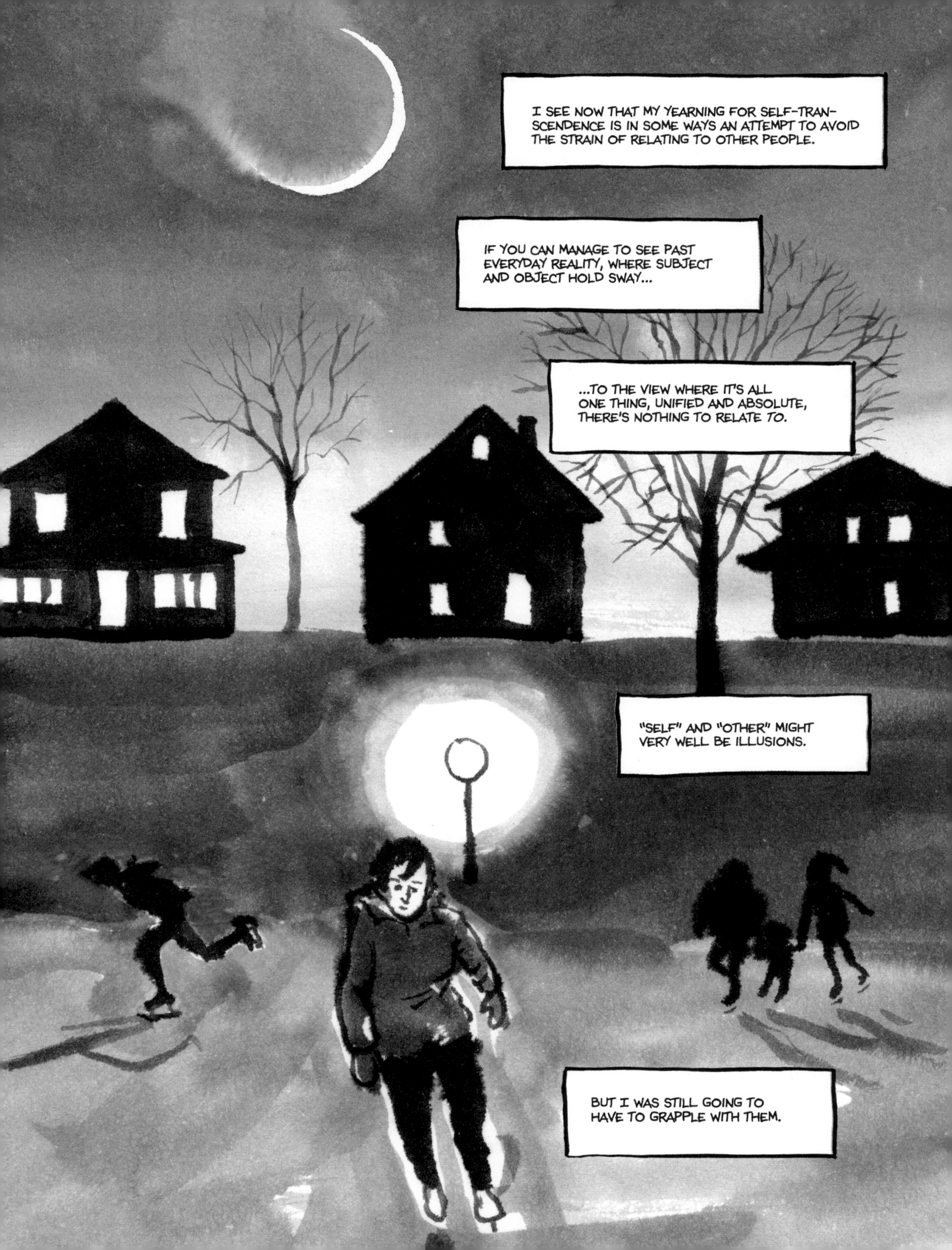
I SEE NOW THAT MY YEARNING FOR SELF-TRANSCENDENCE IS IN SOME WAYS AN ATTEMPT TO AVOID THE STRAIN OF RELATING TO OTHER PEOPLE.
IF YOU CAN MANAGE TO SEE PAST EVERYDAY REALITY, WHERE SUBJECT AND OBJECT HOLD SWAY...
...TO THE VIEW WHERE IT'S ALL ONE THING, UNIFIED AND ABSOLUTE, THERE'S NOTHING TO RELATE *TO*.
"SELF" AND "OTHER" MIGHT VERY WELL BE ILLUSIONS.
BUT I WAS STILL GOING TO HAVE TO GRAPPLE WITH THEM.

1990s

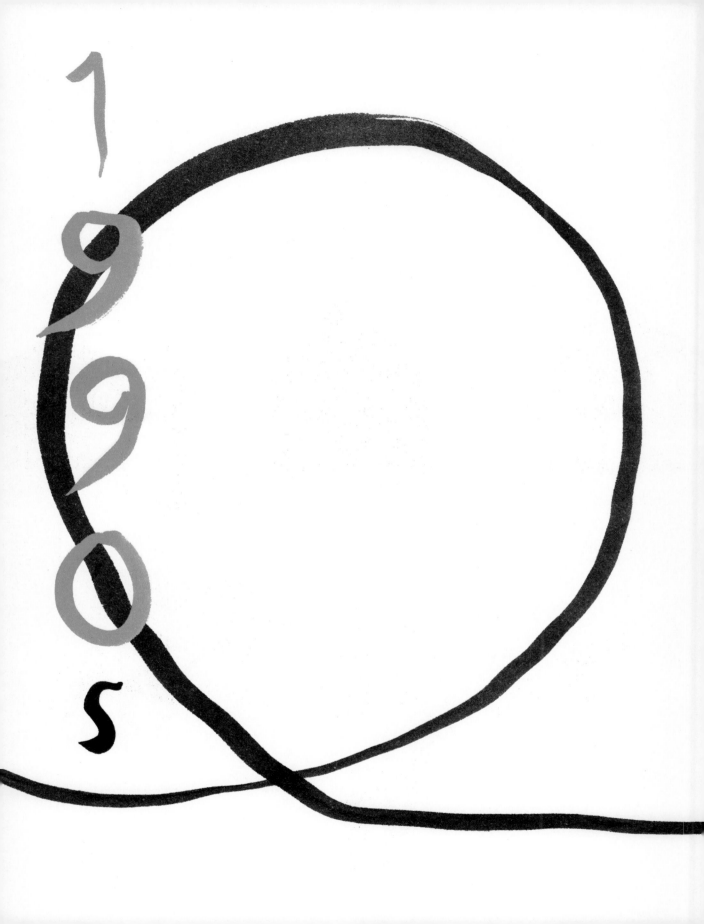

30s

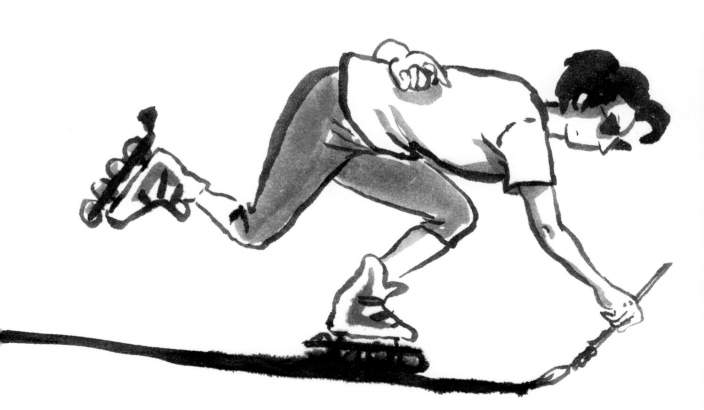

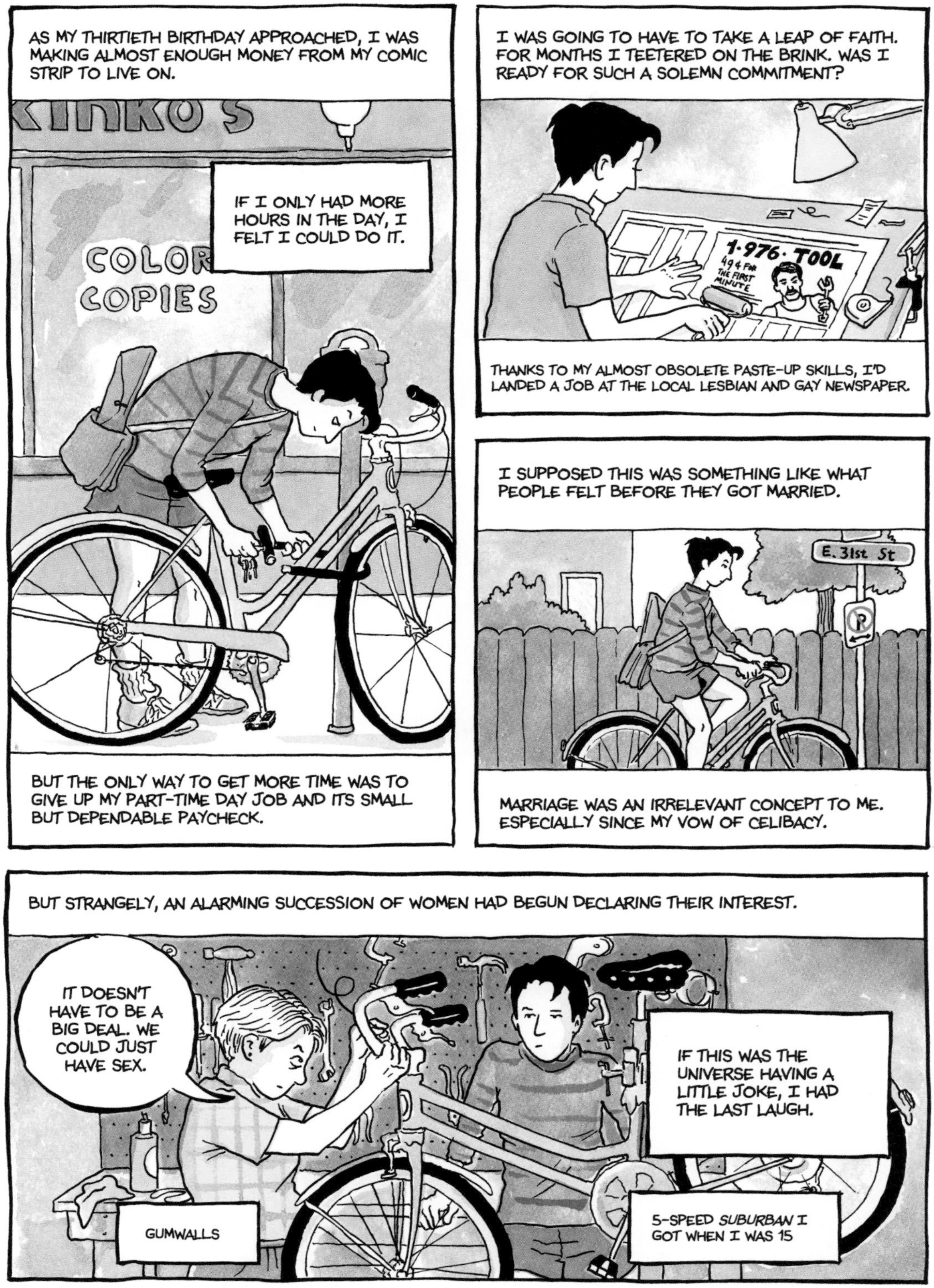
AS MY THIRTIETH BIRTHDAY APPROACHED, I WAS MAKING ALMOST ENOUGH MONEY FROM MY COMIC STRIP TO LIVE ON.
IF I ONLY HAD MORE HOURS IN THE DAY, I FELT I COULD DO IT.
COLOR COPIES
BUT THE ONLY WAY TO GET MORE TIME WAS TO GIVE UP MY PART-TIME DAY JOB AND ITS SMALL BUT DEPENDABLE PAYCHECK.
I WAS GOING TO HAVE TO TAKE A LEAP OF FAITH. FOR MONTHS I TEETERED ON THE BRINK. WAS I READY FOR SUCH A SOLEMN COMMITMENT?
1·976·TOOL
49¢ FOR THE FIRST MINUTE
THANKS TO MY ALMOST OBSOLETE PASTE-UP SKILLS, I'D LANDED A JOB AT THE LOCAL LESBIAN AND GAY NEWSPAPER.
I SUPPOSED THIS WAS SOMETHING LIKE WHAT PEOPLE FELT BEFORE THEY GOT MARRIED.
E. 31st St
MARRIAGE WAS AN IRRELEVANT CONCEPT TO ME. ESPECIALLY SINCE MY VOW OF CELIBACY.
BUT STRANGELY, AN ALARMING SUCCESSION OF WOMEN HAD BEGUN DECLARING THEIR INTEREST.
IT DOESN'T HAVE TO BE A BIG DEAL. WE COULD JUST HAVE SEX.
IF THIS WAS THE UNIVERSE HAVING A LITTLE JOKE, I HAD THE LAST LAUGH.
GUMWALLS
5-SPEED *SUBURBAN* I GOT WHEN I WAS 15

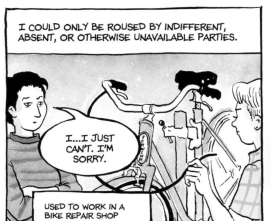

I COULD ONLY BE ROUSED BY INDIFFERENT, ABSENT, OR OTHERWISE UNAVAILABLE PARTIES.

I...I JUST CAN'T. I'M SORRY.

USED TO WORK IN A BIKE REPAIR SHOP

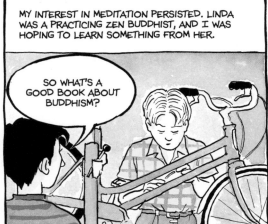

MY INTEREST IN MEDITATION PERSISTED. LINDA WAS A PRACTICING ZEN BUDDHIST, AND I WAS HOPING TO LEARN SOMETHING FROM HER.

SO WHAT'S A GOOD BOOK ABOUT BUDDHISM?

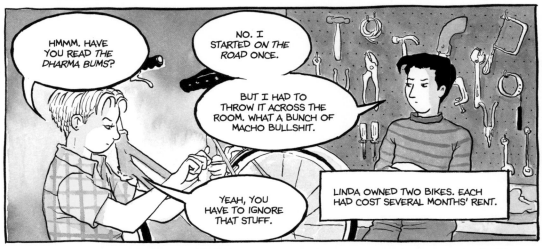

HMMM. HAVE YOU READ *THE DHARMA BUMS*?

NO. I STARTED *ON THE ROAD* ONCE.

BUT I HAD TO THROW IT ACROSS THE ROOM. WHAT A BUNCH OF MACHO BULLSHIT.

YEAH, YOU HAVE TO IGNORE THAT STUFF.

LINDA OWNED TWO BIKES. EACH HAD COST SEVERAL MONTHS' RENT.

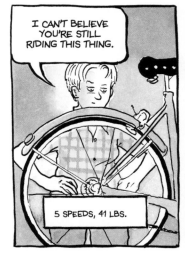

I CAN'T BELIEVE YOU'RE STILL RIDING THIS THING.

5 SPEEDS, 41 LBS.

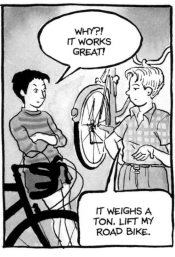

WHY?! IT WORKS GREAT!

IT WEIGHS A TON. LIFT MY ROAD BIKE.

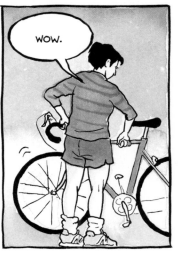

WOW.

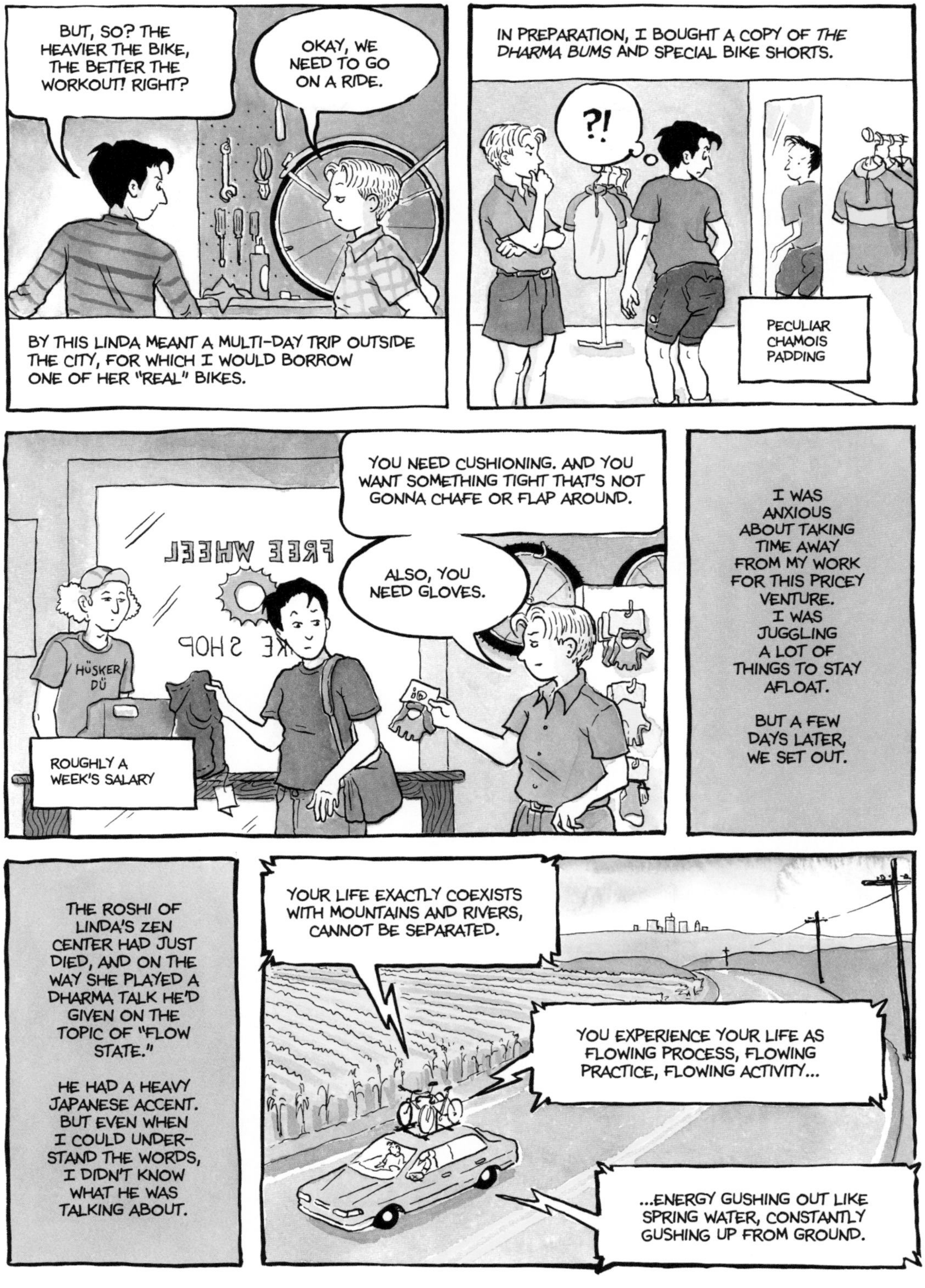

BUT, SO? THE HEAVIER THE BIKE, THE BETTER THE WORKOUT! RIGHT?
OKAY, WE NEED TO GO ON A RIDE.
BY THIS LINDA MEANT A MULTI-DAY TRIP OUTSIDE THE CITY, FOR WHICH I WOULD BORROW ONE OF HER "REAL" BIKES.
IN PREPARATION, I BOUGHT A COPY OF *THE DHARMA BUMS* AND SPECIAL BIKE SHORTS.
?!
PECULIAR CHAMOIS PADDING
YOU NEED CUSHIONING. AND YOU WANT SOMETHING TIGHT THAT'S NOT GONNA CHAFE OR FLAP AROUND.
FREE WHEEL
ALSO, YOU NEED GLOVES.
KE SHOP
HÜSKER DÜ
ROUGHLY A WEEK'S SALARY
I WAS ANXIOUS ABOUT TAKING TIME AWAY FROM MY WORK FOR THIS PRICEY VENTURE. I WAS JUGGLING A LOT OF THINGS TO STAY AFLOAT.
BUT A FEW DAYS LATER, WE SET OUT.
THE ROSHI OF LINDA'S ZEN CENTER HAD JUST DIED, AND ON THE WAY SHE PLAYED A DHARMA TALK HE'D GIVEN ON THE TOPIC OF "FLOW STATE."
HE HAD A HEAVY JAPANESE ACCENT. BUT EVEN WHEN I COULD UNDER-STAND THE WORDS, I DIDN'T KNOW WHAT HE WAS TALKING ABOUT.
YOUR LIFE EXACTLY COEXISTS WITH MOUNTAINS AND RIVERS, CANNOT BE SEPARATED.
YOU EXPERIENCE YOUR LIFE AS FLOWING PROCESS, FLOWING PRACTICE, FLOWING ACTIVITY...
...ENERGY GUSHING OUT LIKE SPRING WATER, CONSTANTLY GUSHING UP FROM GROUND.

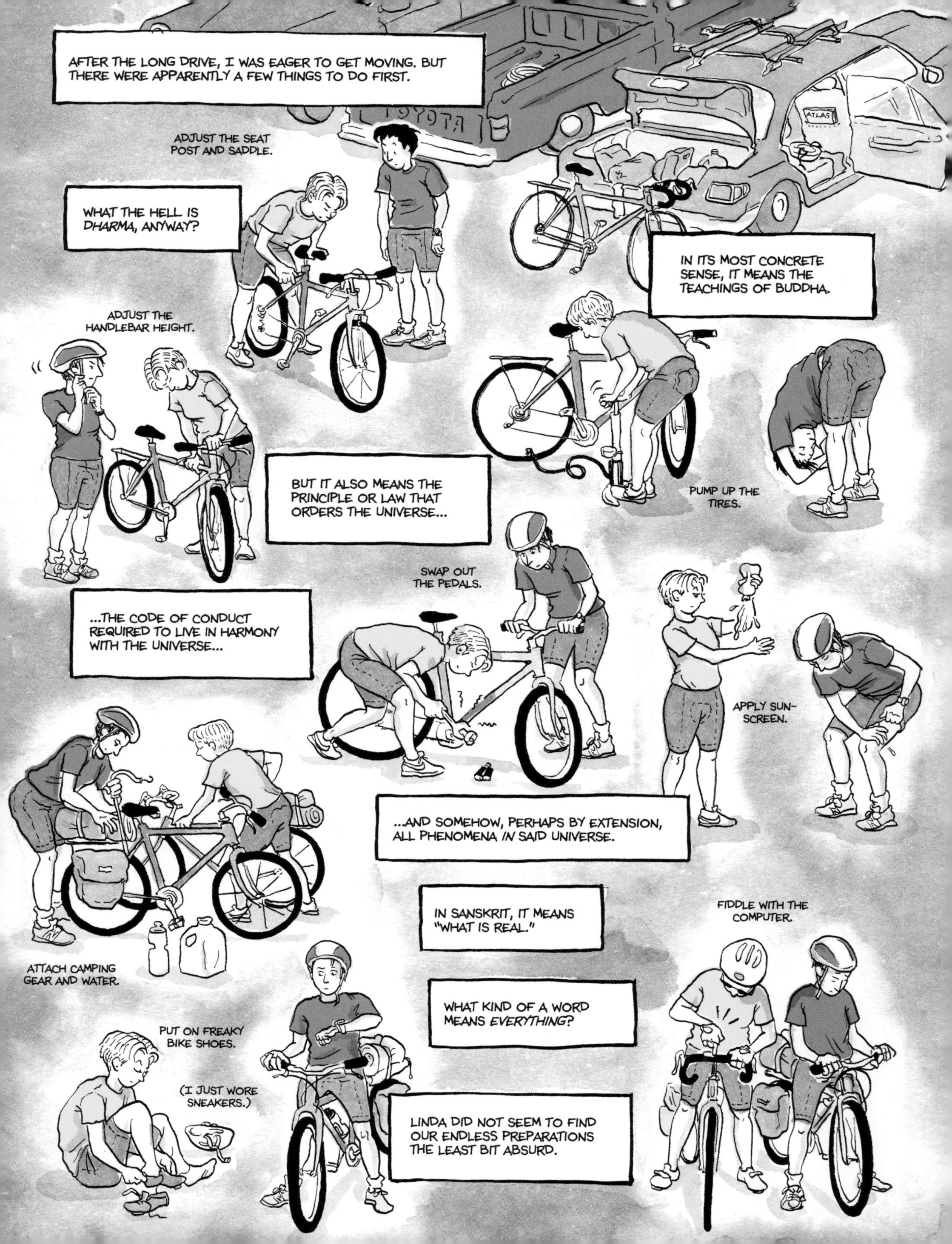

AFTER THE LONG DRIVE, I WAS EAGER TO GET MOVING. BUT THERE WERE APPARENTLY A FEW THINGS TO DO FIRST.
TOYOTA
ATLAS
ADJUST THE SEAT POST AND SADDLE.
WHAT THE HELL IS *DHARMA*, ANYWAY?
IN ITS MOST CONCRETE SENSE, IT MEANS THE TEACHINGS OF BUDDHA.
ADJUST THE HANDLEBAR HEIGHT.
BUT IT ALSO MEANS THE PRINCIPLE OR LAW THAT ORDERS THE UNIVERSE...
PUMP UP THE TIRES.
SWAP OUT THE PEDALS.
...THE CODE OF CONDUCT REQUIRED TO LIVE IN HARMONY WITH THE UNIVERSE...
APPLY SUN-SCREEN.
...AND SOMEHOW, PERHAPS BY EXTENSION, ALL PHENOMENA *IN* SAID UNIVERSE.
IN SANSKRIT, IT MEANS "WHAT IS REAL."
FIDDLE WITH THE COMPUTER.
ATTACH CAMPING GEAR AND WATER.
WHAT KIND OF A WORD MEANS *EVERYTHING*?
PUT ON FREAKY BIKE SHOES.
(I JUST WORE SNEAKERS.)
LINDA DID NOT SEEM TO FIND OUR ENDLESS PREPARATIONS THE LEAST BIT ABSURD.

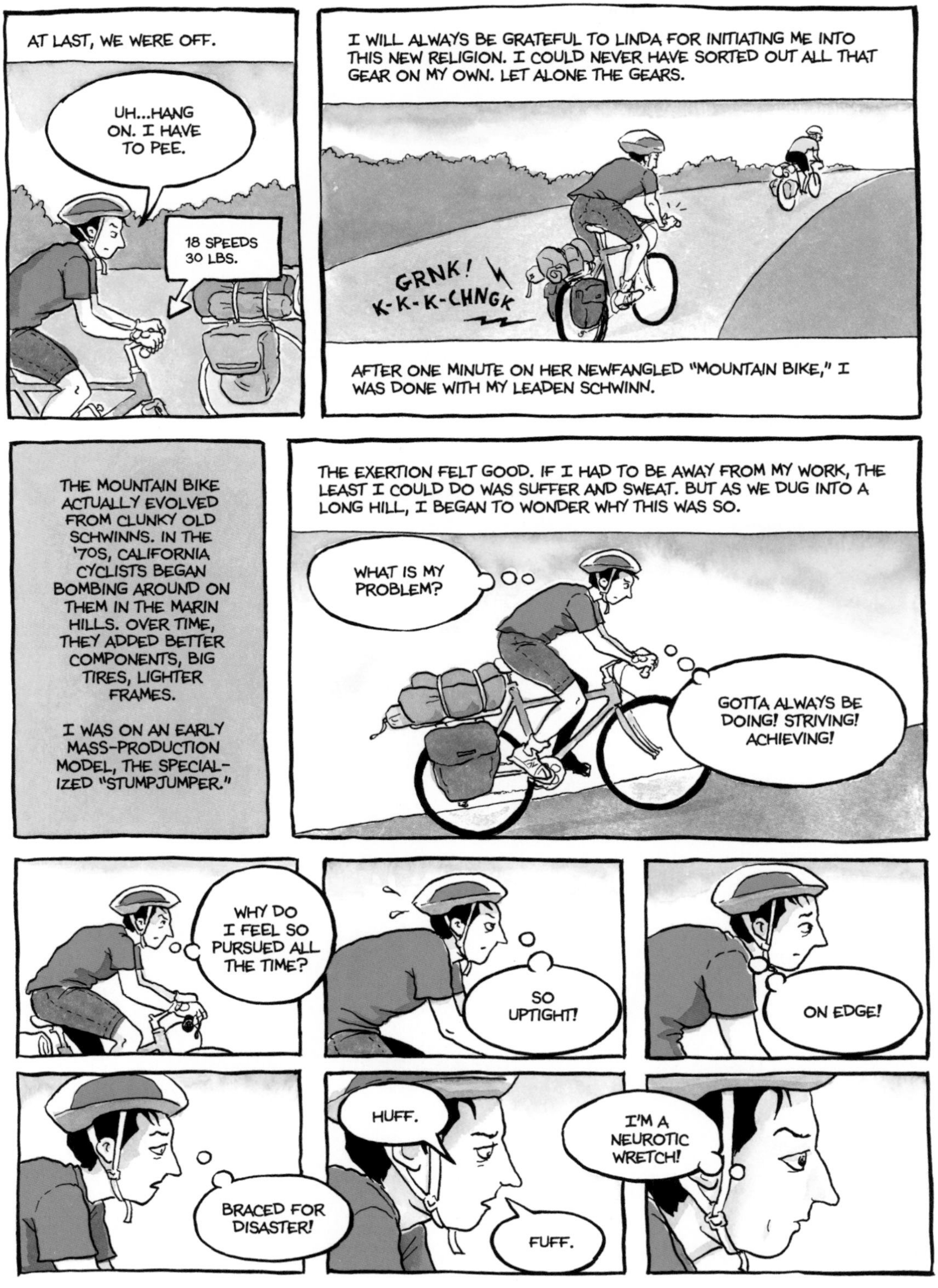

AT LAST, WE WERE OFF.
UH...HANG ON. I HAVE TO PEE.
18 SPEEDS 30 LBS.
I WILL ALWAYS BE GRATEFUL TO LINDA FOR INITIATING ME INTO THIS NEW RELIGION. I COULD NEVER HAVE SORTED OUT ALL THAT GEAR ON MY OWN. LET ALONE THE GEARS.
GRNK! K-K-K-CHNGK
AFTER ONE MINUTE ON HER NEWFANGLED "MOUNTAIN BIKE," I WAS DONE WITH MY LEADEN SCHWINN.
THE MOUNTAIN BIKE ACTUALLY EVOLVED FROM CLUNKY OLD SCHWINNS. IN THE '70S, CALIFORNIA CYCLISTS BEGAN BOMBING AROUND ON THEM IN THE MARIN HILLS. OVER TIME, THEY ADDED BETTER COMPONENTS, BIG TIRES, LIGHTER FRAMES.
I WAS ON AN EARLY MASS-PRODUCTION MODEL, THE SPECIALIZED "STUMPJUMPER."
THE EXERTION FELT GOOD. IF I HAD TO BE AWAY FROM MY WORK, THE LEAST I COULD DO WAS SUFFER AND SWEAT. BUT AS WE DUG INTO A LONG HILL, I BEGAN TO WONDER WHY THIS WAS SO.
WHAT IS MY PROBLEM?
GOTTA ALWAYS BE DOING! STRIVING! ACHIEVING!
WHY DO I FEEL SO PURSUED ALL THE TIME?
SO UPTIGHT!
ON EDGE!
BRACED FOR DISASTER!
HUFF.
FUFF.
I'M A NEUROTIC WRETCH!

SOMETHING BECAME SUDDENLY CLEAR TO ME.

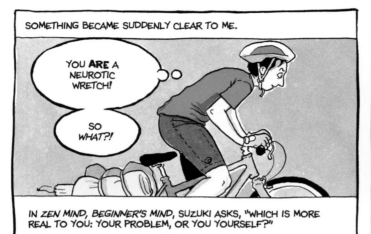

YOU **ARE** A NEUROTIC WRETCH!

SO WHAT?!

IN *ZEN MIND, BEGINNER'S MIND,* SUZUKI ASKS, "WHICH IS MORE REAL TO YOU: YOUR PROBLEM, OR YOU YOURSELF?"

IN MY FLASH OF SELF-COM-PASSION, IF I CAN CALL IT THAT, I GOT A SMALL HIT OF THE MUSHROOM BLISS.

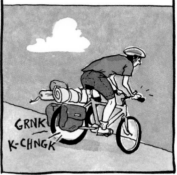

GRNK
K-CHNGK

I HAD ALMOST FORGOTTEN ABOUT THIS SIDE EFFECT OF EXERTION, THIS SLACKENING OF THE EGO'S GRIP.

IN ANY CASE, IT WAS THE MOST PROLONGED AEROBIC WORKOUT I'D HAD SINCE I QUIT KARATE FIVE YEARS EARLIER.

AT THE END OF THE RIDE I WAS STIFF, SADDLESORE, SUNBURNT, SALT-COATED, AND SOMEWHAT SLAPHAPPY.

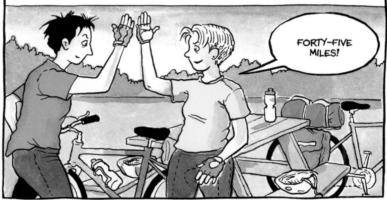

FORTY-FIVE MILES!

I BEGAN READING *THE DHARMA BUMS* THAT NIGHT. KEROUAC DESCRIBES MEETING THE POET GARY SNYDER IN BERKELEY.

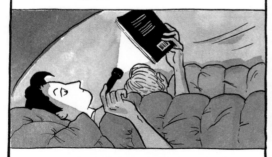

HE USES THINLY DISGUISED PSEUDONYMS. GARY SNYDER IS JAPHY RYDER. KEROUAC IS RAY SMITH. THEIR FRIEND THE POET ALLEN GINSBERG IS ALVAH GOLDBOOK.

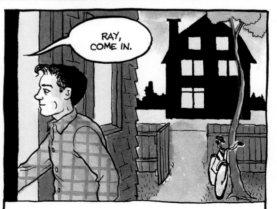

RAY, COME IN.

IT'S 1955. JACK HAD GOTTEN INTO BUDDHISM A YEAR EARLIER. HE'D WRITTEN *ON THE ROAD,* BUT HADN'T FOUND A PUBLISHER YET.

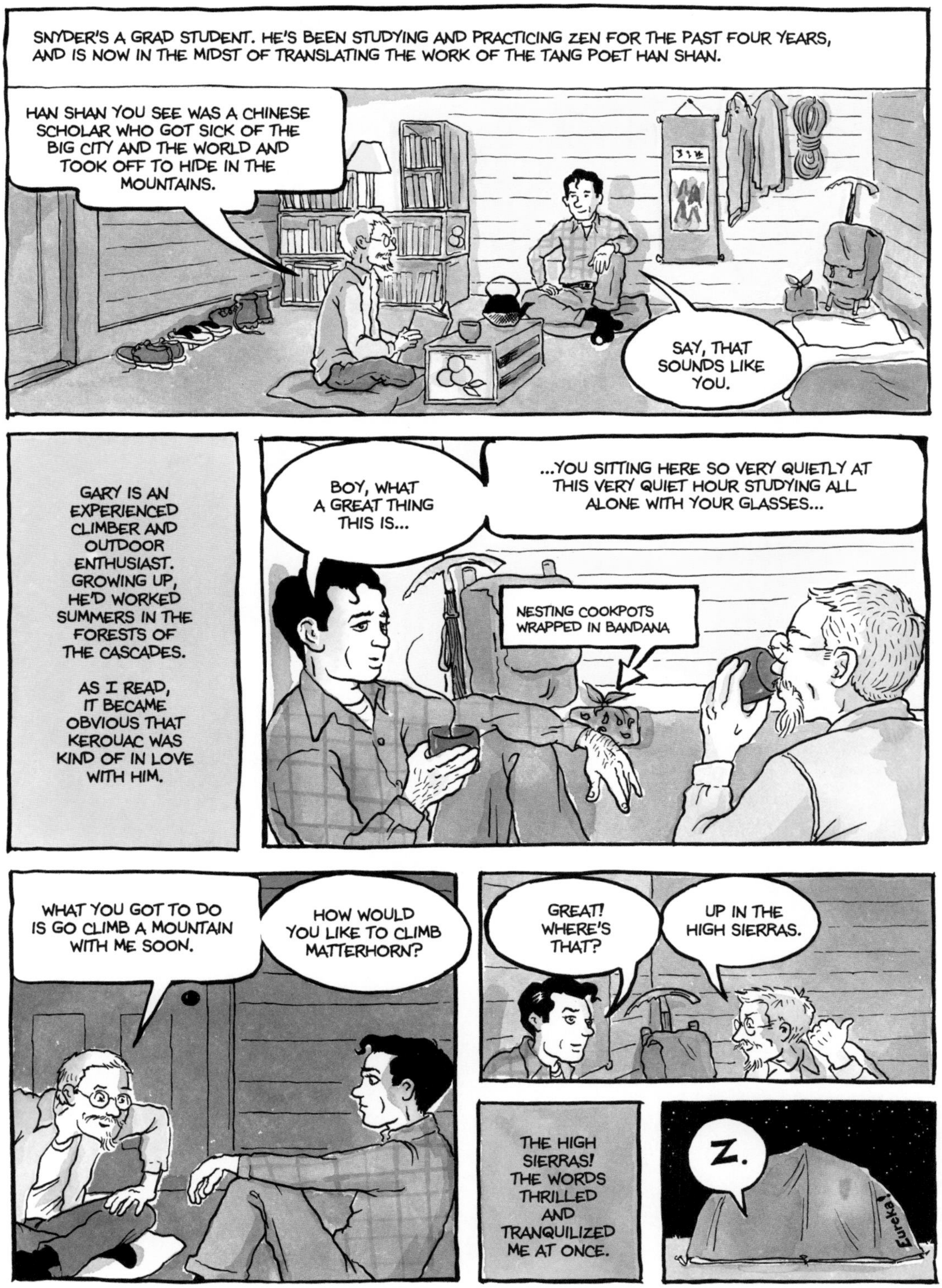
SNYDER'S A GRAD STUDENT. HE'S BEEN STUDYING AND PRACTICING ZEN FOR THE PAST FOUR YEARS, AND IS NOW IN THE MIDST OF TRANSLATING THE WORK OF THE TANG POET HAN SHAN.
HAN SHAN YOU SEE WAS A CHINESE SCHOLAR WHO GOT SICK OF THE BIG CITY AND THE WORLD AND TOOK OFF TO HIDE IN THE MOUNTAINS.
SAY, THAT SOUNDS LIKE YOU.
GARY IS AN EXPERIENCED CLIMBER AND OUTDOOR ENTHUSIAST. GROWING UP, HE'D WORKED SUMMERS IN THE FORESTS OF THE CASCADES.
AS I READ, IT BECAME OBVIOUS THAT KEROUAC WAS KIND OF IN LOVE WITH HIM.
BOY, WHAT A GREAT THING THIS IS...
...YOU SITTING HERE SO VERY QUIETLY AT THIS VERY QUIET HOUR STUDYING ALL ALONE WITH YOUR GLASSES...
NESTING COOKPOTS WRAPPED IN BANDANA
WHAT YOU GOT TO DO IS GO CLIMB A MOUNTAIN WITH ME SOON.
HOW WOULD YOU LIKE TO CLIMB MATTERHORN?
GREAT! WHERE'S THAT?
UP IN THE HIGH SIERRAS.
THE HIGH SIERRAS! THE WORDS THRILLED AND TRANQUILIZED ME AT ONCE.
Z.
Eureka!

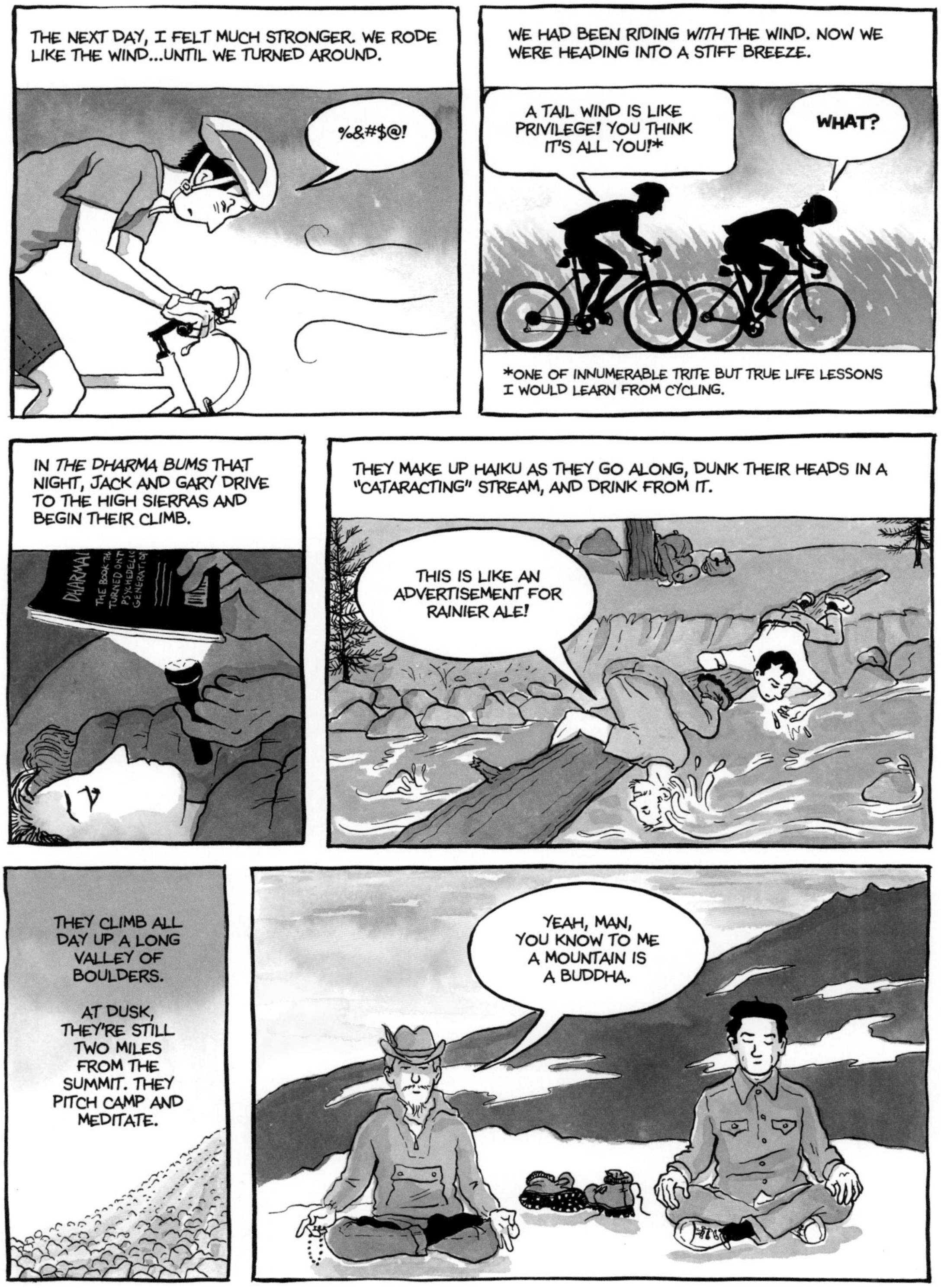
THE NEXT DAY, I FELT MUCH STRONGER. WE RODE LIKE THE WIND...UNTIL WE TURNED AROUND.
%&#$@!
WE HAD BEEN RIDING *WITH* THE WIND. NOW WE WERE HEADING INTO A STIFF BREEZE.
A TAIL WIND IS LIKE PRIVILEGE! YOU THINK IT'S ALL YOU!*
WHAT?
*ONE OF INNUMERABLE TRITE BUT TRUE LIFE LESSONS I WOULD LEARN FROM CYCLING.
IN *THE DHARMA BUMS* THAT NIGHT, JACK AND GARY DRIVE TO THE HIGH SIERRAS AND BEGIN THEIR CLIMB.
THEY MAKE UP HAIKU AS THEY GO ALONG, DUNK THEIR HEADS IN A "CATARACTING" STREAM, AND DRINK FROM IT.
THIS IS LIKE AN ADVERTISEMENT FOR RAINIER ALE!
THEY CLIMB ALL DAY UP A LONG VALLEY OF BOULDERS.
AT DUSK, THEY'RE STILL TWO MILES FROM THE SUMMIT. THEY PITCH CAMP AND MEDITATE.
YEAH, MAN, YOU KNOW TO ME A MOUNTAIN IS A BUDDHA.

JACK HAD BEEN DISAPPOINTED WHEN GARY SAID THEY COULDN'T BRING WINE ALONG. NOW HE'S SURPRISED TO FIND HE DOESN'T WANT IT.

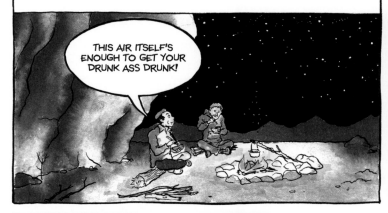

THIS AIR ITSELF'S ENOUGH TO GET YOUR DRUNK ASS DRUNK!

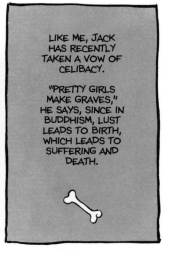

LIKE ME, JACK HAS RECENTLY TAKEN A VOW OF CELIBACY.

"PRETTY GIRLS MAKE GRAVES," HE SAYS, SINCE IN BUDDHISM, LUST LEADS TO BIRTH, WHICH LEADS TO SUFFERING AND DEATH.

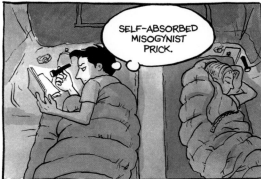

SELF-ABSORBED MISOGYNIST PRICK.

BUT MY OWN VOW WAS EQUALLY SELF-ABSORBED, I SEE NOW. FOR ME, SEX LED TO ENMESHMENT. ALONE, I COULD REMAIN INTACT.

PERHAPS TO DISPEL THE INTIMACY, JACK TELLS A STORY IN WHICH HE MENTIONS HITCHING A RIDE WITH "SOME LITTLE FAGGOT." LATER, HE WATCHES GARY SLEEP.

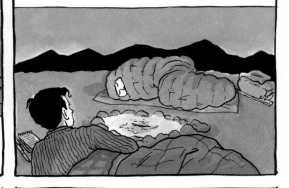

OUR LAST DAY OF RIDING WAS HARD. WHEN WE FINALLY GOT BACK TO THE CAR, I "BONKED."

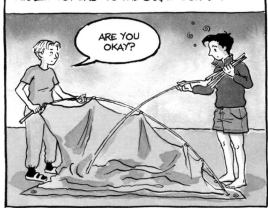

ARE YOU OKAY?

THAT'S ENDURANCE SPORTS LINGO FOR THE PROFOUND EXHAUSTION THAT OCCURS WHEN YOU USE UP ALL YOUR STORED GLYCOGEN.

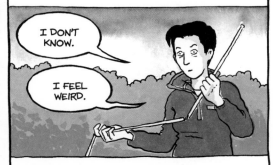

I DON'T KNOW.

I FEEL WEIRD.

IT WAS A BIT LIKE THE FLAT FEELING OF BEING DEPRESSED, WHICH FREAKED ME OUT.

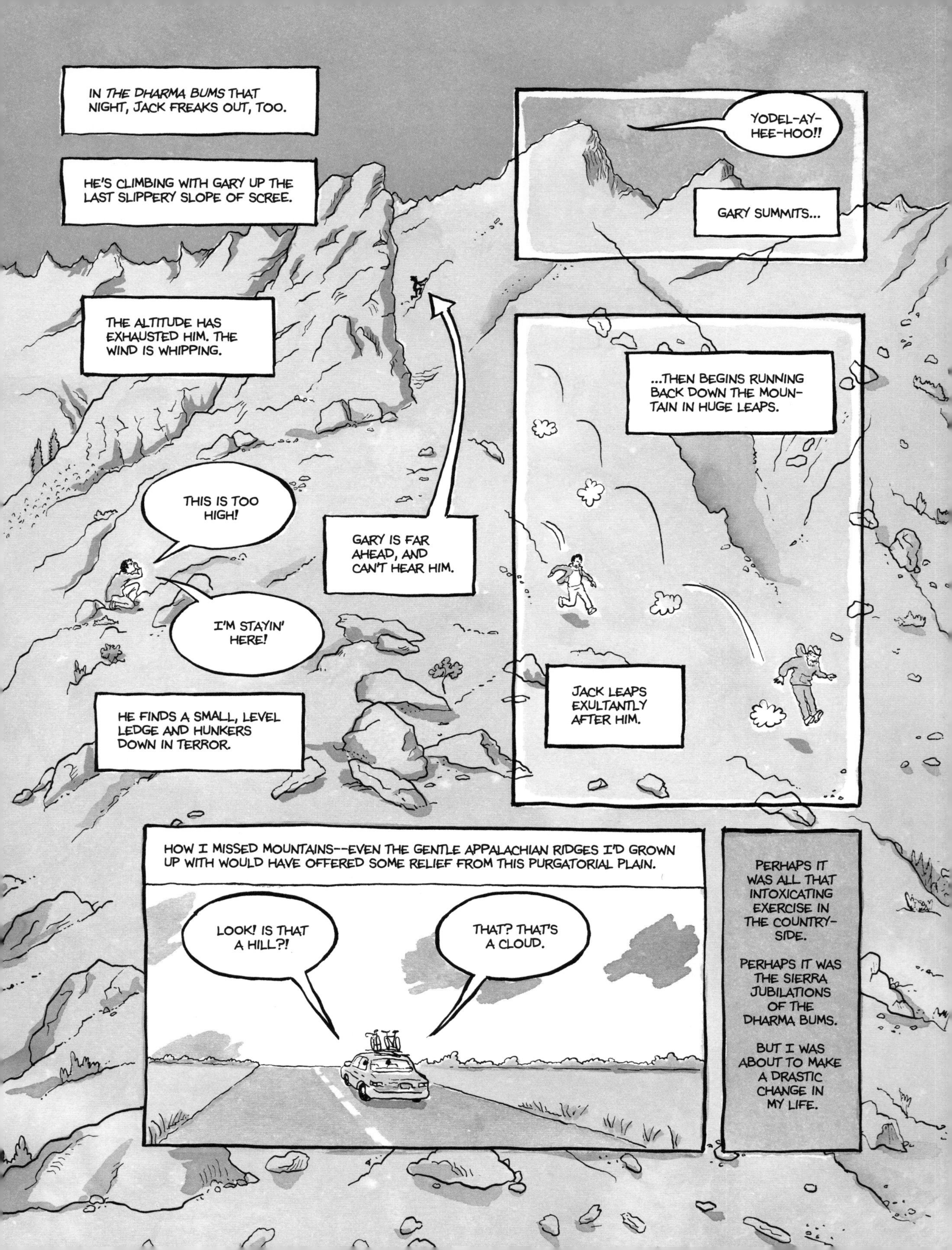

IN *THE DHARMA BUMS* THAT NIGHT, JACK FREAKS OUT, TOO.
HE'S CLIMBING WITH GARY UP THE LAST SLIPPERY SLOPE OF SCREE.
THE ALTITUDE HAS EXHAUSTED HIM. THE WIND IS WHIPPING.
THIS IS TOO HIGH!
I'M STAYIN' HERE!
GARY IS FAR AHEAD, AND CAN'T HEAR HIM.
HE FINDS A SMALL, LEVEL LEDGE AND HUNKERS DOWN IN TERROR.
YODEL-AY-HEE-HOO!!
GARY SUMMITS...
...THEN BEGINS RUNNING BACK DOWN THE MOUNTAIN IN HUGE LEAPS.
JACK LEAPS EXULTANTLY AFTER HIM.
HOW I MISSED MOUNTAINS--EVEN THE GENTLE APPALACHIAN RIDGES I'D GROWN UP WITH WOULD HAVE OFFERED SOME RELIEF FROM THIS PURGATORIAL PLAIN.
LOOK! IS THAT A HILL?!
THAT? THAT'S A CLOUD.
PERHAPS IT WAS ALL THAT INTOXICATING EXERCISE IN THE COUNTRYSIDE.
PERHAPS IT WAS THE SIERRA JUBILATIONS OF THE DHARMA BUMS.
BUT I WAS ABOUT TO MAKE A DRASTIC CHANGE IN MY LIFE.

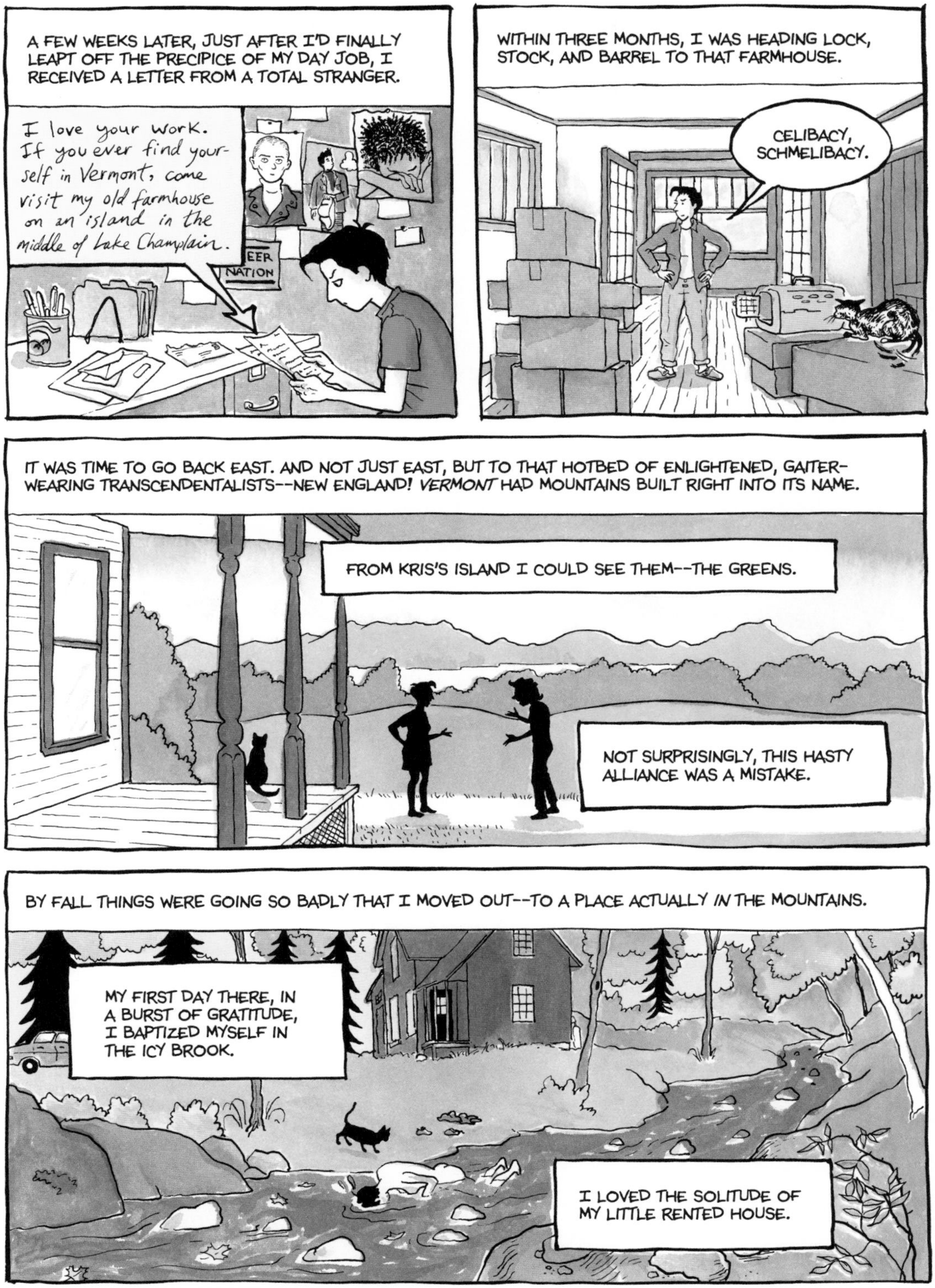
A FEW WEEKS LATER, JUST AFTER I'D FINALLY LEAPT OFF THE PRECIPICE OF MY DAY JOB, I RECEIVED A LETTER FROM A TOTAL STRANGER.
I love your work. If you ever find yourself in Vermont, come visit my old farmhouse on an island in the middle of Lake Champlain.
WITHIN THREE MONTHS, I WAS HEADING LOCK, STOCK, AND BARREL TO THAT FARMHOUSE.
CELIBACY, SCHMELIBACY.
IT WAS TIME TO GO BACK EAST. AND NOT JUST EAST, BUT TO THAT HOTBED OF ENLIGHTENED, GAITER-WEARING TRANSCENDENTALISTS--NEW ENGLAND! *VERMONT* HAD MOUNTAINS BUILT RIGHT INTO ITS NAME.
FROM KRIS'S ISLAND I COULD SEE THEM--THE GREENS.
NOT SURPRISINGLY, THIS HASTY ALLIANCE WAS A MISTAKE.
BY FALL THINGS WERE GOING SO BADLY THAT I MOVED OUT--TO A PLACE ACTUALLY *IN* THE MOUNTAINS.
MY FIRST DAY THERE, IN A BURST OF GRATITUDE, I BAPTIZED MYSELF IN THE ICY BROOK.
I LOVED THE SOLITUDE OF MY LITTLE RENTED HOUSE.

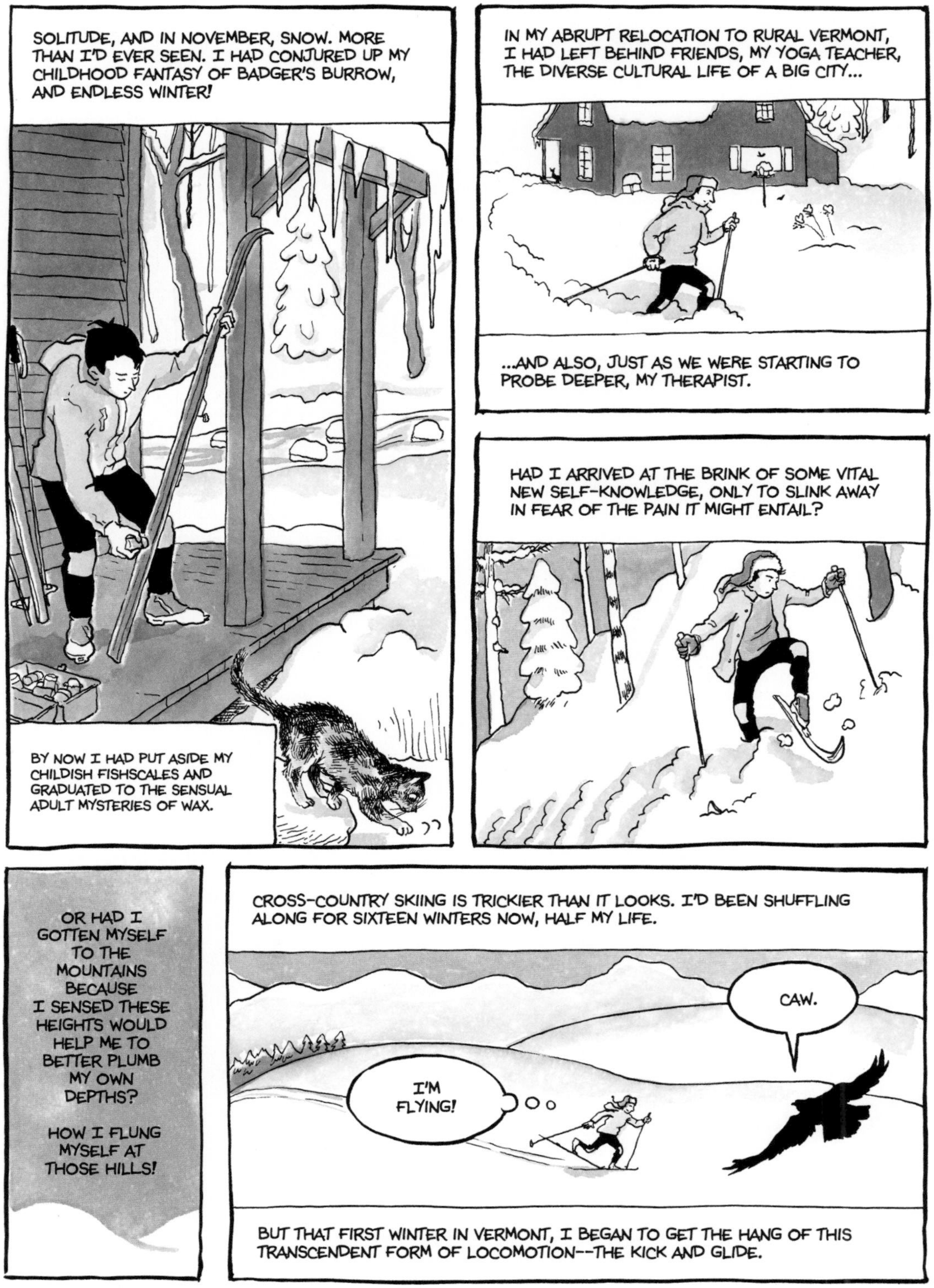

SOLITUDE, AND IN NOVEMBER, SNOW. MORE THAN I'D EVER SEEN. I HAD CONJURED UP MY CHILDHOOD FANTASY OF BADGER'S BURROW, AND ENDLESS WINTER!
BY NOW I HAD PUT ASIDE MY CHILDISH FISHSCALES AND GRADUATED TO THE SENSUAL ADULT MYSTERIES OF WAX.
IN MY ABRUPT RELOCATION TO RURAL VERMONT, I HAD LEFT BEHIND FRIENDS, MY YOGA TEACHER, THE DIVERSE CULTURAL LIFE OF A BIG CITY...
...AND ALSO, JUST AS WE WERE STARTING TO PROBE DEEPER, MY THERAPIST.
HAD I ARRIVED AT THE BRINK OF SOME VITAL NEW SELF-KNOWLEDGE, ONLY TO SLINK AWAY IN FEAR OF THE PAIN IT MIGHT ENTAIL?
OR HAD I GOTTEN MYSELF TO THE MOUNTAINS BECAUSE I SENSED THESE HEIGHTS WOULD HELP ME TO BETTER PLUMB MY OWN DEPTHS?
HOW I FLUNG MYSELF AT THOSE HILLS!
CROSS-COUNTRY SKIING IS TRICKIER THAN IT LOOKS. I'D BEEN SHUFFLING ALONG FOR SIXTEEN WINTERS NOW, HALF MY LIFE.
CAW.
I'M FLYING!
BUT THAT FIRST WINTER IN VERMONT, I BEGAN TO GET THE HANG OF THIS TRANSCENDENT FORM OF LOCOMOTION--THE KICK AND GLIDE.

Panel 1:
IN SPRING, I TOOK TO MY BIKE. THERE WAS NO FLAT TERRAIN. ONE WENT EITHER UP OR DOWN.

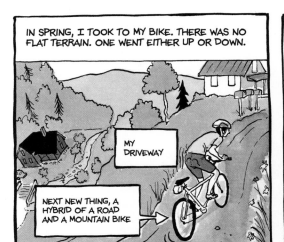

MY DRIVEWAY

NEXT NEW THING, A HYBRID OF A ROAD AND A MOUNTAIN BIKE

Panel 2:
IF I HAD TO CHOOSE BETWEEN ONLY RIDING DOWNHILL OR ONLY RIDING UPHILL FOR THE REST OF MY LIFE--AN EXISTENTIAL QUESTION THAT I PONDERED OFTEN--I WOULD TAKE THE UPHILL.

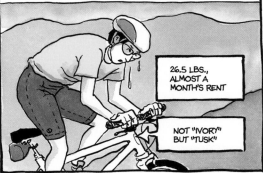

26.5 LBS., ALMOST A MONTH'S RENT

NOT "IVORY" BUT "TUSK"

Panel 3:
IT WAS HARDER, BUT IT WAS A MEASURED DOSE OF PAIN: I WAS IN CONTROL. CAREENING DOWNHILL, WHO KNEW WHAT THE NEXT MOMENT WOULD BRING?

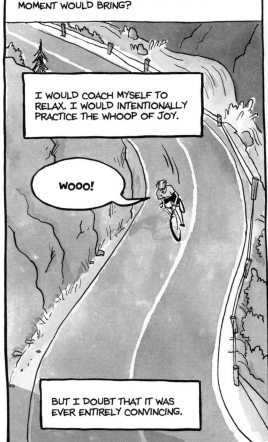

I WOULD COACH MYSELF TO RELAX. I WOULD INTENTIONALLY PRACTICE THE WHOOP OF JOY.

WOOO!

BUT I DOUBT THAT IT WAS EVER ENTIRELY CONVINCING.

Panel 4:
I LOVED THE VERTICALITY OF MY NEW TURF. THE SCOLIOTIC SPINE OF THE GREEN MOUNTAINS RUNS THE LENGTH OF THE STATE.

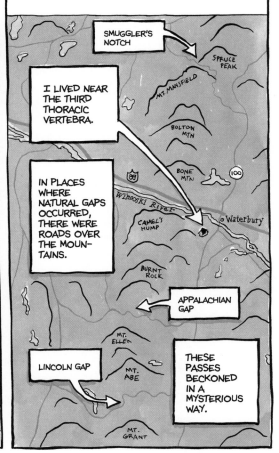

SMUGGLER'S NOTCH

SPRUCE PEAK

MT. MANSFIELD

I LIVED NEAR THE THIRD THORACIC VERTEBRA.

BOLTON MTN

89

BONE MTN

100

Winooski River

o Waterbury

IN PLACES WHERE NATURAL GAPS OCCURRED, THERE WERE ROADS OVER THE MOUNTAINS.

CAMEL'S HUMP

BURNT ROCK

APPALACHIAN GAP

MT. ELLEN

LINCOLN GAP

MT. ABE

THESE PASSES BECKONED IN A MYSTERIOUS WAY.

MT. GRANT

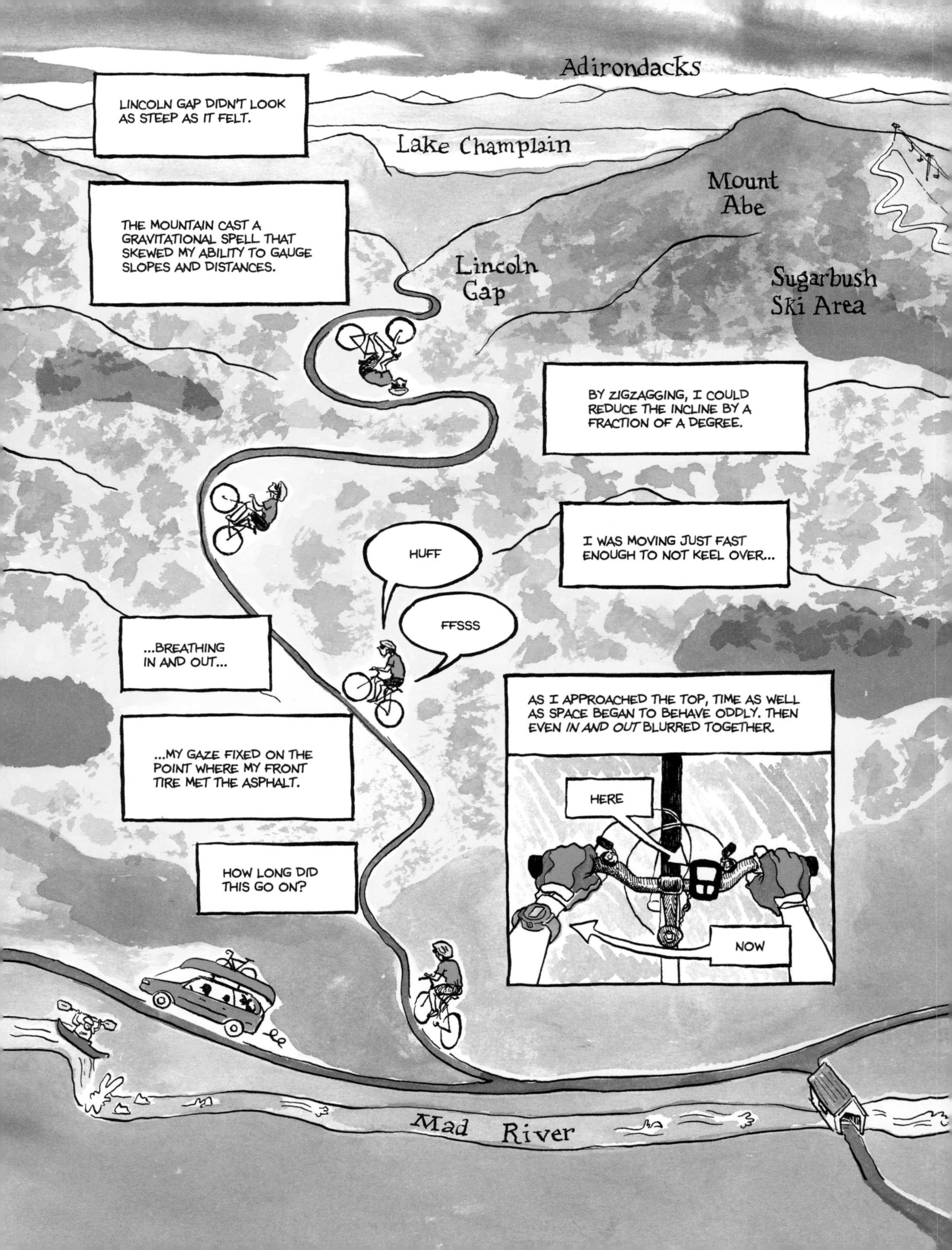
Adirondacks
LINCOLN GAP DIDN'T LOOK AS STEEP AS IT FELT.
Lake Champlain
Mount Abe
THE MOUNTAIN CAST A GRAVITATIONAL SPELL THAT SKEWED MY ABILITY TO GAUGE SLOPES AND DISTANCES.
Lincoln Gap
Sugarbush Ski Area
BY ZIGZAGGING, I COULD REDUCE THE INCLINE BY A FRACTION OF A DEGREE.
I WAS MOVING JUST FAST ENOUGH TO NOT KEEL OVER...
HUFF
FFSSS
...BREATHING IN AND OUT...
...MY GAZE FIXED ON THE POINT WHERE MY FRONT TIRE MET THE ASPHALT.
AS I APPROACHED THE TOP, TIME AS WELL AS SPACE BEGAN TO BEHAVE ODDLY. THEN EVEN *IN AND OUT* BLURRED TOGETHER.
HERE
NOW
HOW LONG DID THIS GO ON?
Mad River

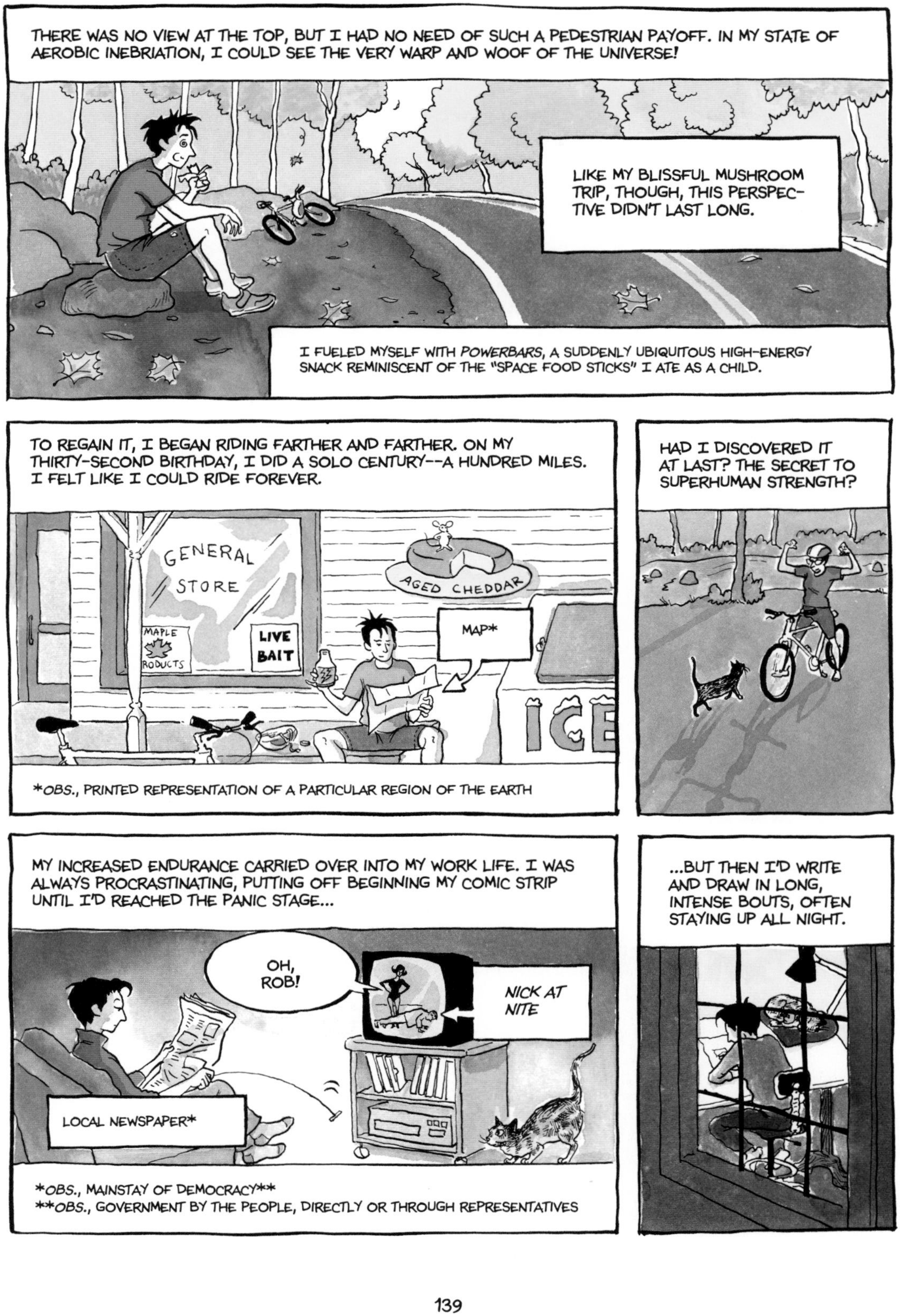
THERE WAS NO VIEW AT THE TOP, BUT I HAD NO NEED OF SUCH A PEDESTRIAN PAYOFF. IN MY STATE OF AEROBIC INEBRIATION, I COULD SEE THE VERY WARP AND WOOF OF THE UNIVERSE!
LIKE MY BLISSFUL MUSHROOM TRIP, THOUGH, THIS PERSPECTIVE DIDN'T LAST LONG.
I FUELED MYSELF WITH *POWERBARS*, A SUDDENLY UBIQUITOUS HIGH-ENERGY SNACK REMINISCENT OF THE "SPACE FOOD STICKS" I ATE AS A CHILD.
TO REGAIN IT, I BEGAN RIDING FARTHER AND FARTHER. ON MY THIRTY-SECOND BIRTHDAY, I DID A SOLO CENTURY--A HUNDRED MILES. I FELT LIKE I COULD RIDE FOREVER.
GENERAL STORE
AGED CHEDDAR
MAPLE PRODUCTS
LIVE BAIT
MAP*
ICE
*OBS., PRINTED REPRESENTATION OF A PARTICULAR REGION OF THE EARTH
HAD I DISCOVERED IT AT LAST? THE SECRET TO SUPERHUMAN STRENGTH?
MY INCREASED ENDURANCE CARRIED OVER INTO MY WORK LIFE. I WAS ALWAYS PROCRASTINATING, PUTTING OFF BEGINNING MY COMIC STRIP UNTIL I'D REACHED THE PANIC STAGE...
OH, ROB!
NICK AT NITE
LOCAL NEWSPAPER*
*OBS., MAINSTAY OF DEMOCRACY**
**OBS., GOVERNMENT BY THE PEOPLE, DIRECTLY OR THROUGH REPRESENTATIVES
...BUT THEN I'D WRITE AND DRAW IN LONG, INTENSE BOUTS, OFTEN STAYING UP ALL NIGHT.

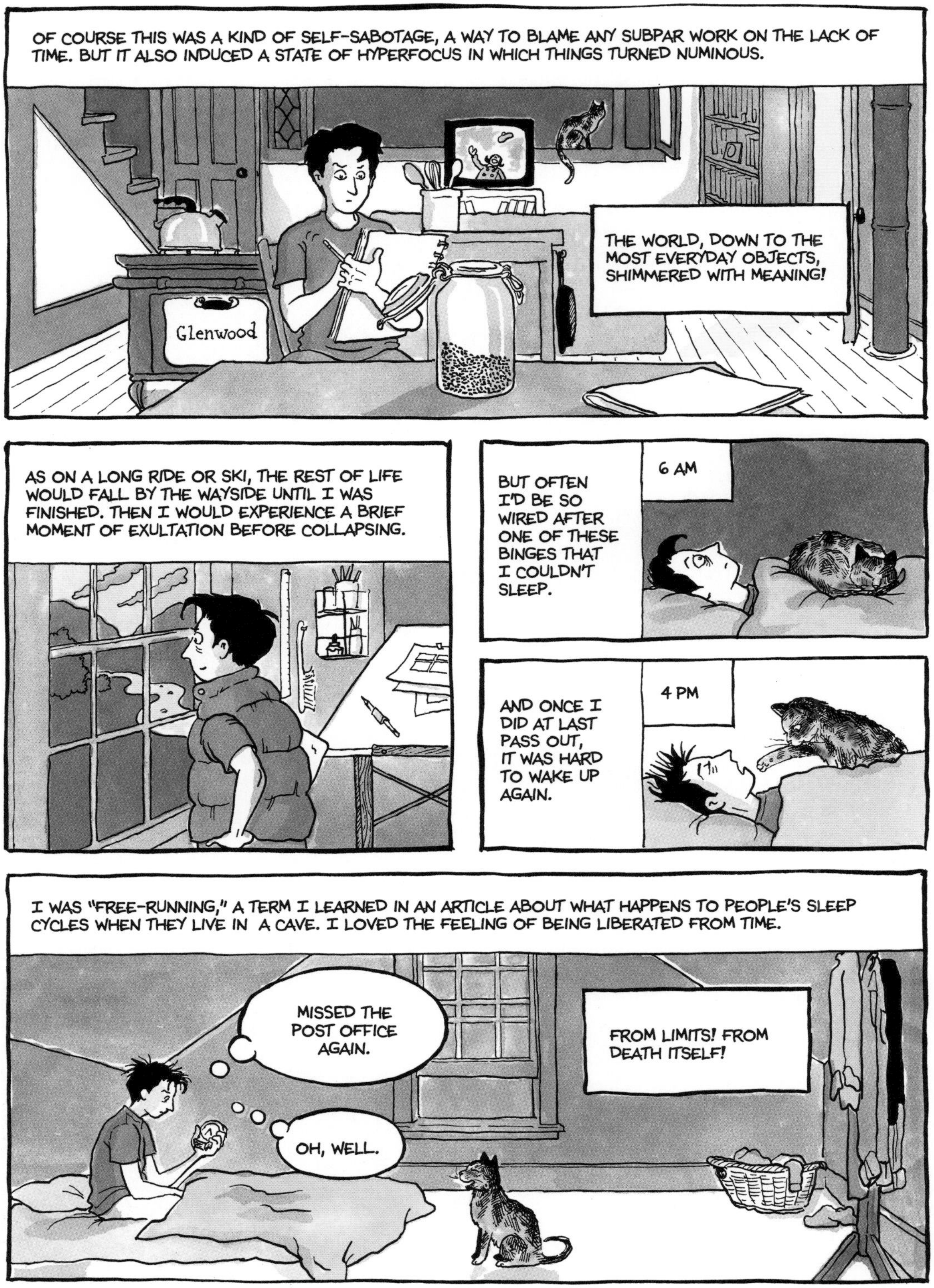
OF COURSE THIS WAS A KIND OF SELF-SABOTAGE, A WAY TO BLAME ANY SUBPAR WORK ON THE LACK OF TIME. BUT IT ALSO INDUCED A STATE OF HYPERFOCUS IN WHICH THINGS TURNED NUMINOUS.
Glenwood
THE WORLD, DOWN TO THE MOST EVERYDAY OBJECTS, SHIMMERED WITH MEANING!
AS ON A LONG RIDE OR SKI, THE REST OF LIFE WOULD FALL BY THE WAYSIDE UNTIL I WAS FINISHED. THEN I WOULD EXPERIENCE A BRIEF MOMENT OF EXULTATION BEFORE COLLAPSING.
BUT OFTEN I'D BE SO WIRED AFTER ONE OF THESE BINGES THAT I COULDN'T SLEEP.
6 AM
AND ONCE I DID AT LAST PASS OUT, IT WAS HARD TO WAKE UP AGAIN.
4 PM
I WAS "FREE-RUNNING," A TERM I LEARNED IN AN ARTICLE ABOUT WHAT HAPPENS TO PEOPLE'S SLEEP CYCLES WHEN THEY LIVE IN A CAVE. I LOVED THE FEELING OF BEING LIBERATED FROM TIME.
MISSED THE POST OFFICE AGAIN.
OH, WELL.
FROM LIMITS! FROM DEATH ITSELF!

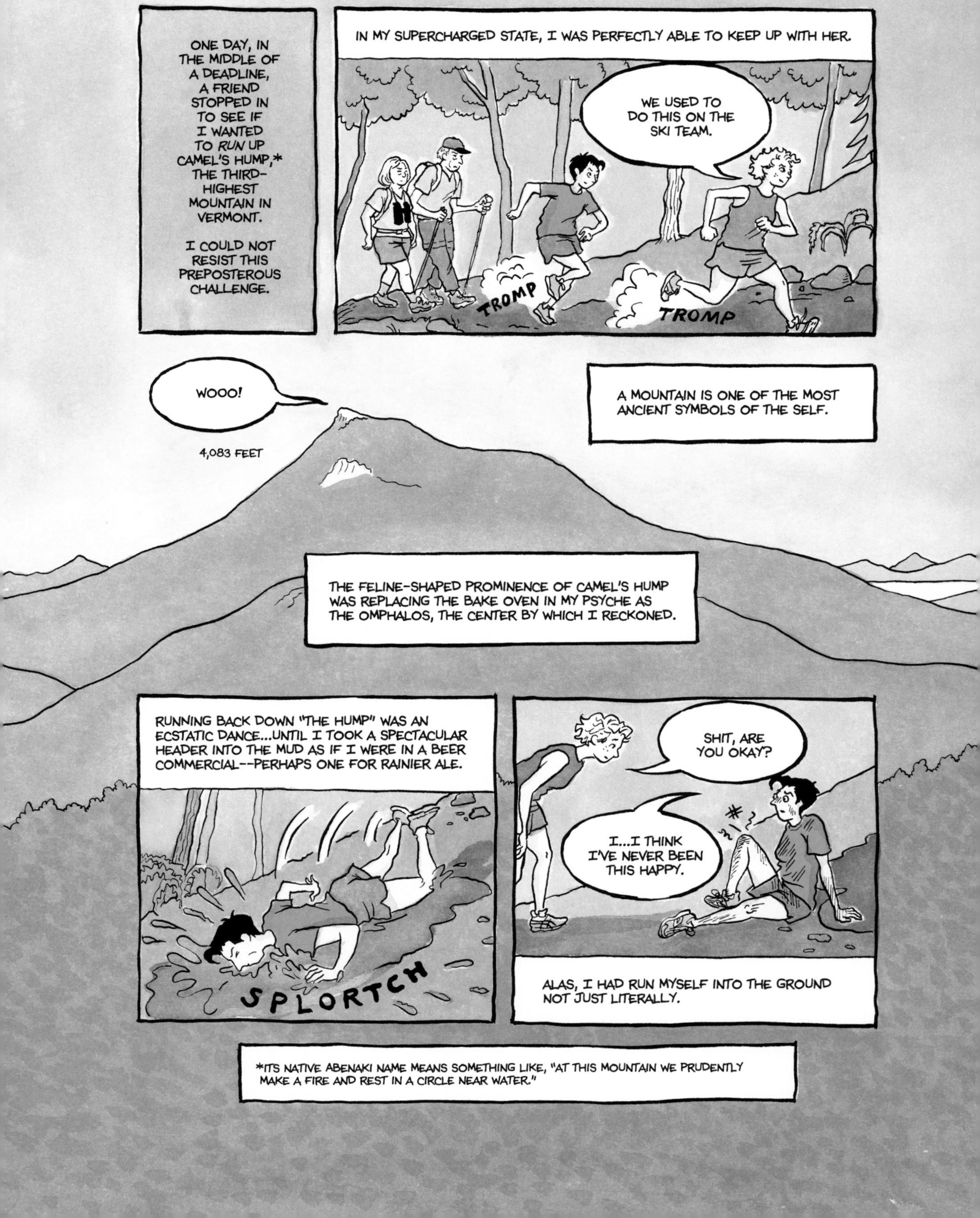

ONE DAY, IN THE MIDDLE OF A DEADLINE, A FRIEND STOPPED IN TO SEE IF I WANTED TO *RUN* UP CAMEL'S HUMP,* THE THIRD-HIGHEST MOUNTAIN IN VERMONT.
I COULD NOT RESIST THIS PREPOSTEROUS CHALLENGE.
IN MY SUPERCHARGED STATE, I WAS PERFECTLY ABLE TO KEEP UP WITH HER.
WE USED TO DO THIS ON THE SKI TEAM.
TROMP
TROMP
WOOO!
4,083 FEET
A MOUNTAIN IS ONE OF THE MOST ANCIENT SYMBOLS OF THE SELF.
THE FELINE-SHAPED PROMINENCE OF CAMEL'S HUMP WAS REPLACING THE BAKE OVEN IN MY PSYCHE AS THE OMPHALOS, THE CENTER BY WHICH I RECKONED.
RUNNING BACK DOWN "THE HUMP" WAS AN ECSTATIC DANCE...UNTIL I TOOK A SPECTACULAR HEADER INTO THE MUD AS IF I WERE IN A BEER COMMERCIAL--PERHAPS ONE FOR RAINIER ALE.
SPLORTCH
SHIT, ARE YOU OKAY?
I...I THINK I'VE NEVER BEEN THIS HAPPY.
ALAS, I HAD RUN MYSELF INTO THE GROUND NOT JUST LITERALLY.
*ITS NATIVE ABENAKI NAME MEANS SOMETHING LIKE, "AT THIS MOUNTAIN WE PRUDENTLY MAKE A FIRE AND REST IN A CIRCLE NEAR WATER."

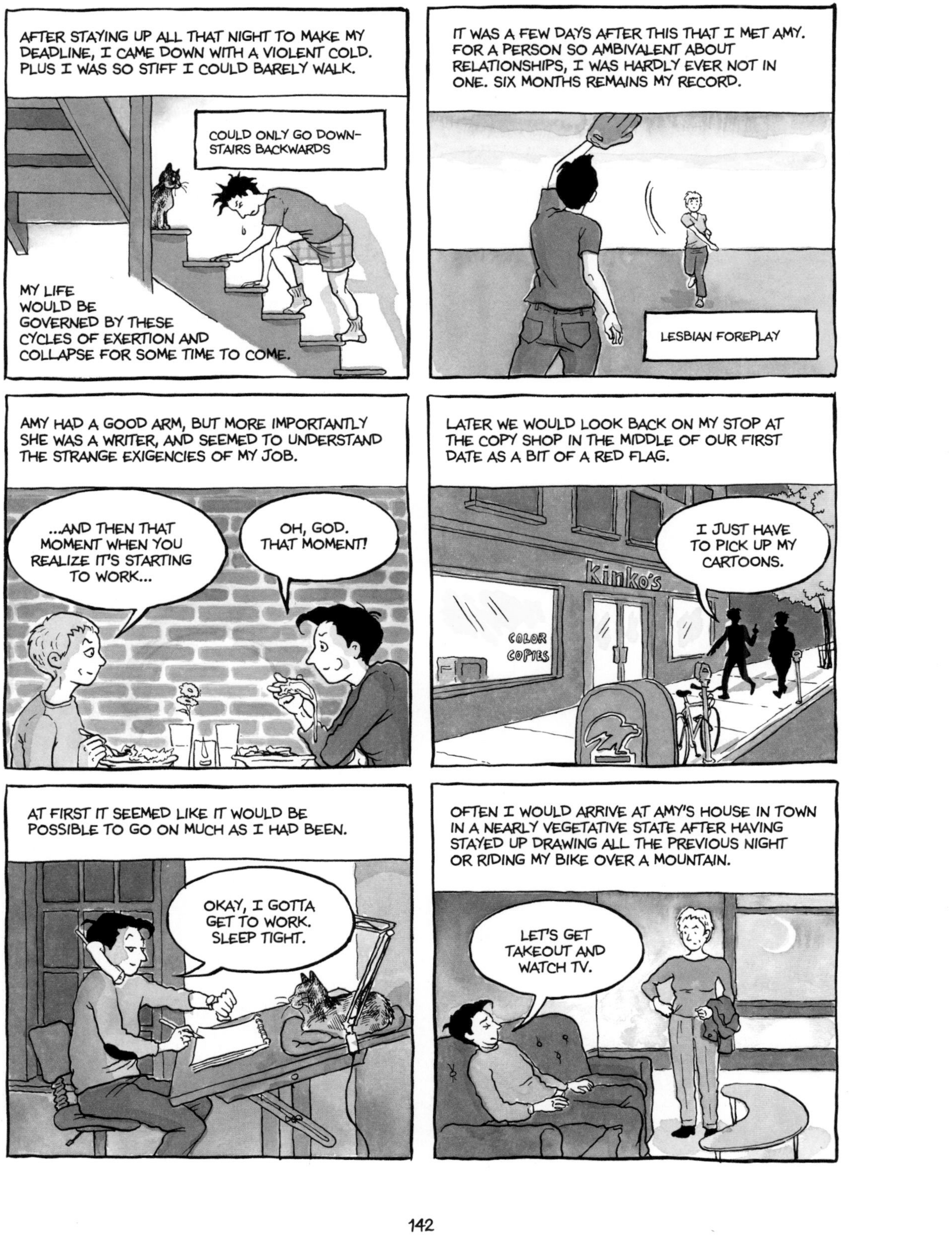
AFTER STAYING UP ALL THAT NIGHT TO MAKE MY DEADLINE, I CAME DOWN WITH A VIOLENT COLD. PLUS I WAS SO STIFF I COULD BARELY WALK.
COULD ONLY GO DOWN-STAIRS BACKWARDS
MY LIFE WOULD BE GOVERNED BY THESE CYCLES OF EXERTION AND COLLAPSE FOR SOME TIME TO COME.
IT WAS A FEW DAYS AFTER THIS THAT I MET AMY. FOR A PERSON SO AMBIVALENT ABOUT RELATIONSHIPS, I WAS HARDLY EVER NOT IN ONE. SIX MONTHS REMAINS MY RECORD.
LESBIAN FOREPLAY
AMY HAD A GOOD ARM, BUT MORE IMPORTANTLY SHE WAS A WRITER, AND SEEMED TO UNDERSTAND THE STRANGE EXIGENCIES OF MY JOB.
...AND THEN THAT MOMENT WHEN YOU REALIZE IT'S STARTING TO WORK...
OH, GOD. THAT MOMENT!
LATER WE WOULD LOOK BACK ON MY STOP AT THE COPY SHOP IN THE MIDDLE OF OUR FIRST DATE AS A BIT OF A RED FLAG.
Kinko's
COLOR COPIES
I JUST HAVE TO PICK UP MY CARTOONS.
AT FIRST IT SEEMED LIKE IT WOULD BE POSSIBLE TO GO ON MUCH AS I HAD BEEN.
OKAY, I GOTTA GET TO WORK. SLEEP TIGHT.
OFTEN I WOULD ARRIVE AT AMY'S HOUSE IN TOWN IN A NEARLY VEGETATIVE STATE AFTER HAVING STAYED UP DRAWING ALL THE PREVIOUS NIGHT OR RIDING MY BIKE OVER A MOUNTAIN.
LET'S GET TAKEOUT AND WATCH TV.

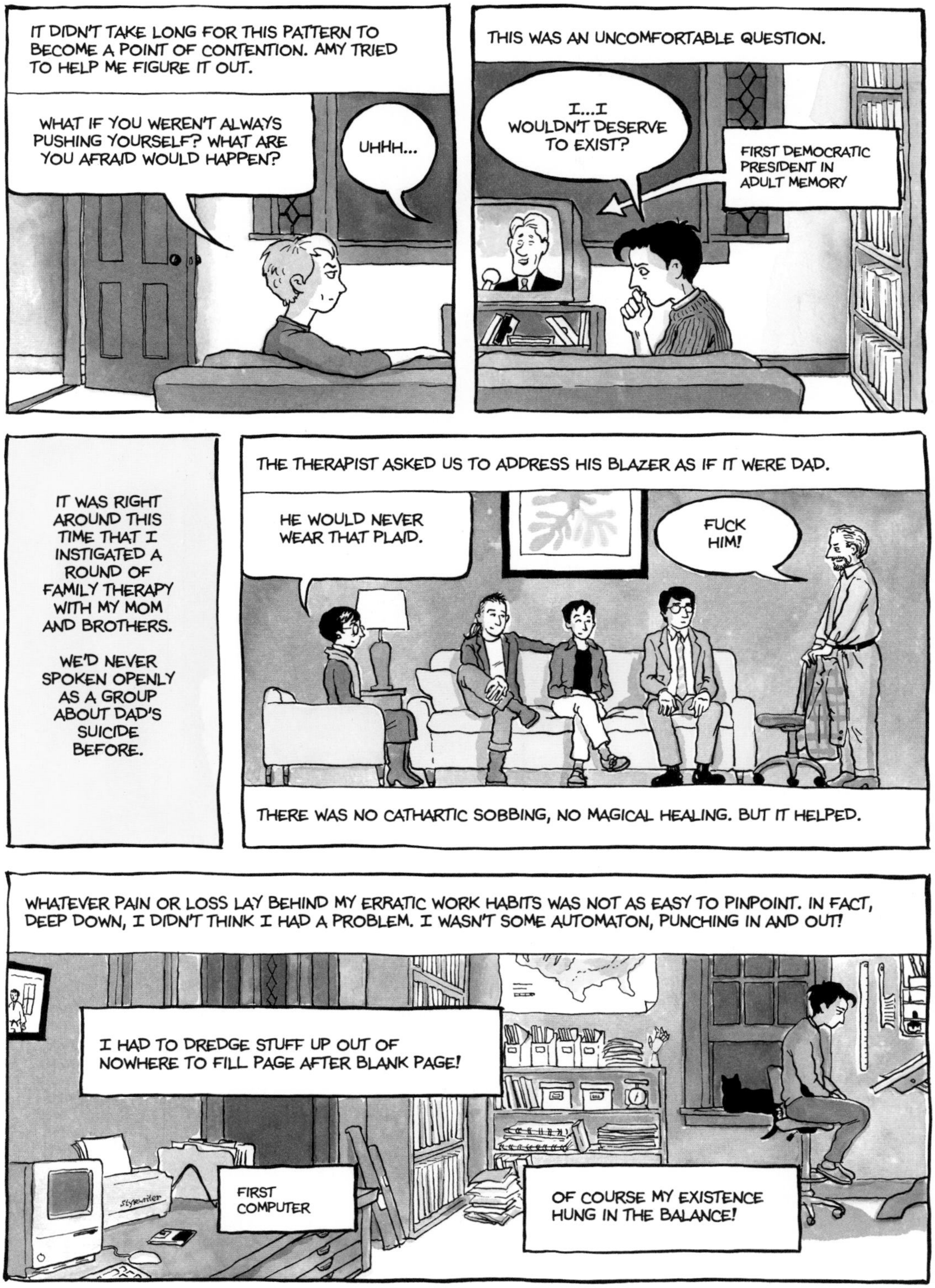

IT DIDN'T TAKE LONG FOR THIS PATTERN TO BECOME A POINT OF CONTENTION. AMY TRIED TO HELP ME FIGURE IT OUT.
WHAT IF YOU WEREN'T ALWAYS PUSHING YOURSELF? WHAT ARE YOU AFRAID WOULD HAPPEN?
UHHH...
THIS WAS AN UNCOMFORTABLE QUESTION.
I...I WOULDN'T DESERVE TO EXIST?
FIRST DEMOCRATIC PRESIDENT IN ADULT MEMORY
IT WAS RIGHT AROUND THIS TIME THAT I INSTIGATED A ROUND OF FAMILY THERAPY WITH MY MOM AND BROTHERS.
WE'D NEVER SPOKEN OPENLY AS A GROUP ABOUT DAD'S SUICIDE BEFORE.
THE THERAPIST ASKED US TO ADDRESS HIS BLAZER AS IF IT WERE DAD.
HE WOULD NEVER WEAR THAT PLAID.
FUCK HIM!
THERE WAS NO CATHARTIC SOBBING, NO MAGICAL HEALING. BUT IT HELPED.
WHATEVER PAIN OR LOSS LAY BEHIND MY ERRATIC WORK HABITS WAS NOT AS EASY TO PINPOINT. IN FACT, DEEP DOWN, I DIDN'T THINK I HAD A PROBLEM. I WASN'T SOME AUTOMATON, PUNCHING IN AND OUT!
I HAD TO DREDGE STUFF UP OUT OF NOWHERE TO FILL PAGE AFTER BLANK PAGE!
FIRST COMPUTER
OF COURSE MY EXISTENCE HUNG IN THE BALANCE!

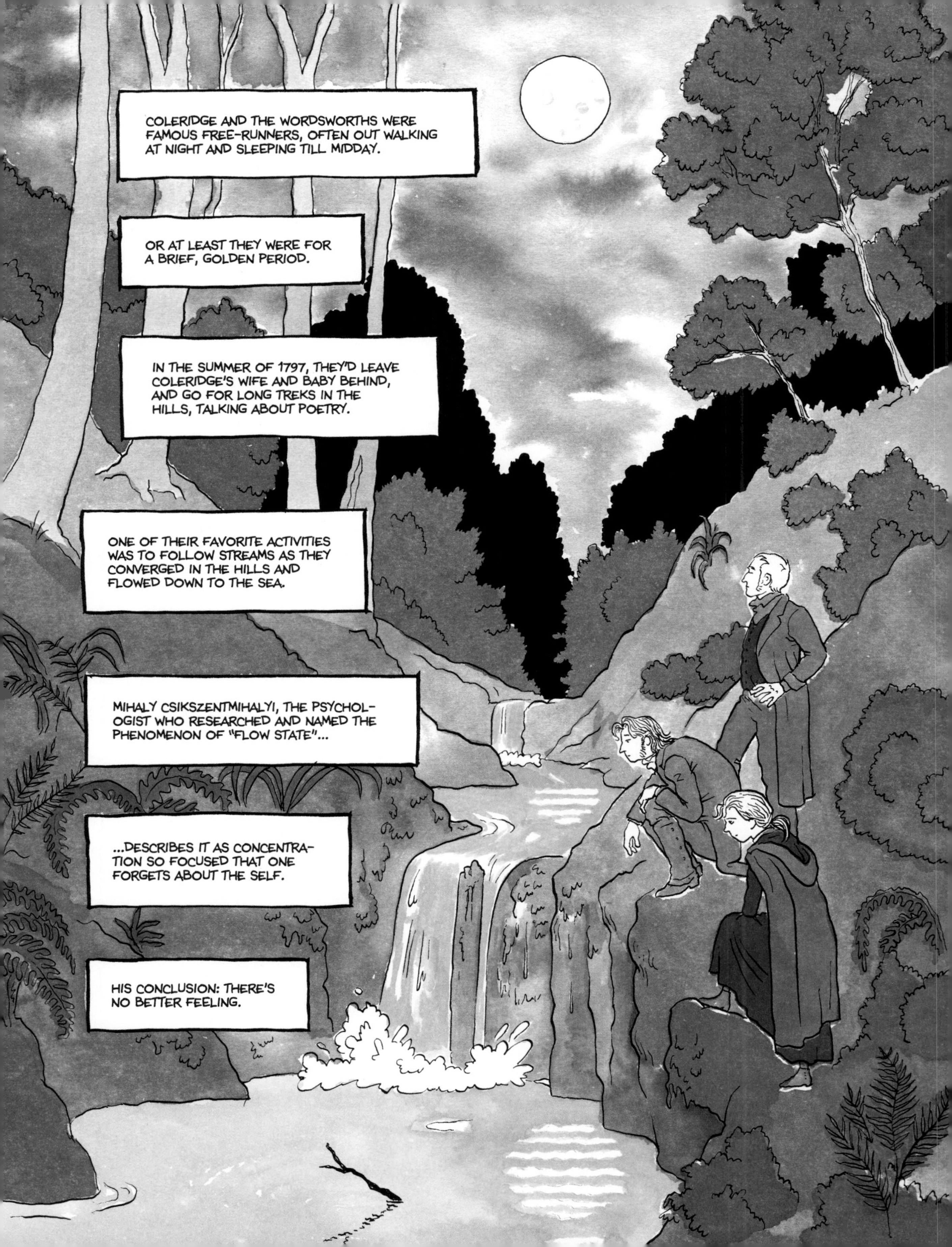
COLERIDGE AND THE WORDSWORTHS WERE FAMOUS FREE-RUNNERS, OFTEN OUT WALKING AT NIGHT AND SLEEPING TILL MIDDAY.
OR AT LEAST THEY WERE FOR A BRIEF, GOLDEN PERIOD.
IN THE SUMMER OF 1797, THEY'D LEAVE COLERIDGE'S WIFE AND BABY BEHIND, AND GO FOR LONG TREKS IN THE HILLS, TALKING ABOUT POETRY.
ONE OF THEIR FAVORITE ACTIVITIES WAS TO FOLLOW STREAMS AS THEY CONVERGED IN THE HILLS AND FLOWED DOWN TO THE SEA.
MIHALY CSIKSZENTMIHALYI, THE PSYCHOLOGIST WHO RESEARCHED AND NAMED THE PHENOMENON OF "FLOW STATE"...
...DESCRIBES IT AS CONCENTRATION SO FOCUSED THAT ONE FORGETS ABOUT THE SELF.
HIS CONCLUSION: THERE'S NO BETTER FEELING.

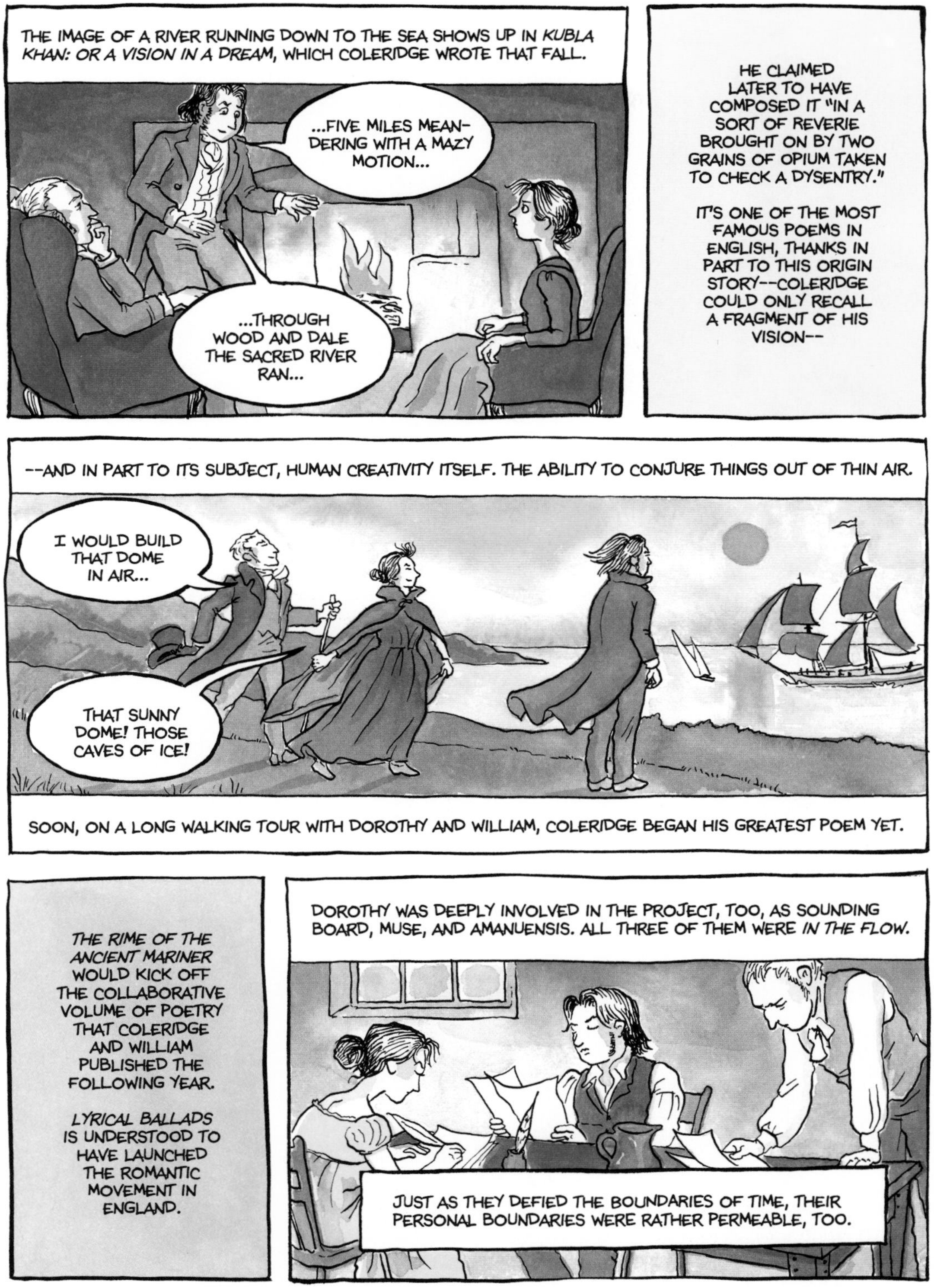

THE IMAGE OF A RIVER RUNNING DOWN TO THE SEA SHOWS UP IN *KUBLA KHAN: OR A VISION IN A DREAM*, WHICH COLERIDGE WROTE THAT FALL.
...FIVE MILES MEAN-DERING WITH A MAZY MOTION...
...THROUGH WOOD AND DALE THE SACRED RIVER RAN...
HE CLAIMED LATER TO HAVE COMPOSED IT "IN A SORT OF REVERIE BROUGHT ON BY TWO GRAINS OF OPIUM TAKEN TO CHECK A DYSENTRY."
IT'S ONE OF THE MOST FAMOUS POEMS IN ENGLISH, THANKS IN PART TO THIS ORIGIN STORY--COLERIDGE COULD ONLY RECALL A FRAGMENT OF HIS VISION--
--AND IN PART TO ITS SUBJECT, HUMAN CREATIVITY ITSELF. THE ABILITY TO CONJURE THINGS OUT OF THIN AIR.
I WOULD BUILD THAT DOME IN AIR...
THAT SUNNY DOME! THOSE CAVES OF ICE!
SOON, ON A LONG WALKING TOUR WITH DOROTHY AND WILLIAM, COLERIDGE BEGAN HIS GREATEST POEM YET.
THE RIME OF THE ANCIENT MARINER WOULD KICK OFF THE COLLABORATIVE VOLUME OF POETRY THAT COLERIDGE AND WILLIAM PUBLISHED THE FOLLOWING YEAR.
LYRICAL BALLADS IS UNDERSTOOD TO HAVE LAUNCHED THE ROMANTIC MOVEMENT IN ENGLAND.
DOROTHY WAS DEEPLY INVOLVED IN THE PROJECT, TOO, AS SOUNDING BOARD, MUSE, AND AMANUENSIS. ALL THREE OF THEM WERE *IN THE FLOW*.
JUST AS THEY DEFIED THE BOUNDARIES OF TIME, THEIR PERSONAL BOUNDARIES WERE RATHER PERMEABLE, TOO.

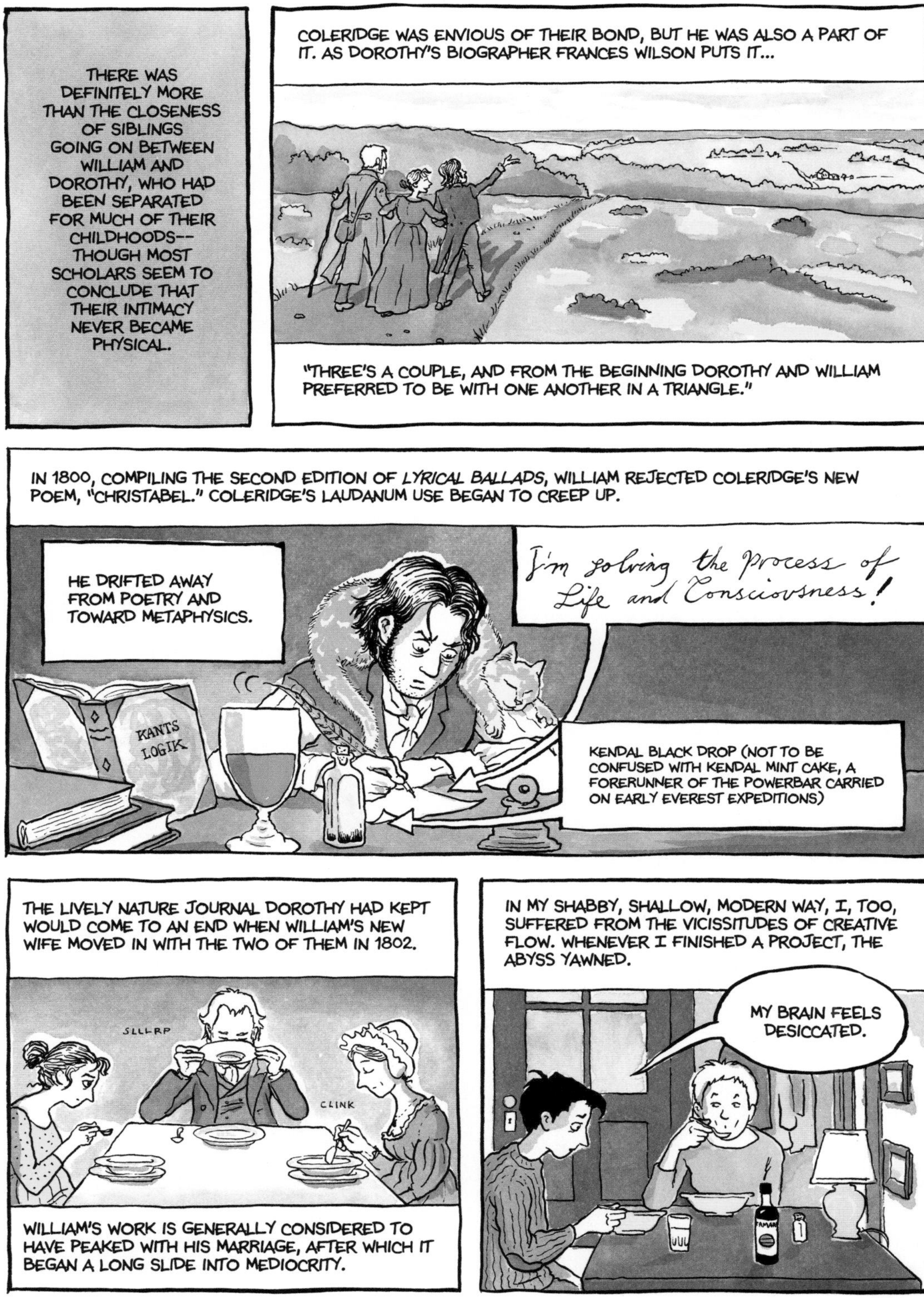
THERE WAS DEFINITELY MORE THAN THE CLOSENESS OF SIBLINGS GOING ON BETWEEN WILLIAM AND DOROTHY, WHO HAD BEEN SEPARATED FOR MUCH OF THEIR CHILDHOODS-- THOUGH MOST SCHOLARS SEEM TO CONCLUDE THAT THEIR INTIMACY NEVER BECAME PHYSICAL.
COLERIDGE WAS ENVIOUS OF THEIR BOND, BUT HE WAS ALSO A PART OF IT. AS DOROTHY'S BIOGRAPHER FRANCES WILSON PUTS IT...
"THREE'S A COUPLE, AND FROM THE BEGINNING DOROTHY AND WILLIAM PREFERRED TO BE WITH ONE ANOTHER IN A TRIANGLE."
IN 1800, COMPILING THE SECOND EDITION OF *LYRICAL BALLADS*, WILLIAM REJECTED COLERIDGE'S NEW POEM, "CHRISTABEL." COLERIDGE'S LAUDANUM USE BEGAN TO CREEP UP.
HE DRIFTED AWAY FROM POETRY AND TOWARD METAPHYSICS.
I'm solving the Process of Life and Consciousness!
KANTS LOGIK
KENDAL BLACK DROP (NOT TO BE CONFUSED WITH KENDAL MINT CAKE, A FORERUNNER OF THE POWERBAR CARRIED ON EARLY EVEREST EXPEDITIONS)
THE LIVELY NATURE JOURNAL DOROTHY HAD KEPT WOULD COME TO AN END WHEN WILLIAM'S NEW WIFE MOVED IN WITH THE TWO OF THEM IN 1802.
SLLLRP
CLINK
WILLIAM'S WORK IS GENERALLY CONSIDERED TO HAVE PEAKED WITH HIS MARRIAGE, AFTER WHICH IT BEGAN A LONG SLIDE INTO MEDIOCRITY.
IN MY SHABBY, SHALLOW, MODERN WAY, I, TOO, SUFFERED FROM THE VICISSITUDES OF CREATIVE FLOW. WHENEVER I FINISHED A PROJECT, THE ABYSS YAWNED.
MY BRAIN FEELS DESICCATED.

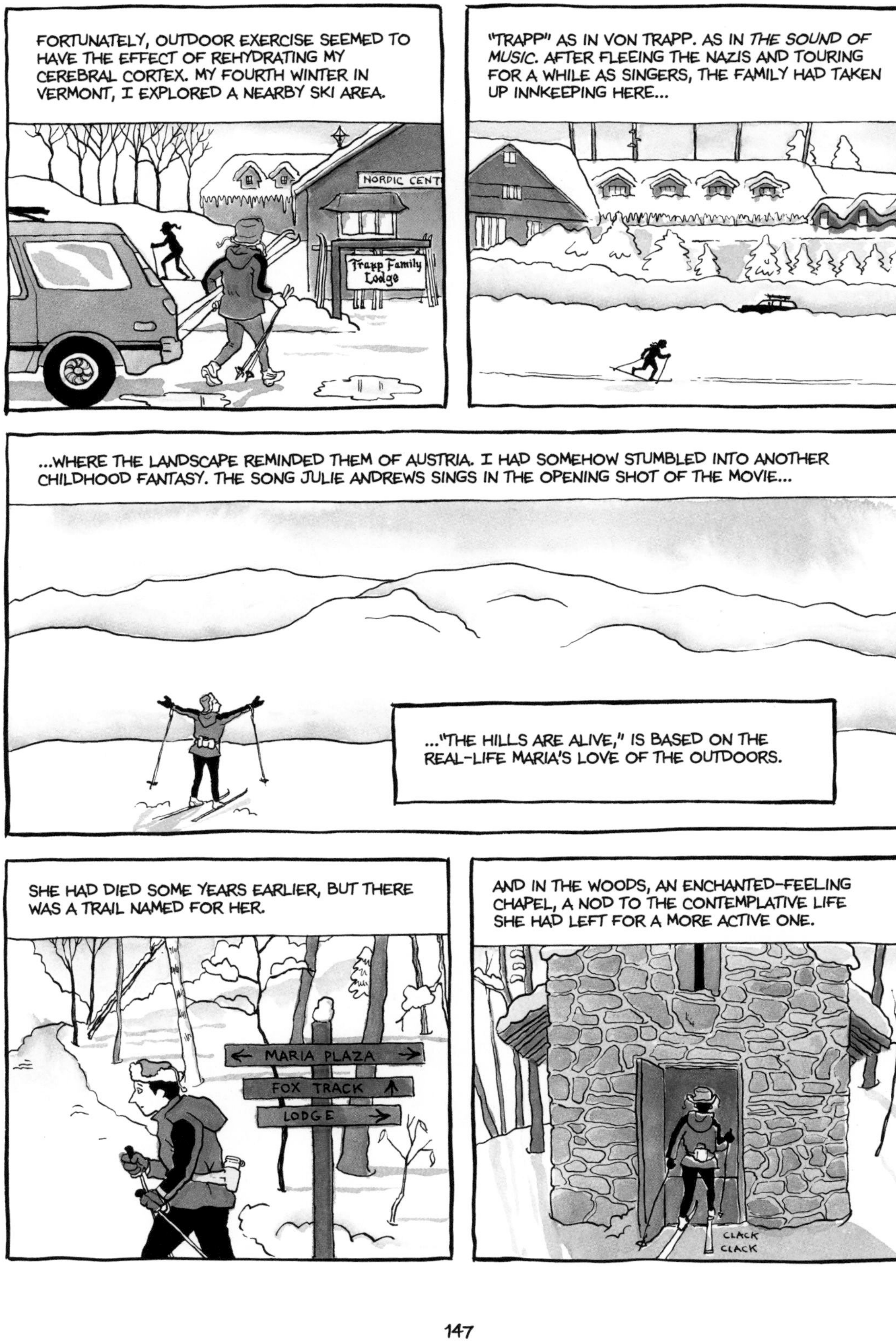
FORTUNATELY, OUTDOOR EXERCISE SEEMED TO HAVE THE EFFECT OF REHYDRATING MY CEREBRAL CORTEX. MY FOURTH WINTER IN VERMONT, I EXPLORED A NEARBY SKI AREA.
NORDIC CENT
Trapp Family Lodge
"TRAPP" AS IN VON TRAPP. AS IN *THE SOUND OF MUSIC*. AFTER FLEEING THE NAZIS AND TOURING FOR A WHILE AS SINGERS, THE FAMILY HAD TAKEN UP INNKEEPING HERE...
...WHERE THE LANDSCAPE REMINDED THEM OF AUSTRIA. I HAD SOMEHOW STUMBLED INTO ANOTHER CHILDHOOD FANTASY. THE SONG JULIE ANDREWS SINGS IN THE OPENING SHOT OF THE MOVIE...
..."THE HILLS ARE ALIVE," IS BASED ON THE REAL-LIFE MARIA'S LOVE OF THE OUTDOORS.
SHE HAD DIED SOME YEARS EARLIER, BUT THERE WAS A TRAIL NAMED FOR HER.
MARIA PLAZA
FOX TRACK
LODGE
AND IN THE WOODS, AN ENCHANTED-FEELING CHAPEL, A NOD TO THE CONTEMPLATIVE LIFE SHE HAD LEFT FOR A MORE ACTIVE ONE.
CLACK
CLACK

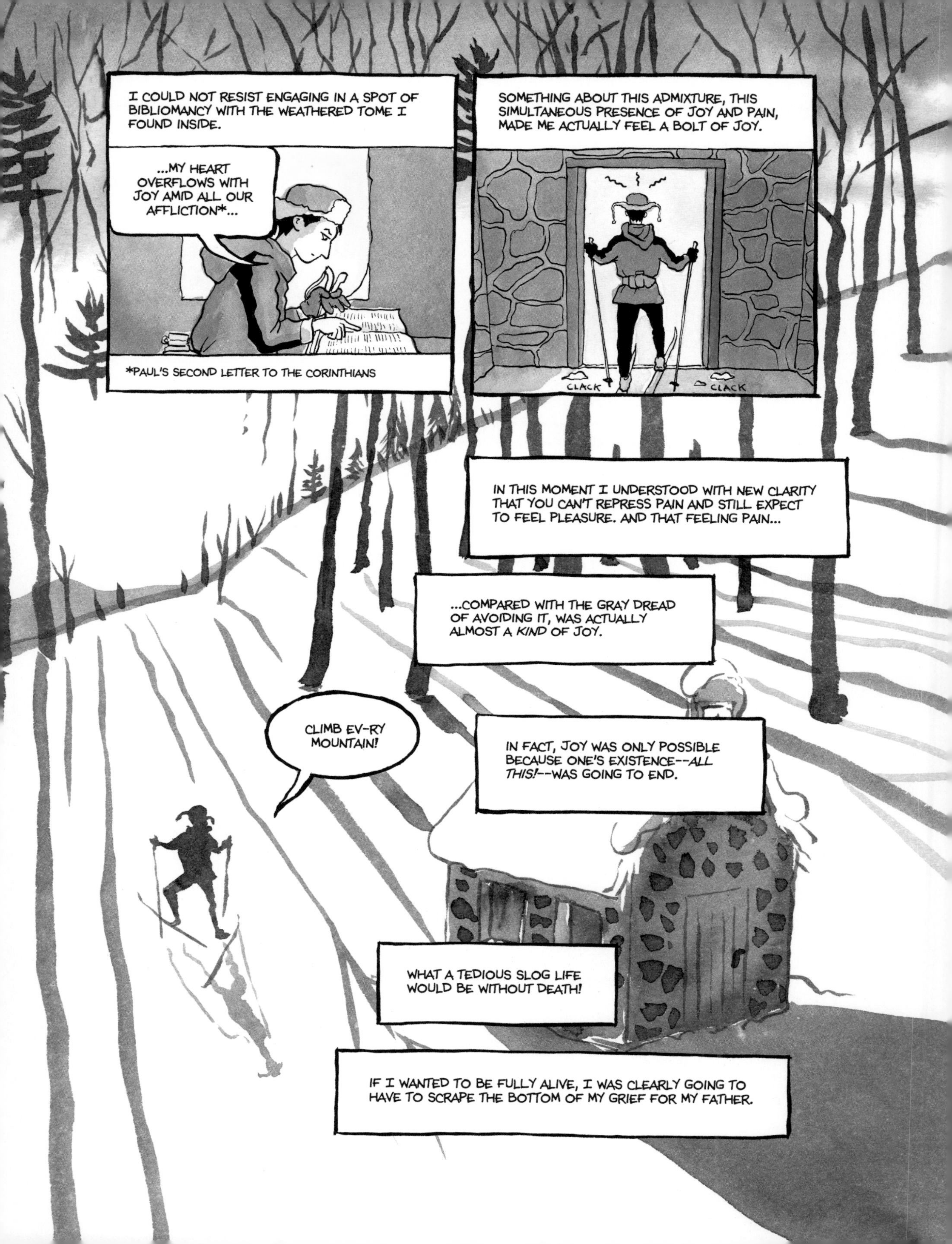

I COULD NOT RESIST ENGAGING IN A SPOT OF BIBLIOMANCY WITH THE WEATHERED TOME I FOUND INSIDE.
...MY HEART OVERFLOWS WITH JOY AMID ALL OUR AFFLICTION*...
*PAUL'S SECOND LETTER TO THE CORINTHIANS
SOMETHING ABOUT THIS ADMIXTURE, THIS SIMULTANEOUS PRESENCE OF JOY AND PAIN, MADE ME ACTUALLY FEEL A BOLT OF JOY.
CLACK
CLACK
IN THIS MOMENT I UNDERSTOOD WITH NEW CLARITY THAT YOU CAN'T REPRESS PAIN AND STILL EXPECT TO FEEL PLEASURE. AND THAT FEELING PAIN...
...COMPARED WITH THE GRAY DREAD OF AVOIDING IT, WAS ACTUALLY ALMOST A *KIND* OF JOY.
CLIMB EV-RY MOUNTAIN!
IN FACT, JOY WAS ONLY POSSIBLE BECAUSE ONE'S EXISTENCE--*ALL THIS!*--WAS GOING TO END.
WHAT A TEDIOUS SLOG LIFE WOULD BE WITHOUT DEATH!
IF I WANTED TO BE FULLY ALIVE, I WAS CLEARLY GOING TO HAVE TO SCRAPE THE BOTTOM OF MY GRIEF FOR MY FATHER.

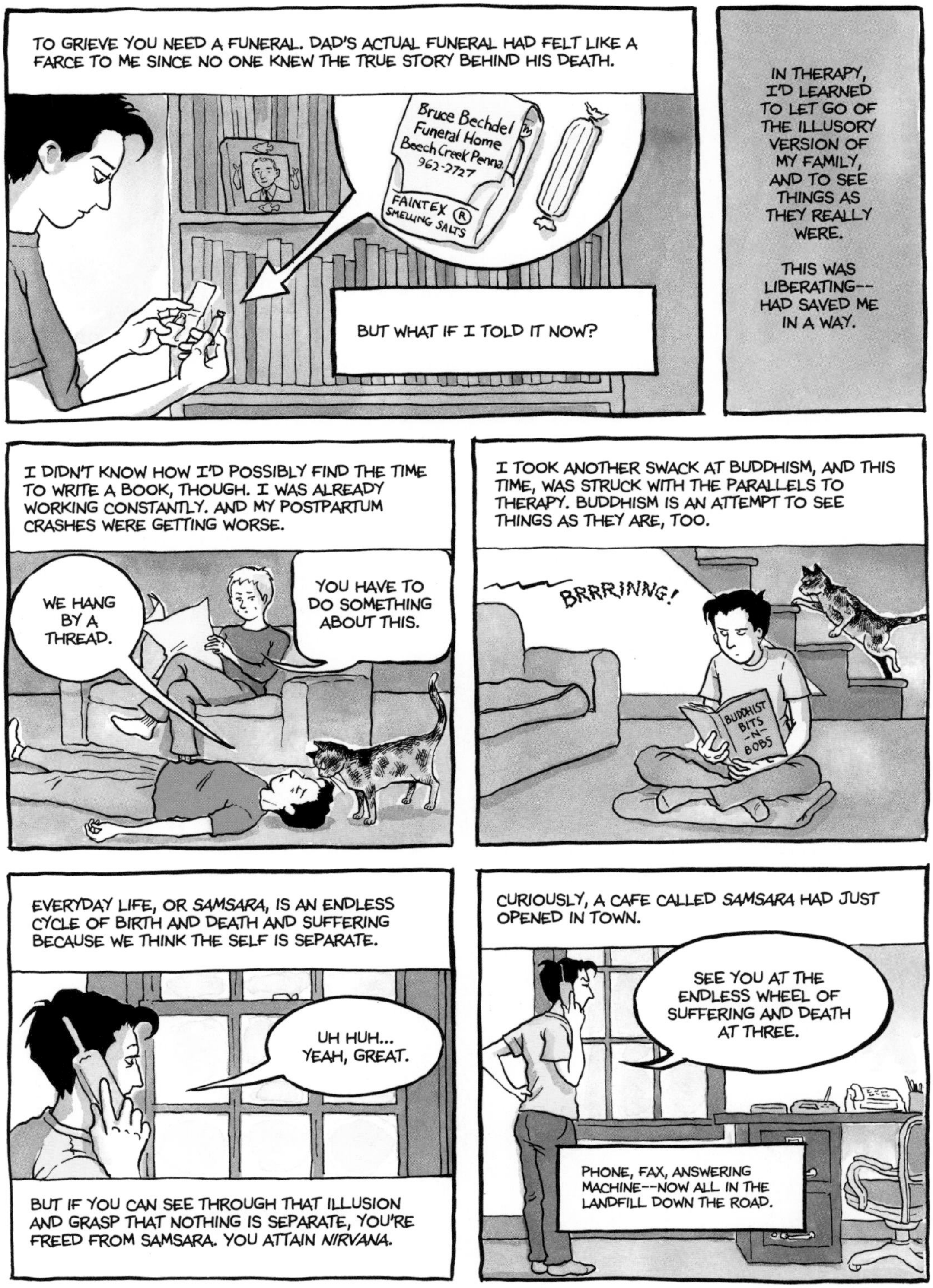
TO GRIEVE YOU NEED A FUNERAL. DAD'S ACTUAL FUNERAL HAD FELT LIKE A FARCE TO ME SINCE NO ONE KNEW THE TRUE STORY BEHIND HIS DEATH.
Bruce Bechdel Funeral Home Beech Creek Penna. 962-2727
FAINTEX ® SMELLING SALTS
BUT WHAT IF I TOLD IT NOW?
IN THERAPY, I'D LEARNED TO LET GO OF THE ILLUSORY VERSION OF MY FAMILY, AND TO SEE THINGS AS THEY REALLY WERE.
THIS WAS LIBERATING-- HAD SAVED ME IN A WAY.
I DIDN'T KNOW HOW I'D POSSIBLY FIND THE TIME TO WRITE A BOOK, THOUGH. I WAS ALREADY WORKING CONSTANTLY. AND MY POSTPARTUM CRASHES WERE GETTING WORSE.
WE HANG BY A THREAD.
YOU HAVE TO DO SOMETHING ABOUT THIS.
I TOOK ANOTHER SWACK AT BUDDHISM, AND THIS TIME, WAS STRUCK WITH THE PARALLELS TO THERAPY. BUDDHISM IS AN ATTEMPT TO SEE THINGS AS THEY ARE, TOO.
BRRRINNG!
BUDDHIST BITS -N- BOBS
EVERYDAY LIFE, OR *SAMSARA*, IS AN ENDLESS CYCLE OF BIRTH AND DEATH AND SUFFERING BECAUSE WE THINK THE SELF IS SEPARATE.
UH HUH... YEAH, GREAT.
BUT IF YOU CAN SEE THROUGH THAT ILLUSION AND GRASP THAT NOTHING IS SEPARATE, YOU'RE FREED FROM SAMSARA. YOU ATTAIN *NIRVANA*.
CURIOUSLY, A CAFE CALLED *SAMSARA* HAD JUST OPENED IN TOWN.
SEE YOU AT THE ENDLESS WHEEL OF SUFFERING AND DEATH AT THREE.
PHONE, FAX, ANSWERING MACHINE--NOW ALL IN THE LANDFILL DOWN THE ROAD.

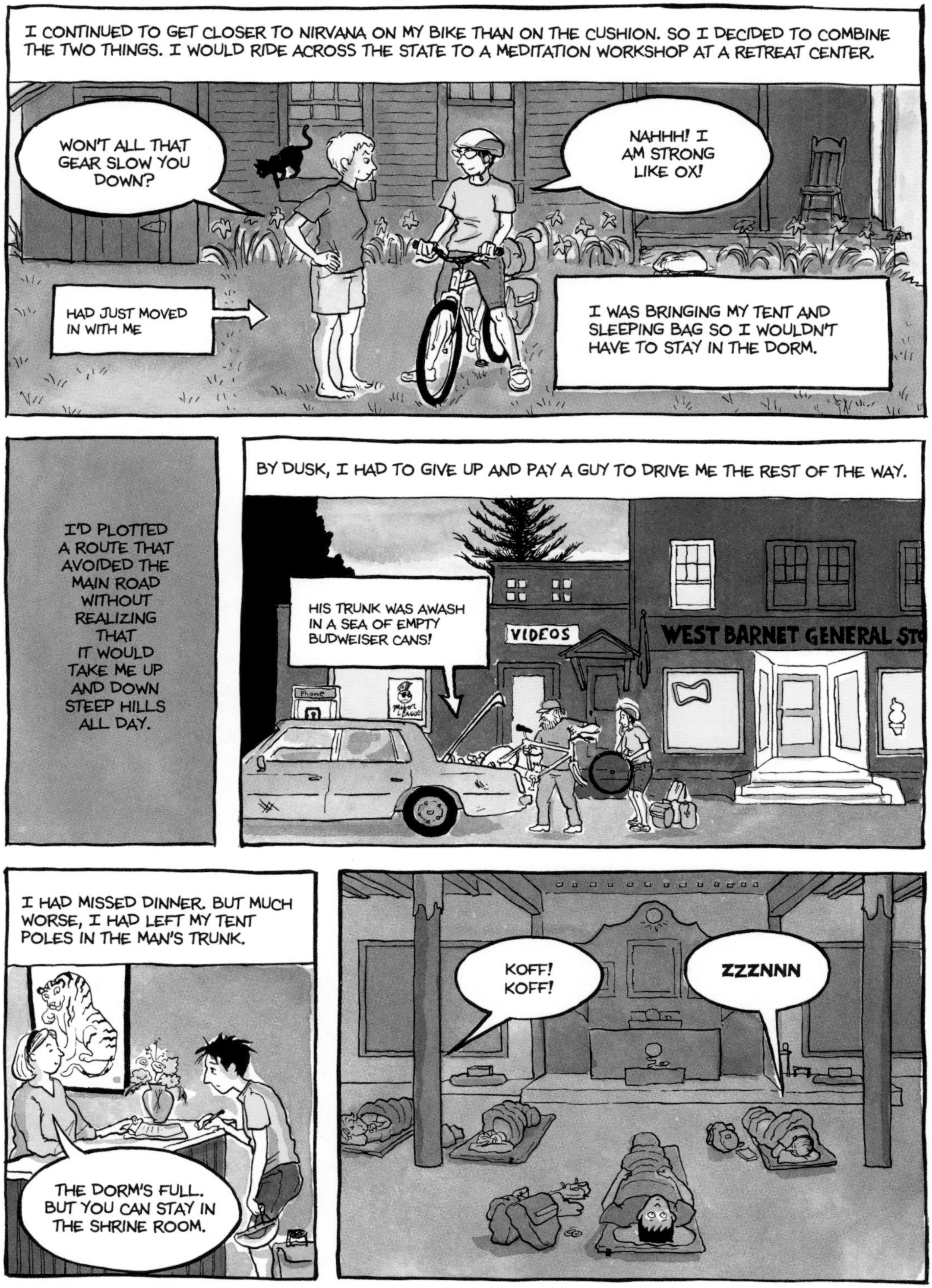

I CONTINUED TO GET CLOSER TO NIRVANA ON MY BIKE THAN ON THE CUSHION. SO I DECIDED TO COMBINE THE TWO THINGS. I WOULD RIDE ACROSS THE STATE TO A MEDITATION WORKSHOP AT A RETREAT CENTER.
WON'T ALL THAT GEAR SLOW YOU DOWN?
NAHHH! I AM STRONG LIKE OX!
HAD JUST MOVED IN WITH ME
I WAS BRINGING MY TENT AND SLEEPING BAG SO I WOULDN'T HAVE TO STAY IN THE DORM.
I'D PLOTTED A ROUTE THAT AVOIDED THE MAIN ROAD WITHOUT REALIZING THAT IT WOULD TAKE ME UP AND DOWN STEEP HILLS ALL DAY.
BY DUSK, I HAD TO GIVE UP AND PAY A GUY TO DRIVE ME THE REST OF THE WAY.
HIS TRUNK WAS AWASH IN A SEA OF EMPTY BUDWEISER CANS!
VIDEOS
WEST BARNET GENERAL ST
I HAD MISSED DINNER. BUT MUCH WORSE, I HAD LEFT MY TENT POLES IN THE MAN'S TRUNK.
THE DORM'S FULL. BUT YOU CAN STAY IN THE SHRINE ROOM.
KOFF! KOFF!
ZZZNNN

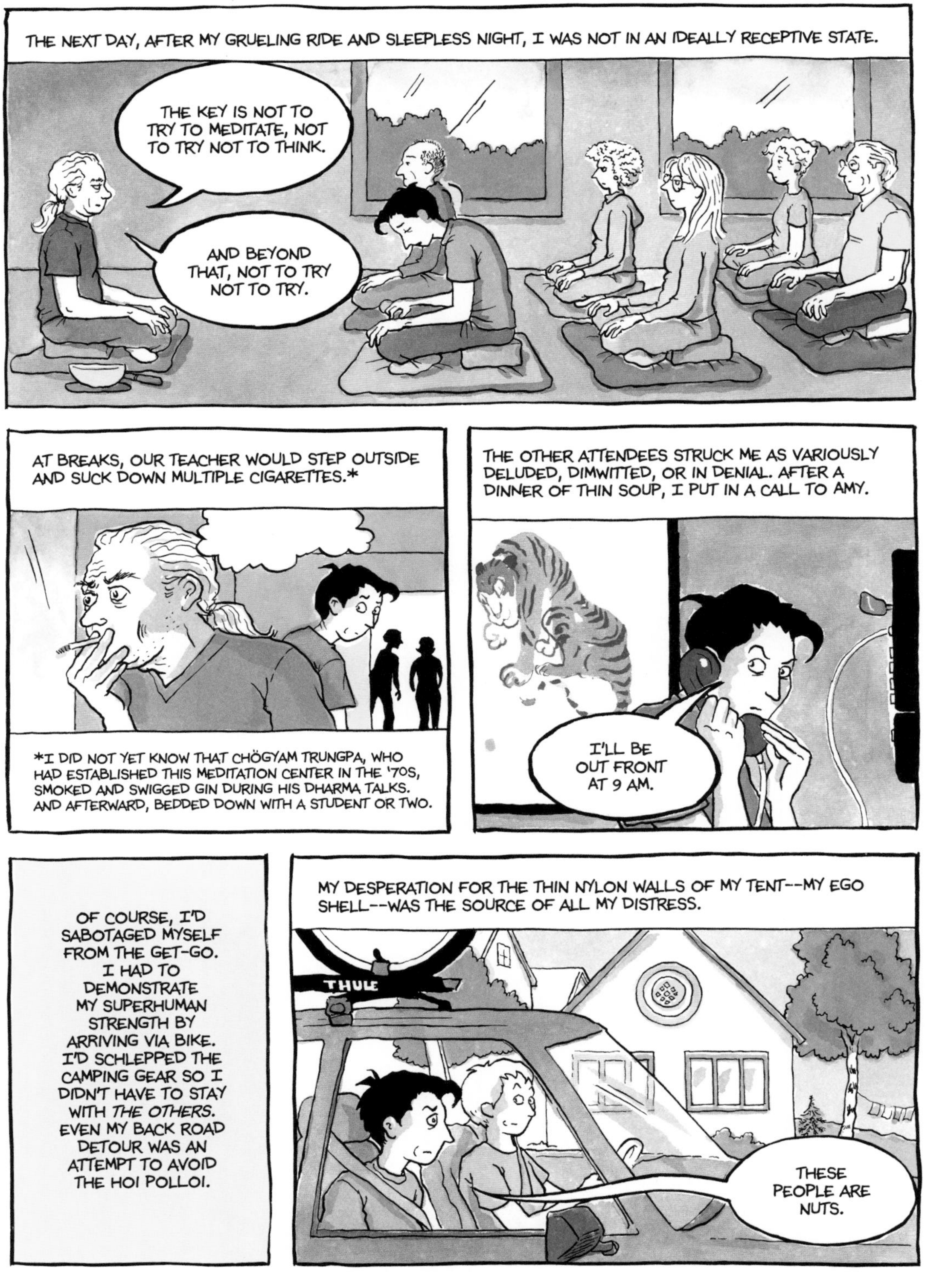
THE NEXT DAY, AFTER MY GRUELING RIDE AND SLEEPLESS NIGHT, I WAS NOT IN AN IDEALLY RECEPTIVE STATE.
THE KEY IS NOT TO TRY TO MEDITATE, NOT TO TRY NOT TO THINK.
AND BEYOND THAT, NOT TO TRY NOT TO TRY.
AT BREAKS, OUR TEACHER WOULD STEP OUTSIDE AND SUCK DOWN MULTIPLE CIGARETTES.*
*I DID NOT YET KNOW THAT CHÖGYAM TRUNGPA, WHO HAD ESTABLISHED THIS MEDITATION CENTER IN THE '70S, SMOKED AND SWIGGED GIN DURING HIS DHARMA TALKS. AND AFTERWARD, BEDDED DOWN WITH A STUDENT OR TWO.
THE OTHER ATTENDEES STRUCK ME AS VARIOUSLY DELUDED, DIMWITTED, OR IN DENIAL. AFTER A DINNER OF THIN SOUP, I PUT IN A CALL TO AMY.
I'LL BE OUT FRONT AT 9 AM.
OF COURSE, I'D SABOTAGED MYSELF FROM THE GET-GO. I HAD TO DEMONSTRATE MY SUPERHUMAN STRENGTH BY ARRIVING VIA BIKE. I'D SCHLEPPED THE CAMPING GEAR SO I DIDN'T HAVE TO STAY WITH *THE OTHERS*. EVEN MY BACK ROAD DETOUR WAS AN ATTEMPT TO AVOID THE HOI POLLOI.
MY DESPERATION FOR THE THIN NYLON WALLS OF MY TENT--MY EGO SHELL--WAS THE SOURCE OF ALL MY DISTRESS.
THULE
THESE PEOPLE ARE NUTS.

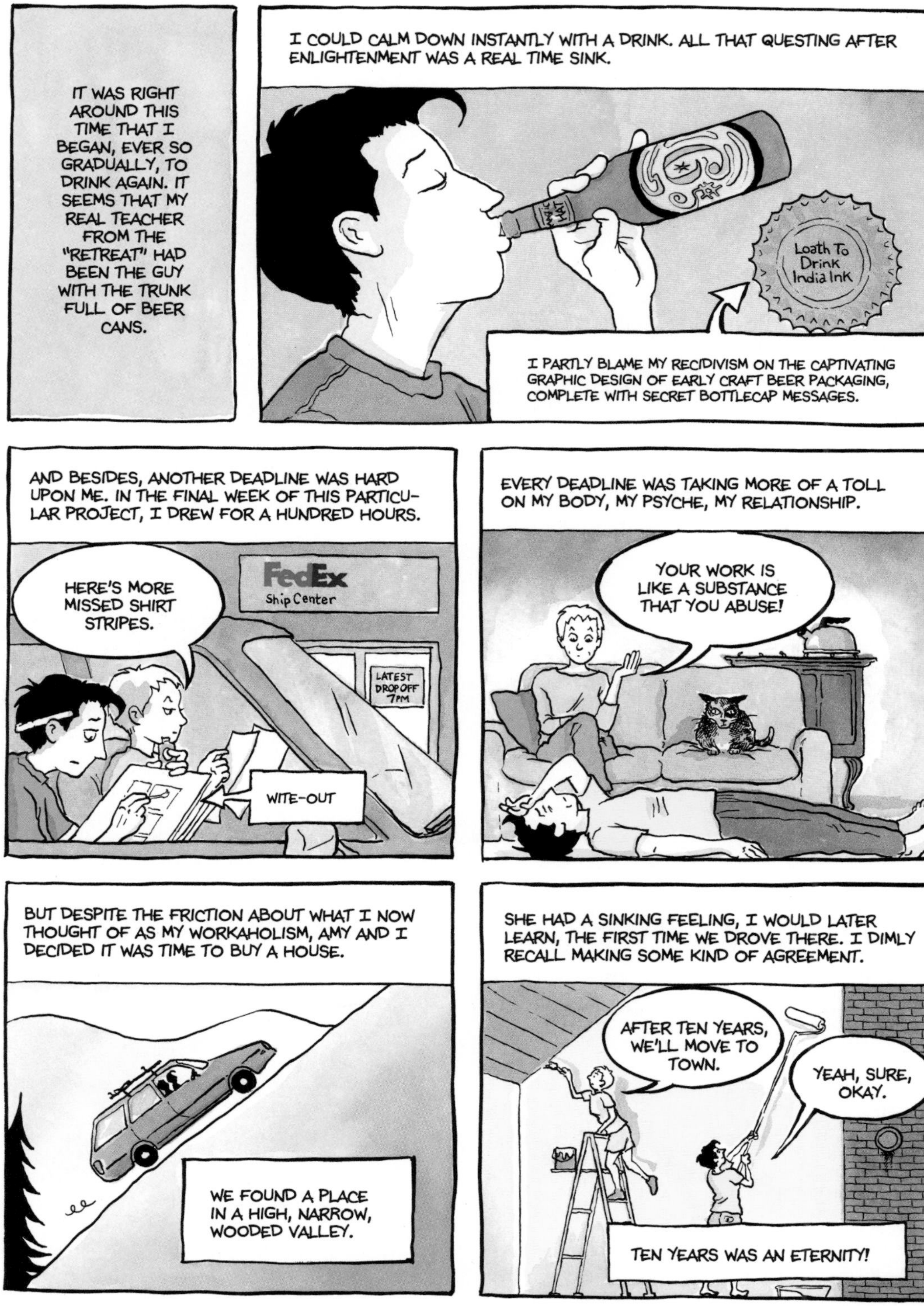
IT WAS RIGHT AROUND THIS TIME THAT I BEGAN, EVER SO GRADUALLY, TO DRINK AGAIN. IT SEEMS THAT MY REAL TEACHER FROM THE "RETREAT" HAD BEEN THE GUY WITH THE TRUNK FULL OF BEER CANS.
I COULD CALM DOWN INSTANTLY WITH A DRINK. ALL THAT QUESTING AFTER ENLIGHTENMENT WAS A REAL TIME SINK.
Loath To Drink India Ink
I PARTLY BLAME MY RECIDIVISM ON THE CAPTIVATING GRAPHIC DESIGN OF EARLY CRAFT BEER PACKAGING, COMPLETE WITH SECRET BOTTLECAP MESSAGES.
AND BESIDES, ANOTHER DEADLINE WAS HARD UPON ME. IN THE FINAL WEEK OF THIS PARTICULAR PROJECT, I DREW FOR A HUNDRED HOURS.
FedEx Ship Center
HERE'S MORE MISSED SHIRT STRIPES.
LATEST DROP OFF 7PM
WITE-OUT
EVERY DEADLINE WAS TAKING MORE OF A TOLL ON MY BODY, MY PSYCHE, MY RELATIONSHIP.
YOUR WORK IS LIKE A SUBSTANCE THAT YOU ABUSE!
BUT DESPITE THE FRICTION ABOUT WHAT I NOW THOUGHT OF AS MY WORKAHOLISM, AMY AND I DECIDED IT WAS TIME TO BUY A HOUSE.
WE FOUND A PLACE IN A HIGH, NARROW, WOODED VALLEY.
SHE HAD A SINKING FEELING, I WOULD LATER LEARN, THE FIRST TIME WE DROVE THERE. I DIMLY RECALL MAKING SOME KIND OF AGREEMENT.
AFTER TEN YEARS, WE'LL MOVE TO TOWN.
YEAH, SURE, OKAY.
TEN YEARS WAS AN ETERNITY!

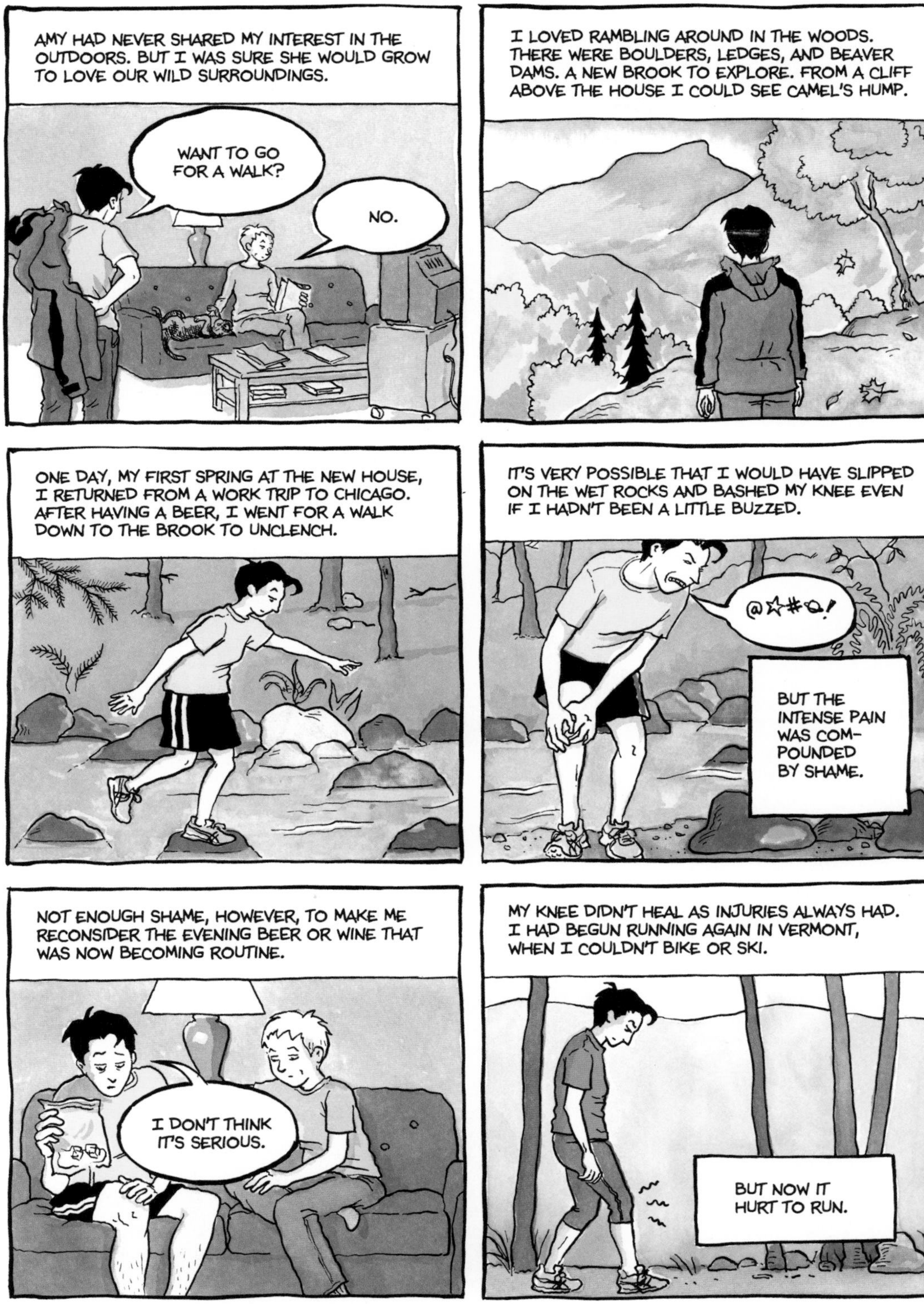
AMY HAD NEVER SHARED MY INTEREST IN THE OUTDOORS. BUT I WAS SURE SHE WOULD GROW TO LOVE OUR WILD SURROUNDINGS.
WANT TO GO FOR A WALK?
NO.
I LOVED RAMBLING AROUND IN THE WOODS. THERE WERE BOULDERS, LEDGES, AND BEAVER DAMS. A NEW BROOK TO EXPLORE. FROM A CLIFF ABOVE THE HOUSE I COULD SEE CAMEL'S HUMP.
ONE DAY, MY FIRST SPRING AT THE NEW HOUSE, I RETURNED FROM A WORK TRIP TO CHICAGO. AFTER HAVING A BEER, I WENT FOR A WALK DOWN TO THE BROOK TO UNCLENCH.
IT'S VERY POSSIBLE THAT I WOULD HAVE SLIPPED ON THE WET ROCKS AND BASHED MY KNEE EVEN IF I HADN'T BEEN A LITTLE BUZZED.
@☆#!
BUT THE INTENSE PAIN WAS COMPOUNDED BY SHAME.
NOT ENOUGH SHAME, HOWEVER, TO MAKE ME RECONSIDER THE EVENING BEER OR WINE THAT WAS NOW BECOMING ROUTINE.
I DON'T THINK IT'S SERIOUS.
MY KNEE DIDN'T HEAL AS INJURIES ALWAYS HAD. I HAD BEGUN RUNNING AGAIN IN VERMONT, WHEN I COULDN'T BIKE OR SKI.
BUT NOW IT HURT TO RUN.

INCREASINGLY, OTHER BODILY LIMITATIONS WERE ASSERTING THEMSELVES. I HAD PERIODIC HEADACHES THAT WOULD RENDER ME USELESS FOR AN ENTIRE DAY, SOMETIMES TWO.

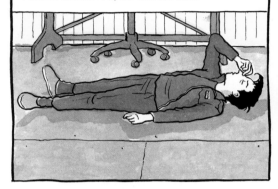

THE BOUTS OF EXERCISE-INDUCED TACHYCARDIA THAT HAD STARTED UP IN MY TWENTIES WERE LASTING LONGER AND LEAVING ME WEAKER.

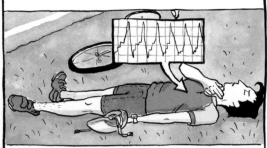

(I HAD ALWAYS ESCHEWED FANCY BIKE JERSEYS AS A WASTE OF MONEY. THEN I TRIED ONE AND RUED EVERY SECOND I'D SPENT IN A SODDEN COTTON T-SHIRT.)

BUT I DIDN'T CONSIDER ANY OF THESE THINGS REAL PROBLEMS. IN GENERAL, I STILL FELT STRONG LIKE OX.

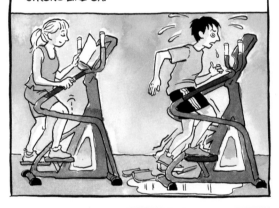

I HAD JOINED THE Y TO STAY IN SHAPE DURING STICK SEASON.* ONCE OR TWICE A WEEK I'D DO THE STAIRMASTER AND LIFT SOME WEIGHTS.

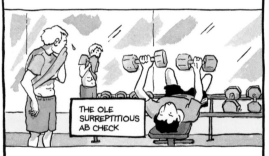

THE OLE SURREPTITIOUS AB CHECK

*THAT BLEAK AND LENGTHENING STRETCH WHEN IT'S TOO COLD TO BIKE BUT THERE'S NO SNOW TO SKI ON

EVENTUALLY, I MET WITH A TRAINER TO VARY MY WORKOUT.

CHEAT BY JUMPING UP TO THE BAR, THEN LOWER YOURSELF.

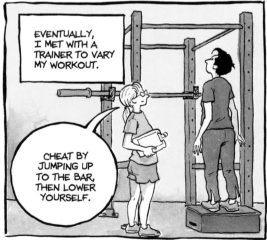

BODYWEIGHT EXERCISES WERE NOW ALL THE RAGE. CHIN-UPS WERE IMPOSSIBLE AT FIRST, SO SHE HAD ME START WITH "NEGATIVES."

IT'S THE SAME RANGE OF MOTION AS GOING UP, BUT EASIER.

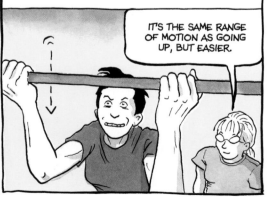

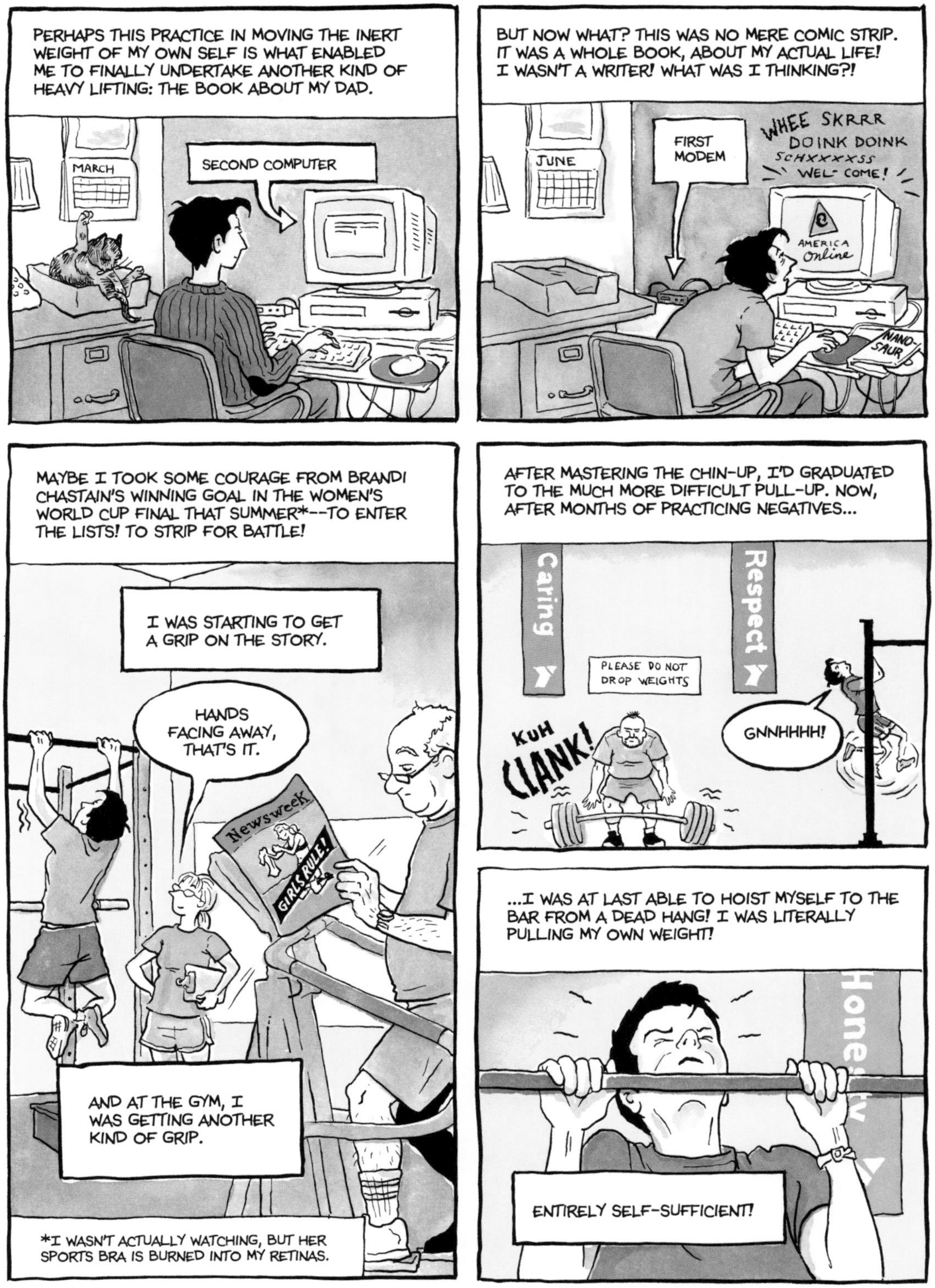
PERHAPS THIS PRACTICE IN MOVING THE INERT WEIGHT OF MY OWN SELF IS WHAT ENABLED ME TO FINALLY UNDERTAKE ANOTHER KIND OF HEAVY LIFTING: THE BOOK ABOUT MY DAD.
MARCH
SECOND COMPUTER
BUT NOW WHAT? THIS WAS NO MERE COMIC STRIP. IT WAS A WHOLE BOOK, ABOUT MY ACTUAL LIFE! I WASN'T A WRITER! WHAT WAS I THINKING?!
JUNE
FIRST MODEM
WHEE SKRRR
DOINK DOINK
SCHXXXXXSS
WEL- COME!
AMERICA Online
NANO-SAUR
MAYBE I TOOK SOME COURAGE FROM BRANDI CHASTAIN'S WINNING GOAL IN THE WOMEN'S WORLD CUP FINAL THAT SUMMER*--TO ENTER THE LISTS! TO STRIP FOR BATTLE!
I WAS STARTING TO GET A GRIP ON THE STORY.
HANDS FACING AWAY, THAT'S IT.
Newsweek
GIRLS RULE!
AND AT THE GYM, I WAS GETTING ANOTHER KIND OF GRIP.
*I WASN'T ACTUALLY WATCHING, BUT HER SPORTS BRA IS BURNED INTO MY RETINAS.
AFTER MASTERING THE CHIN-UP, I'D GRADUATED TO THE MUCH MORE DIFFICULT PULL-UP. NOW, AFTER MONTHS OF PRACTICING NEGATIVES...
Caring
Respect
PLEASE DO NOT DROP WEIGHTS
KUH CLANK!
GNHHHHH!
...I WAS AT LAST ABLE TO HOIST MYSELF TO THE BAR FROM A DEAD HANG! I WAS LITERALLY PULLING MY OWN WEIGHT!
Honesty
ENTIRELY SELF-SUFFICIENT!

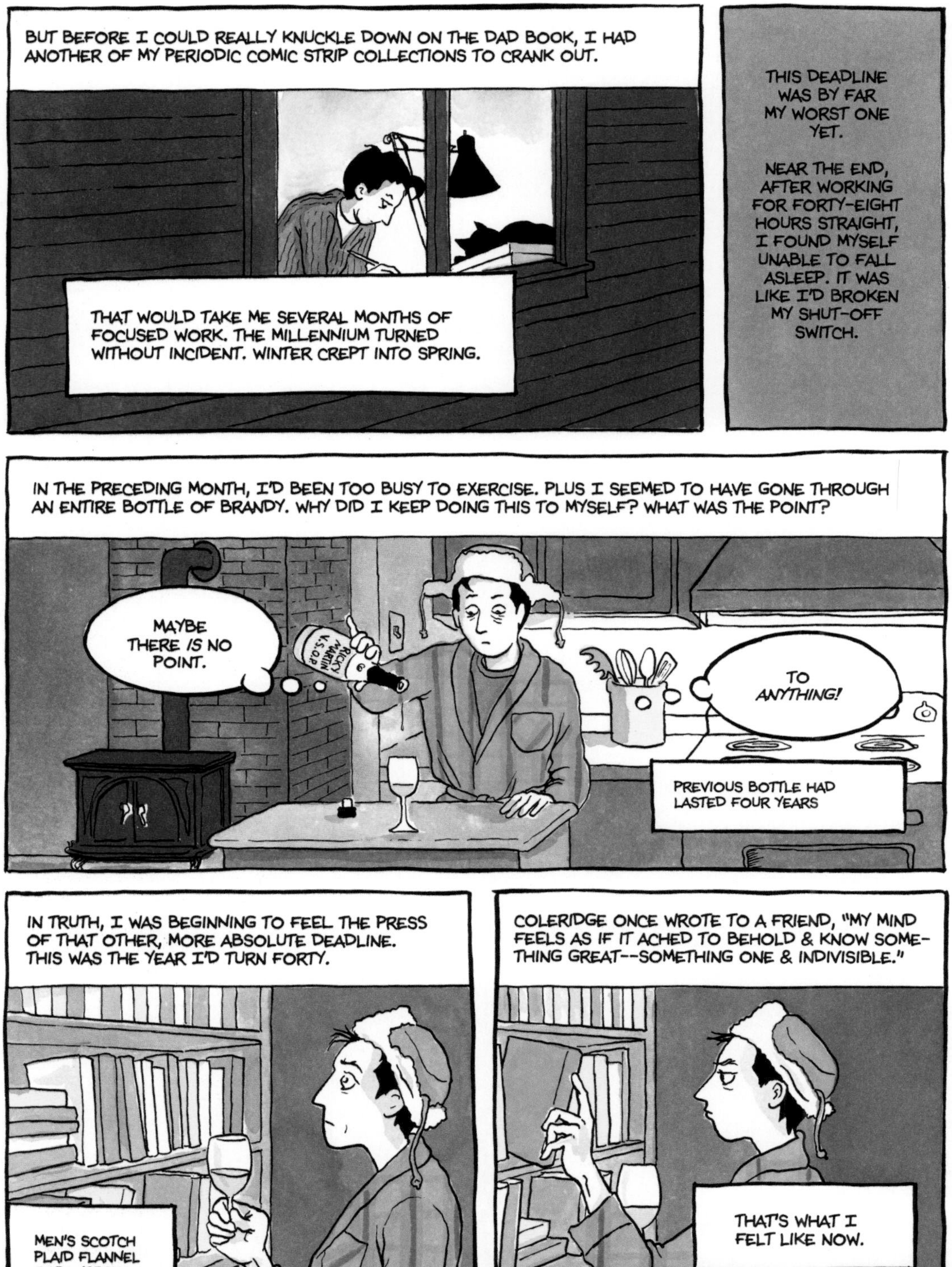

BUT BEFORE I COULD REALLY KNUCKLE DOWN ON THE DAD BOOK, I HAD ANOTHER OF MY PERIODIC COMIC STRIP COLLECTIONS TO CRANK OUT.
THAT WOULD TAKE ME SEVERAL MONTHS OF FOCUSED WORK. THE MILLENNIUM TURNED WITHOUT INCIDENT. WINTER CREPT INTO SPRING.
THIS DEADLINE WAS BY FAR MY WORST ONE YET.
NEAR THE END, AFTER WORKING FOR FORTY-EIGHT HOURS STRAIGHT, I FOUND MYSELF UNABLE TO FALL ASLEEP. IT WAS LIKE I'D BROKEN MY SHUT-OFF SWITCH.
IN THE PRECEDING MONTH, I'D BEEN TOO BUSY TO EXERCISE. PLUS I SEEMED TO HAVE GONE THROUGH AN ENTIRE BOTTLE OF BRANDY. WHY DID I KEEP DOING THIS TO MYSELF? WHAT WAS THE POINT?
MAYBE THERE *IS* NO POINT.
RICKY MARTIN V.S.O.P.
TO *ANYTHING!*
PREVIOUS BOTTLE HAD LASTED FOUR YEARS
IN TRUTH, I WAS BEGINNING TO FEEL THE PRESS OF THAT OTHER, MORE ABSOLUTE DEADLINE. THIS WAS THE YEAR I'D TURN FORTY.
MEN'S SCOTCH PLAID FLANNEL ROBE 1653K
COLERIDGE ONCE WROTE TO A FRIEND, "MY MIND FEELS AS IF IT ACHED TO BEHOLD & KNOW SOME-THING GREAT--SOMETHING ONE & INDIVISIBLE."
THAT'S WHAT I FELT LIKE NOW.

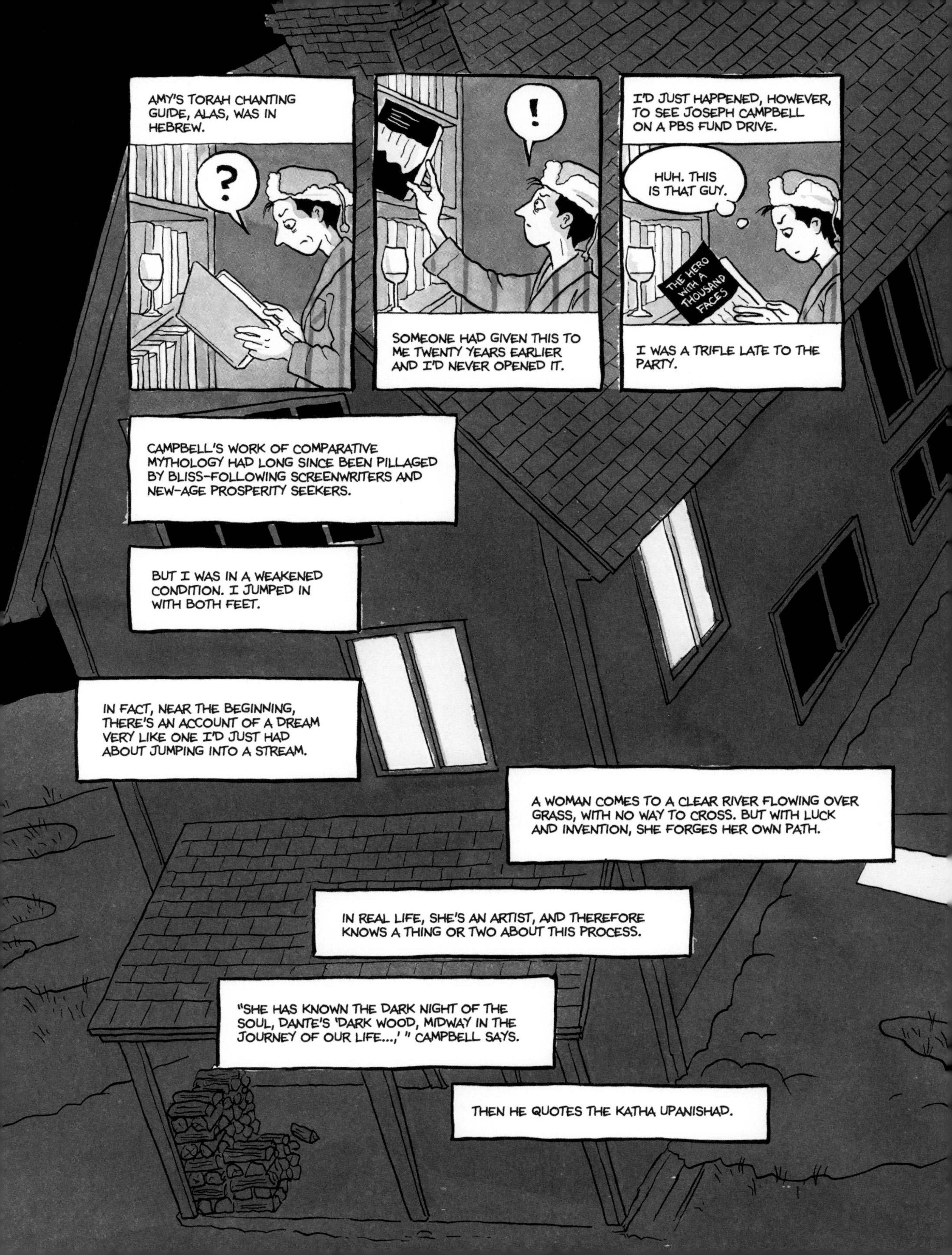
AMY'S TORAH CHANTING GUIDE, ALAS, WAS IN HEBREW.
?
!
SOMEONE HAD GIVEN THIS TO ME TWENTY YEARS EARLIER AND I'D NEVER OPENED IT.
I'D JUST HAPPENED, HOWEVER, TO SEE JOSEPH CAMPBELL ON A PBS FUND DRIVE.
HUH. THIS IS THAT GUY.
THE HERO WITH A THOUSAND FACES
I WAS A TRIFLE LATE TO THE PARTY.
CAMPBELL'S WORK OF COMPARATIVE MYTHOLOGY HAD LONG SINCE BEEN PILLAGED BY BLISS-FOLLOWING SCREENWRITERS AND NEW-AGE PROSPERITY SEEKERS.
BUT I WAS IN A WEAKENED CONDITION. I JUMPED IN WITH BOTH FEET.
IN FACT, NEAR THE BEGINNING, THERE'S AN ACCOUNT OF A DREAM VERY LIKE ONE I'D JUST HAD ABOUT JUMPING INTO A STREAM.
A WOMAN COMES TO A CLEAR RIVER FLOWING OVER GRASS, WITH NO WAY TO CROSS. BUT WITH LUCK AND INVENTION, SHE FORGES HER OWN PATH.
IN REAL LIFE, SHE'S AN ARTIST, AND THEREFORE KNOWS A THING OR TWO ABOUT THIS PROCESS.
"SHE HAS KNOWN THE DARK NIGHT OF THE SOUL, DANTE'S 'DARK WOOD, MIDWAY IN THE JOURNEY OF OUR LIFE...,' " CAMPBELL SAYS.
THEN HE QUOTES THE KATHA UPANISHAD.

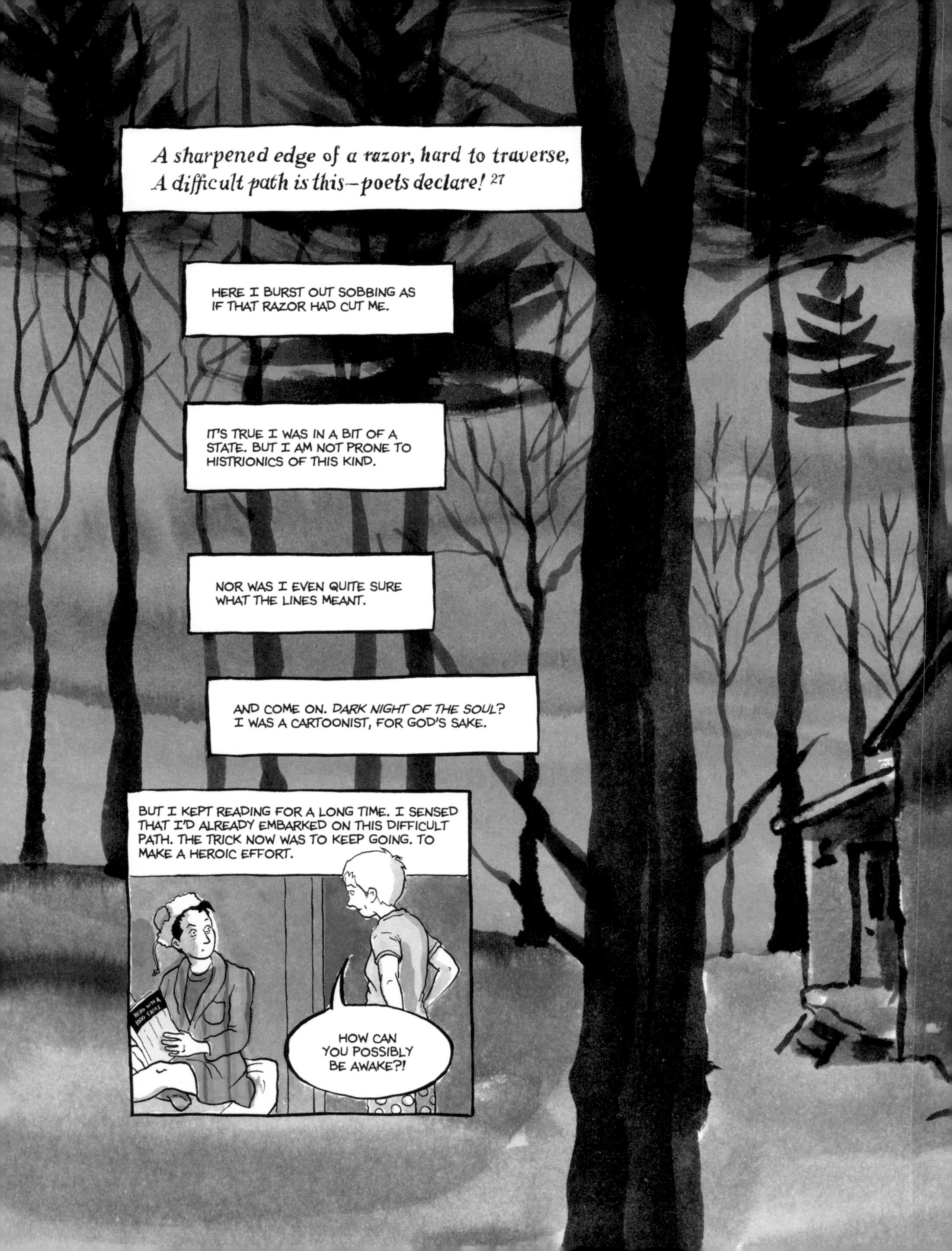
A sharpened edge of a razor, hard to traverse,
A difficult path is this—poets declare! 27
HERE I BURST OUT SOBBING AS IF THAT RAZOR HAD CUT ME.
IT'S TRUE I WAS IN A BIT OF A STATE. BUT I AM NOT PRONE TO HISTRIONICS OF THIS KIND.
NOR WAS I EVEN QUITE SURE WHAT THE LINES MEANT.
AND COME ON. DARK NIGHT OF THE SOUL? I WAS A CARTOONIST, FOR GOD'S SAKE.
BUT I KEPT READING FOR A LONG TIME. I SENSED THAT I'D ALREADY EMBARKED ON THIS DIFFICULT PATH. THE TRICK NOW WAS TO KEEP GOING. TO MAKE A HEROIC EFFORT.
HERO WITH A 1000 FACES
HOW CAN YOU POSSIBLY BE AWAKE?!

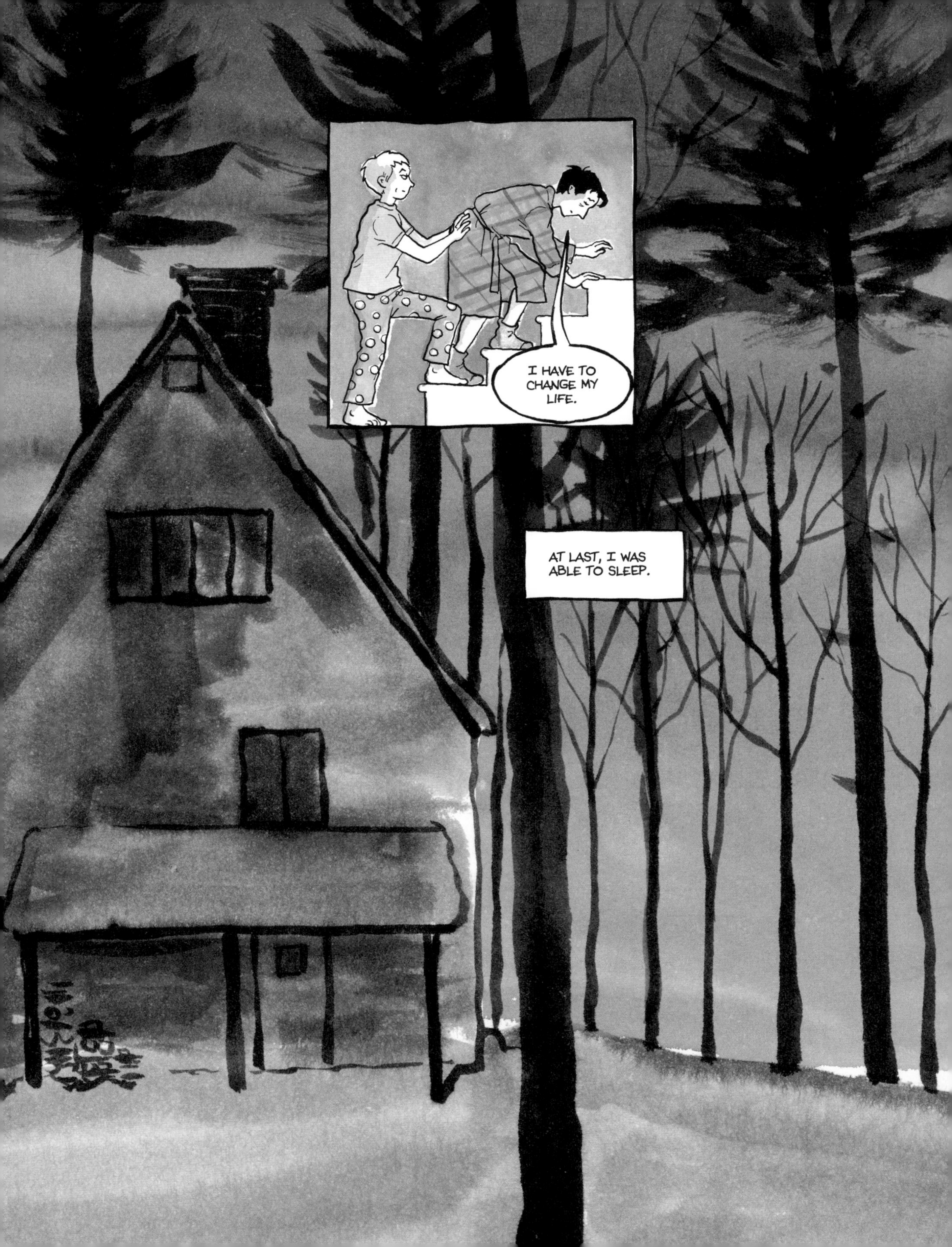
I HAVE TO CHANGE MY LIFE.
AT LAST, I WAS ABLE TO SLEEP.

2000s

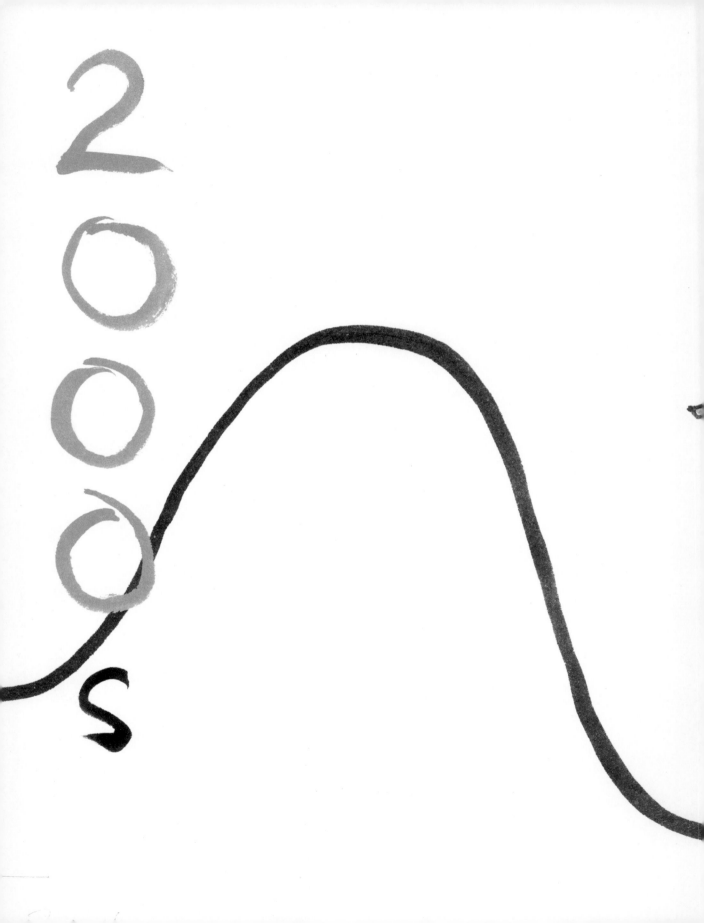

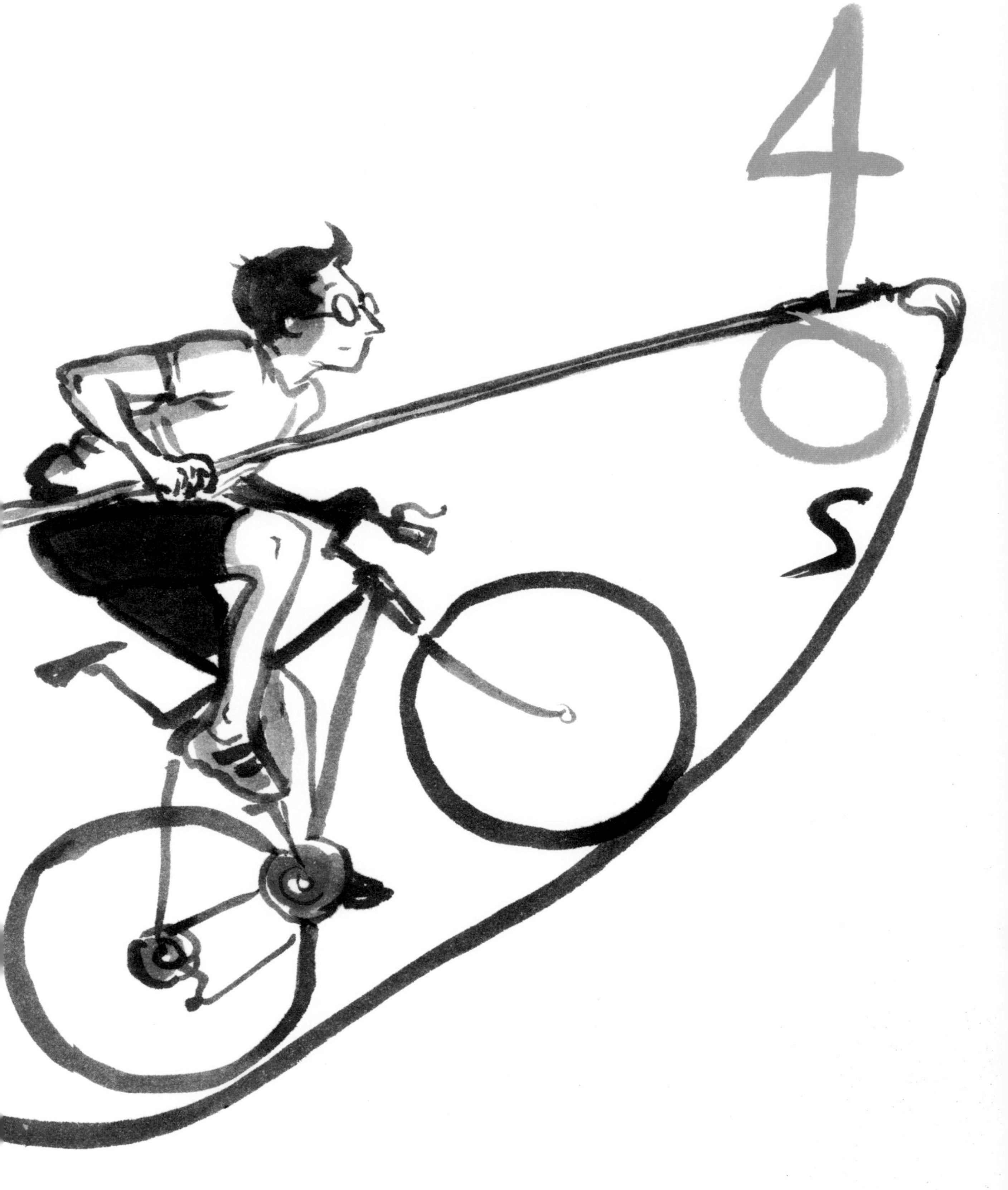
4
o
s

THE THING ABOUT CHANGING YOUR LIFE IS THAT CHANGE MEANS MOVING ON, AND MOVING ON LEADS ESSENTIALLY TO ONE PLACE--THE GRAVE.

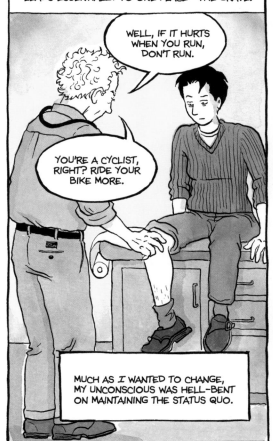

WELL, IF IT HURTS WHEN YOU RUN, DON'T RUN.

YOU'RE A CYCLIST, RIGHT? RIDE YOUR BIKE MORE.

MUCH AS *I* WANTED TO CHANGE, MY UNCONSCIOUS WAS HELL-BENT ON MAINTAINING THE STATUS QUO.

I MET WITH MY DOCTOR THE VERY DAY AFTER MY DARK NIGHT OF THE SOUL. THE KNEE I'D INJURED TWO YEARS EARLIER WAS NOT IMPROVING.

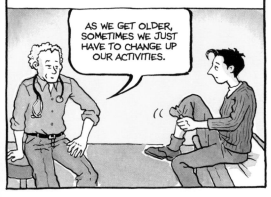

AS WE GET OLDER, SOMETIMES WE JUST HAVE TO CHANGE UP OUR ACTIVITIES.

FOR SOME REASON, HIS ADVICE DID NOT UPSET ME. I DID LIKE BIKING MORE THAN RUNNING. RUNNING WAS HARD.

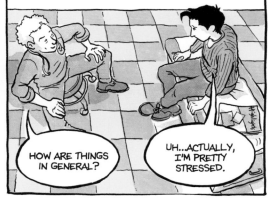

HOW ARE THINGS IN GENERAL?

UH...ACTUALLY, I'M PRETTY STRESSED.

MY INSOMNIA ATTACK THE NIGHT BEFORE HAD BEEN A LITERAL WAKE-UP CALL, AND I WAS DETERMINED TO HEED IT.

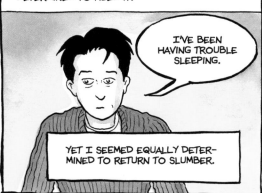

I'VE BEEN HAVING TROUBLE SLEEPING.

YET I SEEMED EQUALLY DETER-MINED TO RETURN TO SLUMBER.

I LEFT THE DOCTOR'S OFFICE THAT DAY WITH TEN SMALL, RED, SOPORIFIC CAPSULES, WHICH HE WARNED WERE JUST A SHORT-TERM FIX.

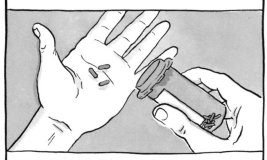

BUT I HAD NO PROBLEM RENEWING THE PRESCRIPTION. FOR THE NEXT FIFTEEN YEARS.

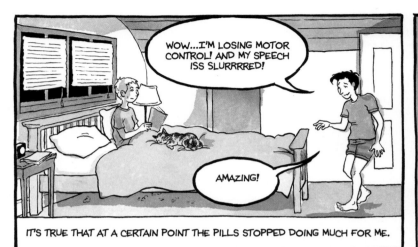

WOW...I'M LOSING MOTOR CONTROL! AND MY SPEECH ISS SLURRRRED!

AMAZING!

IT'S TRUE THAT AT A CERTAIN POINT THE PILLS STOPPED DOING MUCH FOR ME.

BUT IN THOSE EARLY DAYS THEY SENT ME ALMOST INSTANTLY INTO VELVETY BLACK OBLIVION.

WHILE MY HABIT WOULD BE NOWHERE NEAR AS DESTRUCTIVE AS COLERIDGE'S LAUDANUM ADDICTION, I, TOO, WAS ATTEMPTING TO DOSE SOME SORT OF PAIN.

MEANWHILE, IF I WAS GOING TO BIKE MORE, IT WAS TIME TO GET A REAL BIKE. A ROAD BIKE. I COULDN'T AFFORD A NEW ONE, BUT IN EARLY MAY I CHECKED OUT SOME USED MODELS.

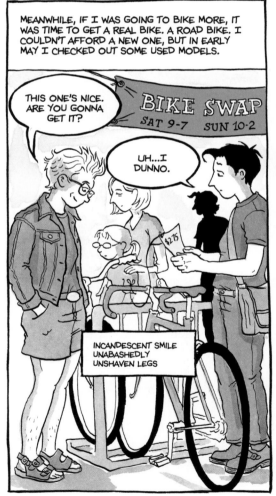

THIS ONE'S NICE. ARE YOU GONNA GET IT?

UH...I DUNNO.

BIKE SWAP
SAT 9-7   SUN 10-2

$2.75

INCANDESCENT SMILE
UNABASHEDLY
UNSHAVEN LEGS

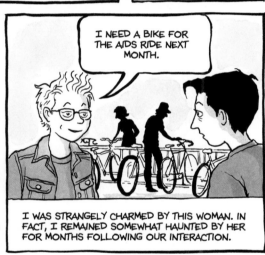

I NEED A BIKE FOR THE AIDS RIDE NEXT MONTH.

I WAS STRANGELY CHARMED BY THIS WOMAN. IN FACT, I REMAINED SOMEWHAT HAUNTED BY HER FOR MONTHS FOLLOWING OUR INTERACTION.

BUT I WASN'T GOING TO HAVE SOME BANAL MID-LIFE CRISIS AFFAIR. THOSE WERE FOR WRETCHES WHO DIDN'T LIVE AS INTENTIONALLY AS I DID.

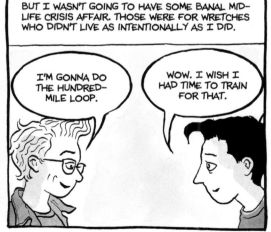

I'M GONNA DO THE HUNDRED-MILE LOOP.

WOW. I WISH I HAD TIME TO TRAIN FOR THAT.

I WOULD SEE THE BIKE-SWAP WOMAN AROUND OCCASIONALLY AFTER THIS. BUT I WOULDN'T TALK TO HER AGAIN FOR ANOTHER SEVEN YEARS--SOME TIME AFTER AMY AND I HAD BROKEN UP.

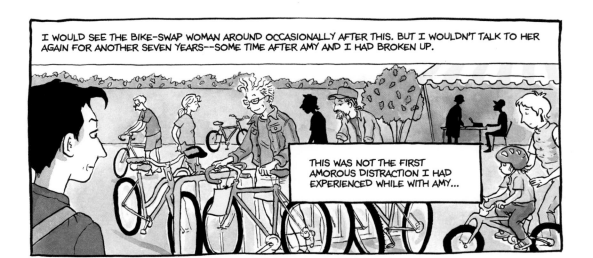

THIS WAS NOT THE FIRST AMOROUS DISTRACTION I HAD EXPERIENCED WHILE WITH AMY...

...NOR WOULD IT BE THE LAST. WITHIN THE YEAR, ANOTHER ONE WOULD PROVOKE A SPATE OF PROFESSIONAL INTERVENTIONS. I STARTED SEEING A NEW THERAPIST...

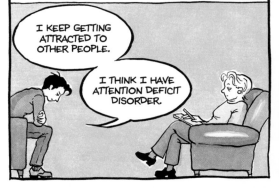

I KEEP GETTING ATTRACTED TO OTHER PEOPLE.

I THINK I HAVE ATTENTION DEFICIT DISORDER.

...AND AN ACUPUNCTURIST. I'D ACTUALLY COME TO HIM ABOUT MY HEADACHES, WHICH I HAD BEGUN TO SUSPECT WERE MIGRAINES.

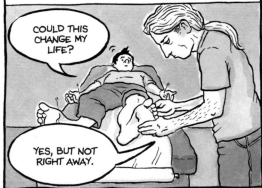

COULD THIS CHANGE MY LIFE?

YES, BUT NOT RIGHT AWAY.

I NOW TOOK IT FOR GRANTED THAT EMOTIONAL AND PHYSICAL ISSUES WERE CONNECTED, SO THIS MULTIPRONGED APPROACH SEEMED PRUDENT.

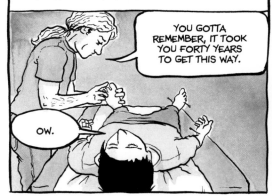

YOU GOTTA REMEMBER, IT TOOK YOU FORTY YEARS TO GET THIS WAY.

OW.

AND I MADE ANOTHER CONCERTED EFFORT AT MEDITATION. THAT SEEMED OBLIGATORY IF I WAS SERIOUS ABOUT THIS MYSTERIOUS *PATH*.

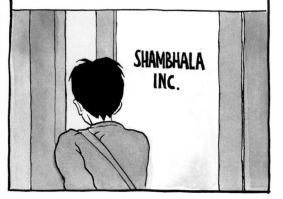

SHAMBHALA INC.

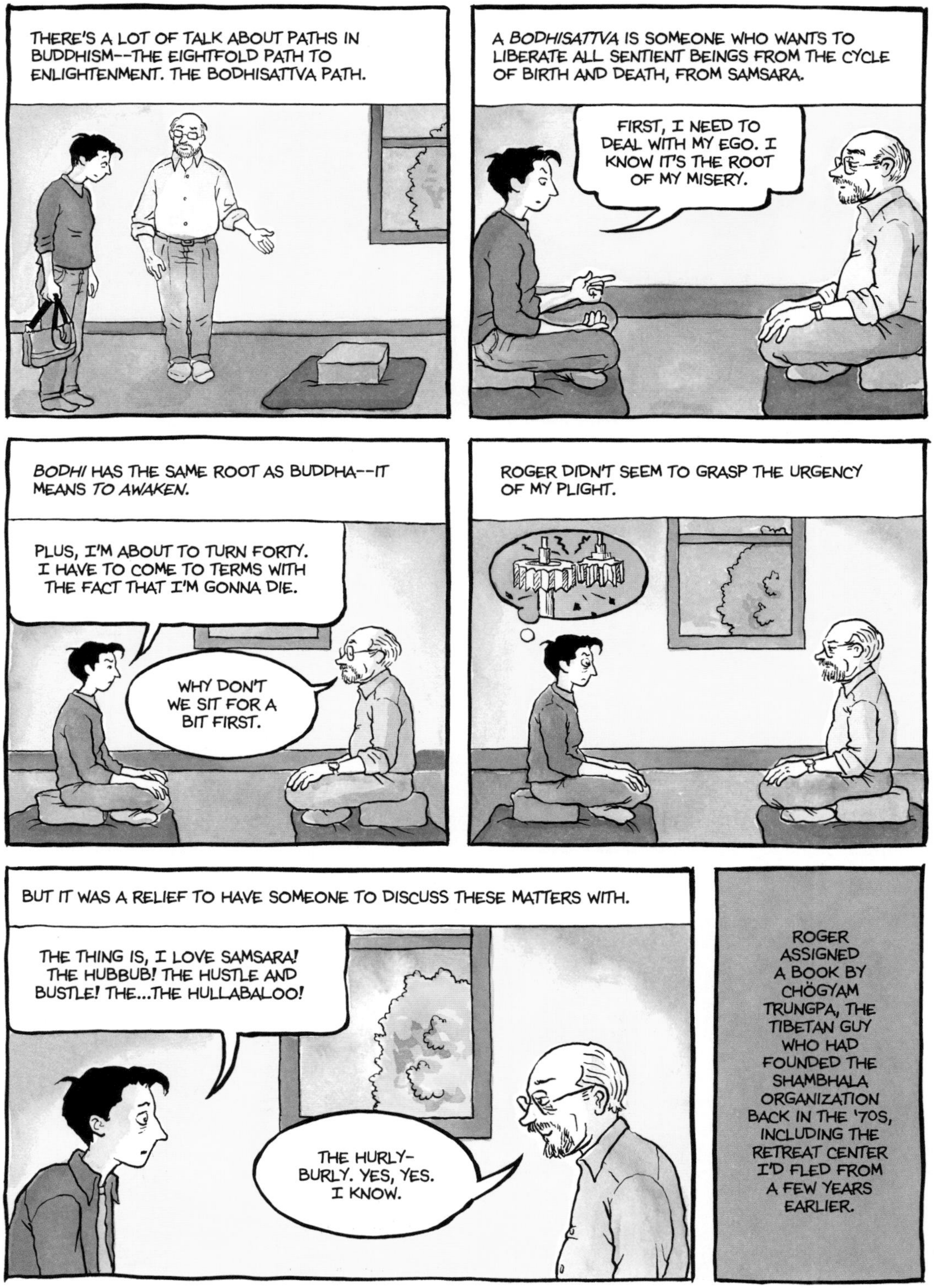
THERE'S A LOT OF TALK ABOUT PATHS IN BUDDHISM--THE EIGHTFOLD PATH TO ENLIGHTENMENT. THE BODHISATTVA PATH.
A *BODHISATTVA* IS SOMEONE WHO WANTS TO LIBERATE ALL SENTIENT BEINGS FROM THE CYCLE OF BIRTH AND DEATH, FROM SAMSARA.
FIRST, I NEED TO DEAL WITH MY EGO. I KNOW IT'S THE ROOT OF MY MISERY.
BODHI HAS THE SAME ROOT AS BUDDHA--IT MEANS *TO AWAKEN.*
PLUS, I'M ABOUT TO TURN FORTY. I HAVE TO COME TO TERMS WITH THE FACT THAT I'M GONNA DIE.
WHY DON'T WE SIT FOR A BIT FIRST.
ROGER DIDN'T SEEM TO GRASP THE URGENCY OF MY PLIGHT.
BUT IT WAS A RELIEF TO HAVE SOMEONE TO DISCUSS THESE MATTERS WITH.
THE THING IS, I LOVE SAMSARA! THE HUBBUB! THE HUSTLE AND BUSTLE! THE...THE HULLABALOO!
THE HURLY-BURLY. YES, YES. I KNOW.
ROGER ASSIGNED A BOOK BY CHÖGYAM TRUNGPA, THE TIBETAN GUY WHO HAD FOUNDED THE SHAMBHALA ORGANIZATION BACK IN THE '70S, INCLUDING THE RETREAT CENTER I'D FLED FROM A FEW YEARS EARLIER.

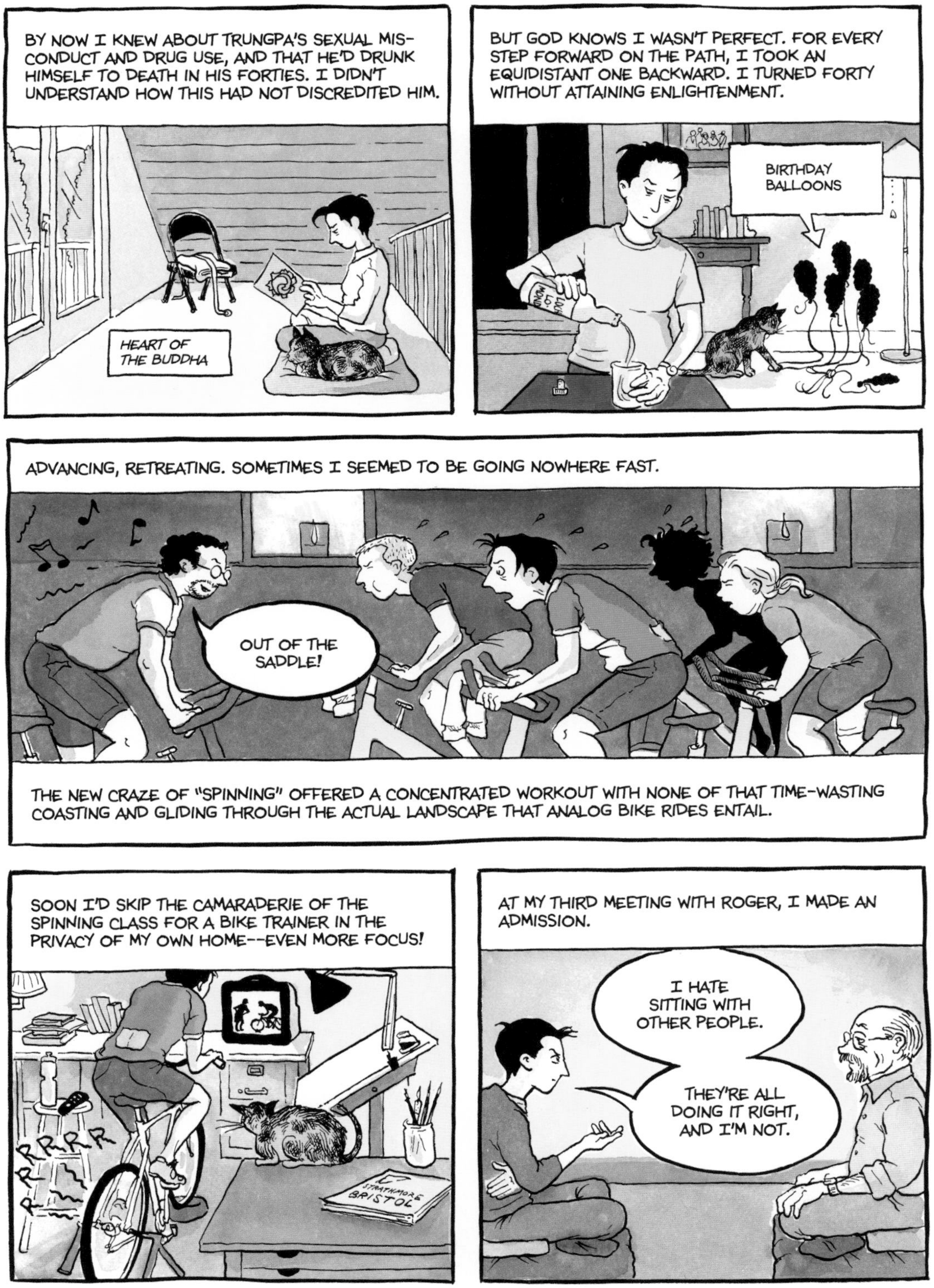
BY NOW I KNEW ABOUT TRUNGPA'S SEXUAL MISCONDUCT AND DRUG USE, AND THAT HE'D DRUNK HIMSELF TO DEATH IN HIS FORTIES. I DIDN'T UNDERSTAND HOW THIS HAD NOT DISCREDITED HIM.
HEART OF THE BUDDHA
BUT GOD KNOWS I WASN'T PERFECT. FOR EVERY STEP FORWARD ON THE PATH, I TOOK AN EQUIDISTANT ONE BACKWARD. I TURNED FORTY WITHOUT ATTAINING ENLIGHTENMENT.
BIRTHDAY BALLOONS
ADVANCING, RETREATING. SOMETIMES I SEEMED TO BE GOING NOWHERE FAST.
OUT OF THE SADDLE!
THE NEW CRAZE OF "SPINNING" OFFERED A CONCENTRATED WORKOUT WITH NONE OF THAT TIME-WASTING COASTING AND GLIDING THROUGH THE ACTUAL LANDSCAPE THAT ANALOG BIKE RIDES ENTAIL.
SOON I'D SKIP THE CAMARADERIE OF THE SPINNING CLASS FOR A BIKE TRAINER IN THE PRIVACY OF MY OWN HOME--EVEN MORE FOCUS!
STRATHMORE BRISTOL
AT MY THIRD MEETING WITH ROGER, I MADE AN ADMISSION.
I HATE SITTING WITH OTHER PEOPLE.
THEY'RE ALL DOING IT RIGHT, AND I'M NOT.

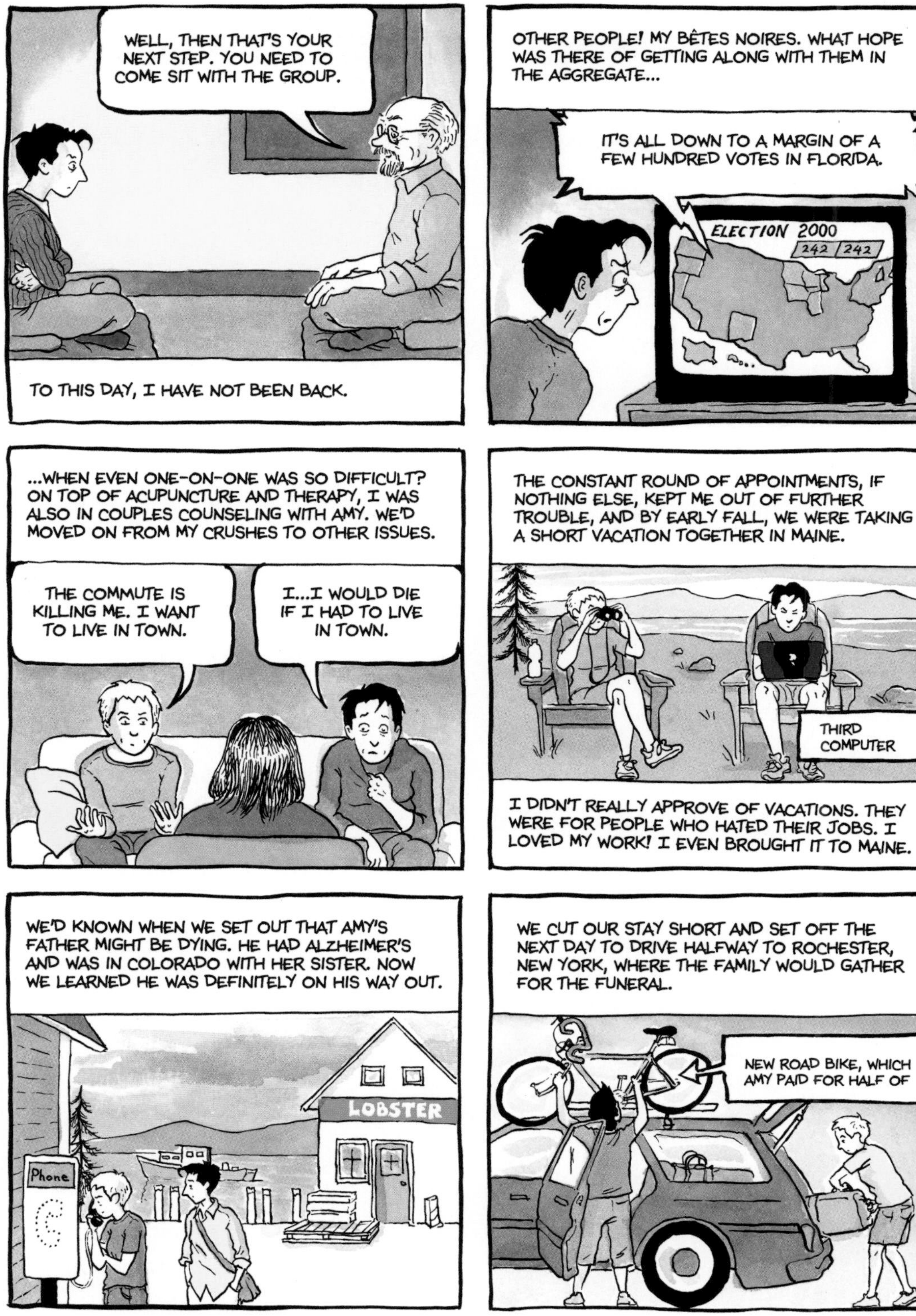
WELL, THEN THAT'S YOUR NEXT STEP. YOU NEED TO COME SIT WITH THE GROUP.
TO THIS DAY, I HAVE NOT BEEN BACK.
OTHER PEOPLE! MY BÊTES NOIRES. WHAT HOPE WAS THERE OF GETTING ALONG WITH THEM IN THE AGGREGATE...
IT'S ALL DOWN TO A MARGIN OF A FEW HUNDRED VOTES IN FLORIDA.
ELECTION 2000
242
242
...WHEN EVEN ONE-ON-ONE WAS SO DIFFICULT? ON TOP OF ACUPUNCTURE AND THERAPY, I WAS ALSO IN COUPLES COUNSELING WITH AMY. WE'D MOVED ON FROM MY CRUSHES TO OTHER ISSUES.
THE COMMUTE IS KILLING ME. I WANT TO LIVE IN TOWN.
I...I WOULD DIE IF I HAD TO LIVE IN TOWN.
THE CONSTANT ROUND OF APPOINTMENTS, IF NOTHING ELSE, KEPT ME OUT OF FURTHER TROUBLE, AND BY EARLY FALL, WE WERE TAKING A SHORT VACATION TOGETHER IN MAINE.
THIRD COMPUTER
I DIDN'T REALLY APPROVE OF VACATIONS. THEY WERE FOR PEOPLE WHO HATED THEIR JOBS. I LOVED MY WORK! I EVEN BROUGHT IT TO MAINE.
WE'D KNOWN WHEN WE SET OUT THAT AMY'S FATHER MIGHT BE DYING. HE HAD ALZHEIMER'S AND WAS IN COLORADO WITH HER SISTER. NOW WE LEARNED HE WAS DEFINITELY ON HIS WAY OUT.
LOBSTER
Phone
WE CUT OUR STAY SHORT AND SET OFF THE NEXT DAY TO DRIVE HALFWAY TO ROCHESTER, NEW YORK, WHERE THE FAMILY WOULD GATHER FOR THE FUNERAL.
NEW ROAD BIKE, WHICH AMY PAID FOR HALF OF

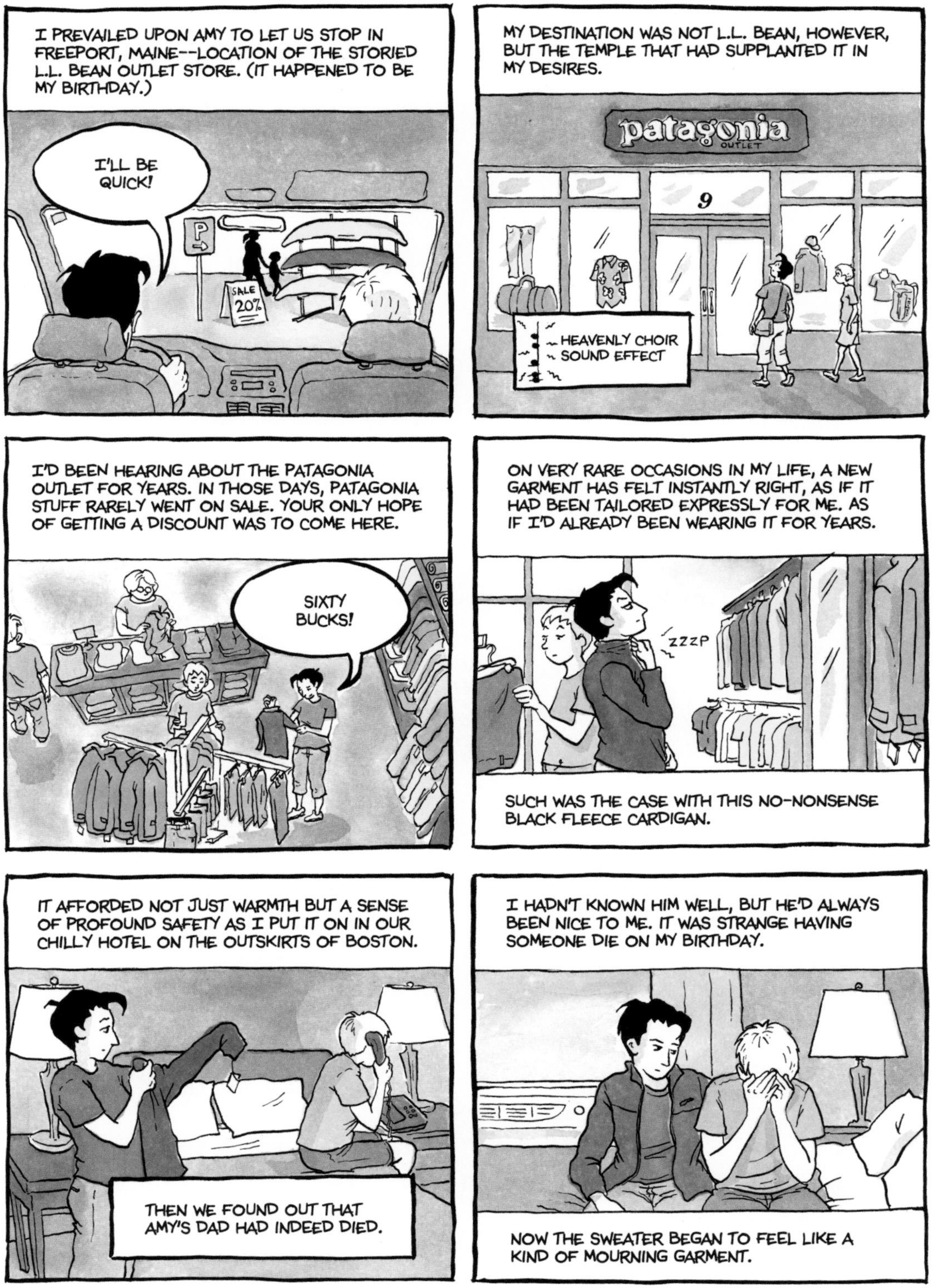
I PREVAILED UPON AMY TO LET US STOP IN FREEPORT, MAINE--LOCATION OF THE STORIED L.L. BEAN OUTLET STORE. (IT HAPPENED TO BE MY BIRTHDAY.)
I'LL BE QUICK!
SALE 20%
MY DESTINATION WAS NOT L.L. BEAN, HOWEVER, BUT THE TEMPLE THAT HAD SUPPLANTED IT IN MY DESIRES.
patagonia OUTLET
9
HEAVENLY CHOIR SOUND EFFECT
I'D BEEN HEARING ABOUT THE PATAGONIA OUTLET FOR YEARS. IN THOSE DAYS, PATAGONIA STUFF RARELY WENT ON SALE. YOUR ONLY HOPE OF GETTING A DISCOUNT WAS TO COME HERE.
SIXTY BUCKS!
ON VERY RARE OCCASIONS IN MY LIFE, A NEW GARMENT HAS FELT INSTANTLY RIGHT, AS IF IT HAD BEEN TAILORED EXPRESSLY FOR ME. AS IF I'D ALREADY BEEN WEARING IT FOR YEARS.
ZZZP
SUCH WAS THE CASE WITH THIS NO-NONSENSE BLACK FLEECE CARDIGAN.
IT AFFORDED NOT JUST WARMTH BUT A SENSE OF PROFOUND SAFETY AS I PUT IT ON IN OUR CHILLY HOTEL ON THE OUTSKIRTS OF BOSTON.
THEN WE FOUND OUT THAT AMY'S DAD HAD INDEED DIED.
I HADN'T KNOWN HIM WELL, BUT HE'D ALWAYS BEEN NICE TO ME. IT WAS STRANGE HAVING SOMEONE DIE ON MY BIRTHDAY.
NOW THE SWEATER BEGAN TO FEEL LIKE A KIND OF MOURNING GARMENT.

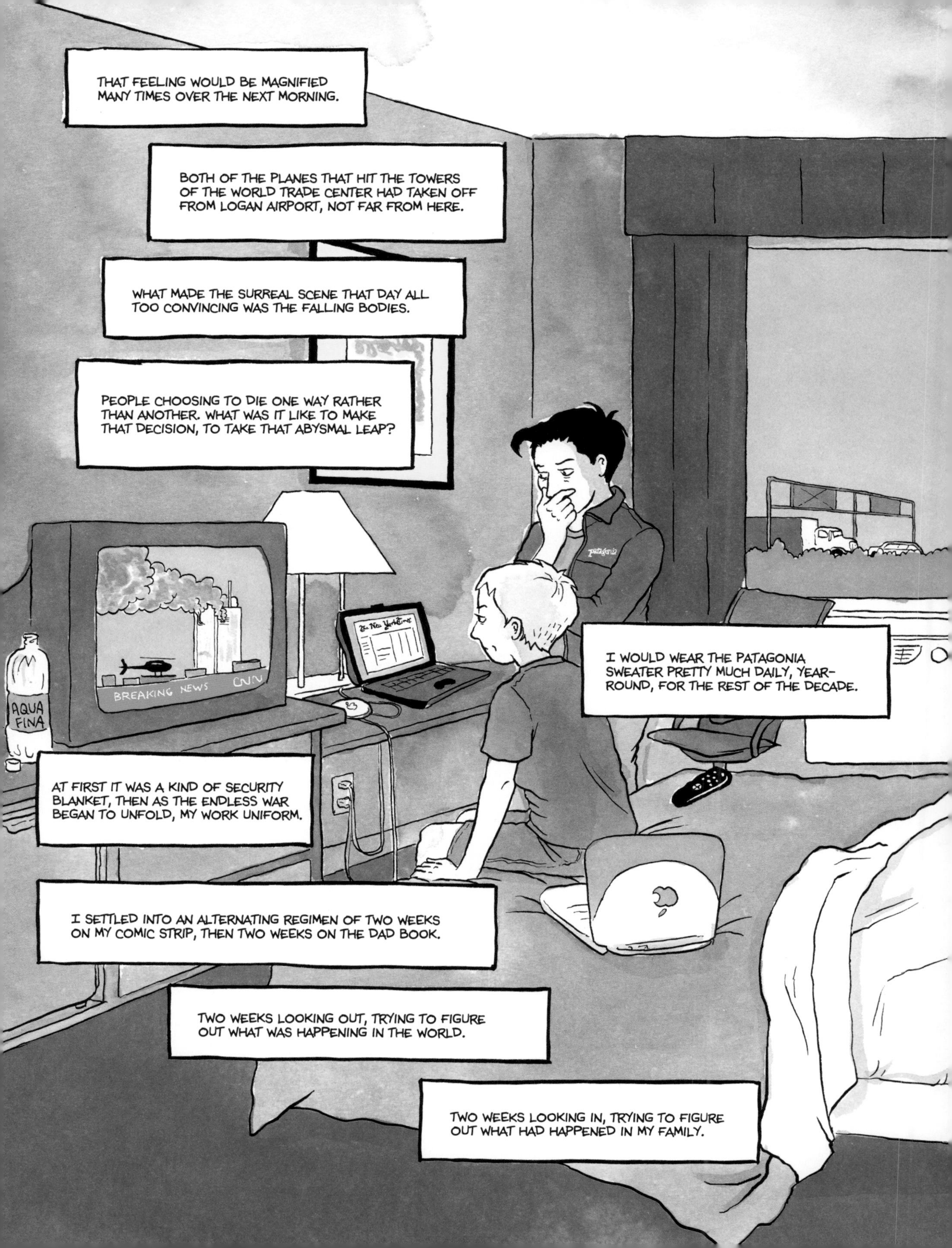
THAT FEELING WOULD BE MAGNIFIED MANY TIMES OVER THE NEXT MORNING.
BOTH OF THE PLANES THAT HIT THE TOWERS OF THE WORLD TRADE CENTER HAD TAKEN OFF FROM LOGAN AIRPORT, NOT FAR FROM HERE.
WHAT MADE THE SURREAL SCENE THAT DAY ALL TOO CONVINCING WAS THE FALLING BODIES.
PEOPLE CHOOSING TO DIE ONE WAY RATHER THAN ANOTHER. WHAT WAS IT LIKE TO MAKE THAT DECISION, TO TAKE THAT ABYSMAL LEAP?
BREAKING NEWS
CNN
AQUA FINA
patagonia
I WOULD WEAR THE PATAGONIA SWEATER PRETTY MUCH DAILY, YEAR-ROUND, FOR THE REST OF THE DECADE.
AT FIRST IT WAS A KIND OF SECURITY BLANKET, THEN AS THE ENDLESS WAR BEGAN TO UNFOLD, MY WORK UNIFORM.
I SETTLED INTO AN ALTERNATING REGIMEN OF TWO WEEKS ON MY COMIC STRIP, THEN TWO WEEKS ON THE DAD BOOK.
TWO WEEKS LOOKING OUT, TRYING TO FIGURE OUT WHAT WAS HAPPENING IN THE WORLD.
TWO WEEKS LOOKING IN, TRYING TO FIGURE OUT WHAT HAD HAPPENED IN MY FAMILY.

I HAD WANTED TO FACE MORTALITY. WAS I HAPPY NOW?

NO, I WAS NOT.

BOTH THE INSIDE AND OUTSIDE WORLDS WERE MAKING ME VERY ANXIOUS, AND IT WAS NO COMFORT TO REALIZE THAT BOTH REALMS OPERATED ACCORDING TO THE SAME PSYCHIC LAWS.

I WAS PARTICULARLY FASCINATED BY THAT CURIOUS CONFUSION OF INSIDE AND OUTSIDE, OF SELF AND OTHER, KNOWN AS "PROJECTION."

STATES LIKE THESE AND THEIR TERRORIST ALLIES CONSTITUTE AN AXIS OF *EVIL*, ARMING TO THREATEN THE PEACE OF THE WORLD.

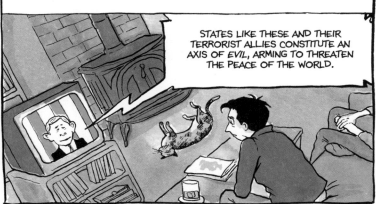

MY TENSION WAS SOMEWHAT RELIEVED BY MOVING HEAVY WEIGHTS, WHETHER IRON PLATES OR MY OWN BODY.

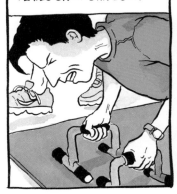

ON DAYS I'D GONE TO THE GYM, I COULD USUALLY FALL RIGHT TO SLEEP. BUT I ONLY HAD TIME FOR THE GYM ONCE A WEEK. FOR A WHILE I WAS ABLE TO SOOTHE MYSELF TO SLEEP BY REPLAYING HOW I'D FIXED A FRIEND'S FLAT ON A BIKE RIDE ONE DAY...

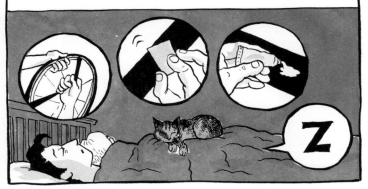

Z

...THE ONLY INDISPUTABLY CONSTRUCTIVE THING I'D ACHIEVED IN QUITE SOME TIME. BUT AFTER A COUPLE MONTHS I HAD WORN OUT THE SCENARIO'S CALMING POWER.

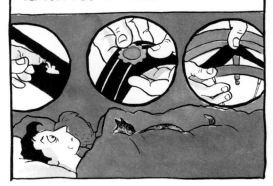

YET DESPITE MY ANXIETY, I WAS SINKING INTO A STATE OF UNUSUALLY DEEP CONCENTRATION ON THE DAD BOOK.

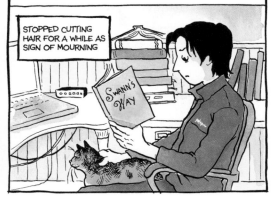

STOPPED CUTTING HAIR FOR A WHILE AS SIGN OF MOURNING

SWANN'S WAY

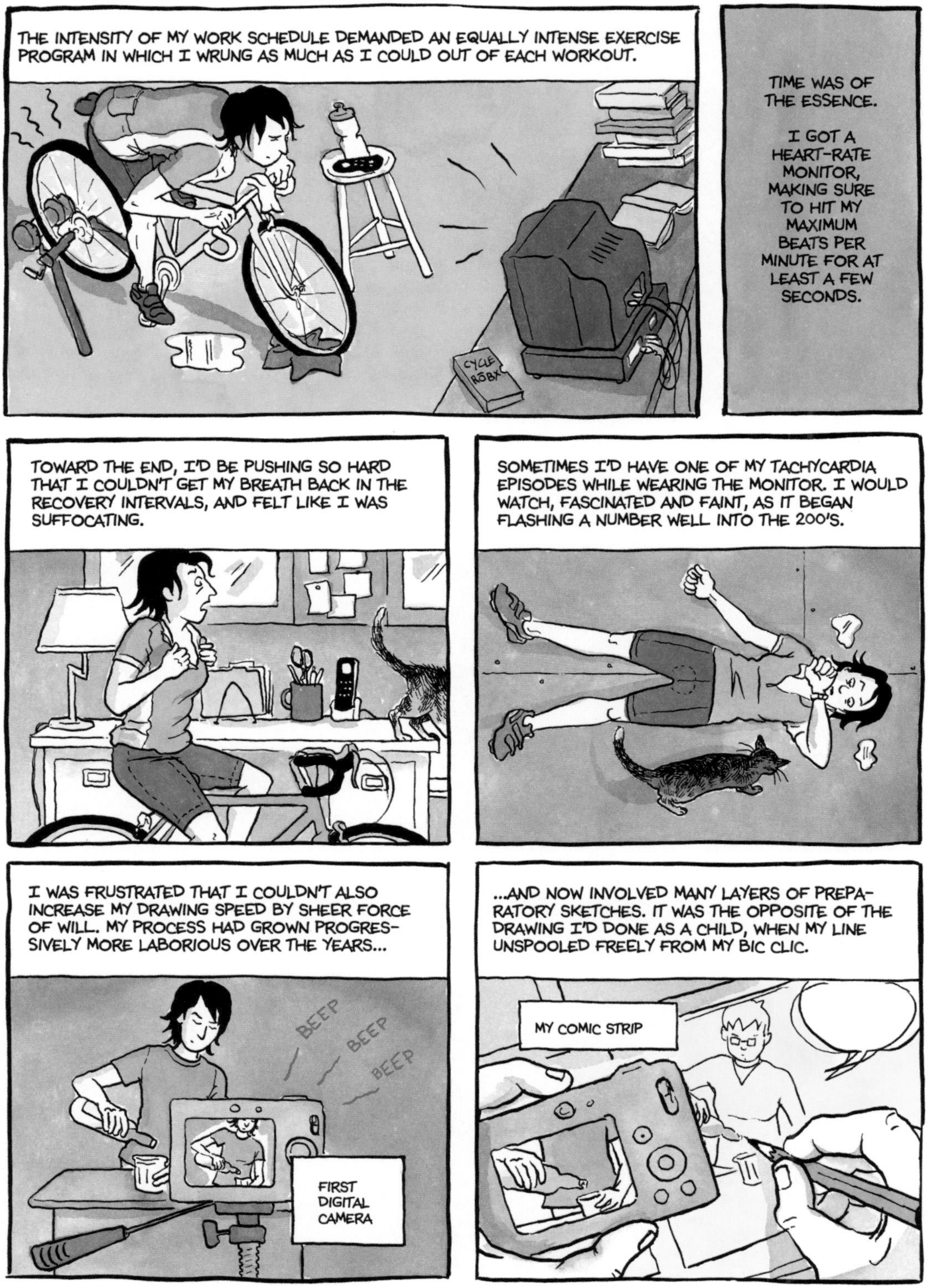
THE INTENSITY OF MY WORK SCHEDULE DEMANDED AN EQUALLY INTENSE EXERCISE PROGRAM IN WHICH I WRUNG AS MUCH AS I COULD OUT OF EACH WORKOUT.
CYCLE RŌBX
TIME WAS OF THE ESSENCE.
I GOT A HEART-RATE MONITOR, MAKING SURE TO HIT MY MAXIMUM BEATS PER MINUTE FOR AT LEAST A FEW SECONDS.
TOWARD THE END, I'D BE PUSHING SO HARD THAT I COULDN'T GET MY BREATH BACK IN THE RECOVERY INTERVALS, AND FELT LIKE I WAS SUFFOCATING.
SOMETIMES I'D HAVE ONE OF MY TACHYCARDIA EPISODES WHILE WEARING THE MONITOR. I WOULD WATCH, FASCINATED AND FAINT, AS IT BEGAN FLASHING A NUMBER WELL INTO THE 200'S.
I WAS FRUSTRATED THAT I COULDN'T ALSO INCREASE MY DRAWING SPEED BY SHEER FORCE OF WILL. MY PROCESS HAD GROWN PROGRESSIVELY MORE LABORIOUS OVER THE YEARS...
BEEP
BEEP
BEEP
FIRST DIGITAL CAMERA
...AND NOW INVOLVED MANY LAYERS OF PREPARATORY SKETCHES. IT WAS THE OPPOSITE OF THE DRAWING I'D DONE AS A CHILD, WHEN MY LINE UNSPOOLED FREELY FROM MY BIC CLIC.
MY COMIC STRIP

I WAS AMPED IN THOSE DAYS. JUST THE IDEA OF "RELAXING" MADE ME WANT TO JUMP OUT OF MY SKIN.

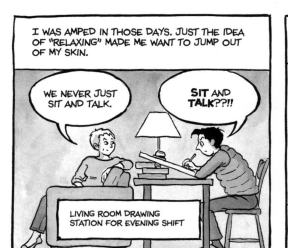

WE NEVER JUST SIT AND TALK.

SIT AND TALK??!!

LIVING ROOM DRAWING STATION FOR EVENING SHIFT

I'D WORK AS LONG AS I COULD, THEN HAVE A NIGHTCAP AS A WAY OF SLAMMING ON THE BRAKES.

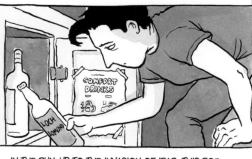

COMFORT DRINKS

LOCH LOMOND

IN THE RUN-UP TO THE INVASION OF IRAQ, THIS ROZ CHAST CARTOON CAME OUT. THE "HOME SECURITY" CALLED FOR "1/2 CUP VANILLA PUDDING, 4 OZ. GIN."

I DIDN'T WANT TO WIND DOWN. I WANTED TO SHUT OFF. TO FEEL NOTHING. THIS WAS NOT UNCONNECTED, I SEE NOW, TO MY WAYWARD AFFECTIONS.

THE BUDDHA CALLED THESE TWO URGES "THE CRAVING FOR EXISTENCE AND NONEXISTENCE."

THE DESIRE FOR A SENSE OF THE SELF AS SOLID, JUST FOR A MOMENT, WHETHER IT'S ATTAINED WITH MERGER OR OBLITERATION.

TORTUOUSLY VEILED EMAIL FLIRTATION

THAT'S WHY YOU NEED TO GET ON THE EIGHT-FOLD PATH--THAT DIFFICULT PATH...

The Nation

FOUR MORE YEARS

Patagonia WINTER 2004

(AT SOME POINT I LEARNED TO COMBINE THE SLEEPING PILL, ACTUALLY AN ANXIOLYTIC CALLED OXAZEPAM, WITH A SLUG OF SCOTCH.)

...LIKE A SHARPENED EDGE OF A RAZOR-- WHICH WILL EVENTUALLY REVEAL TO YOU THAT THE SELF IS EMPTY.

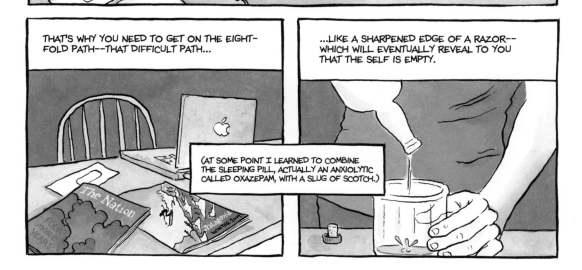

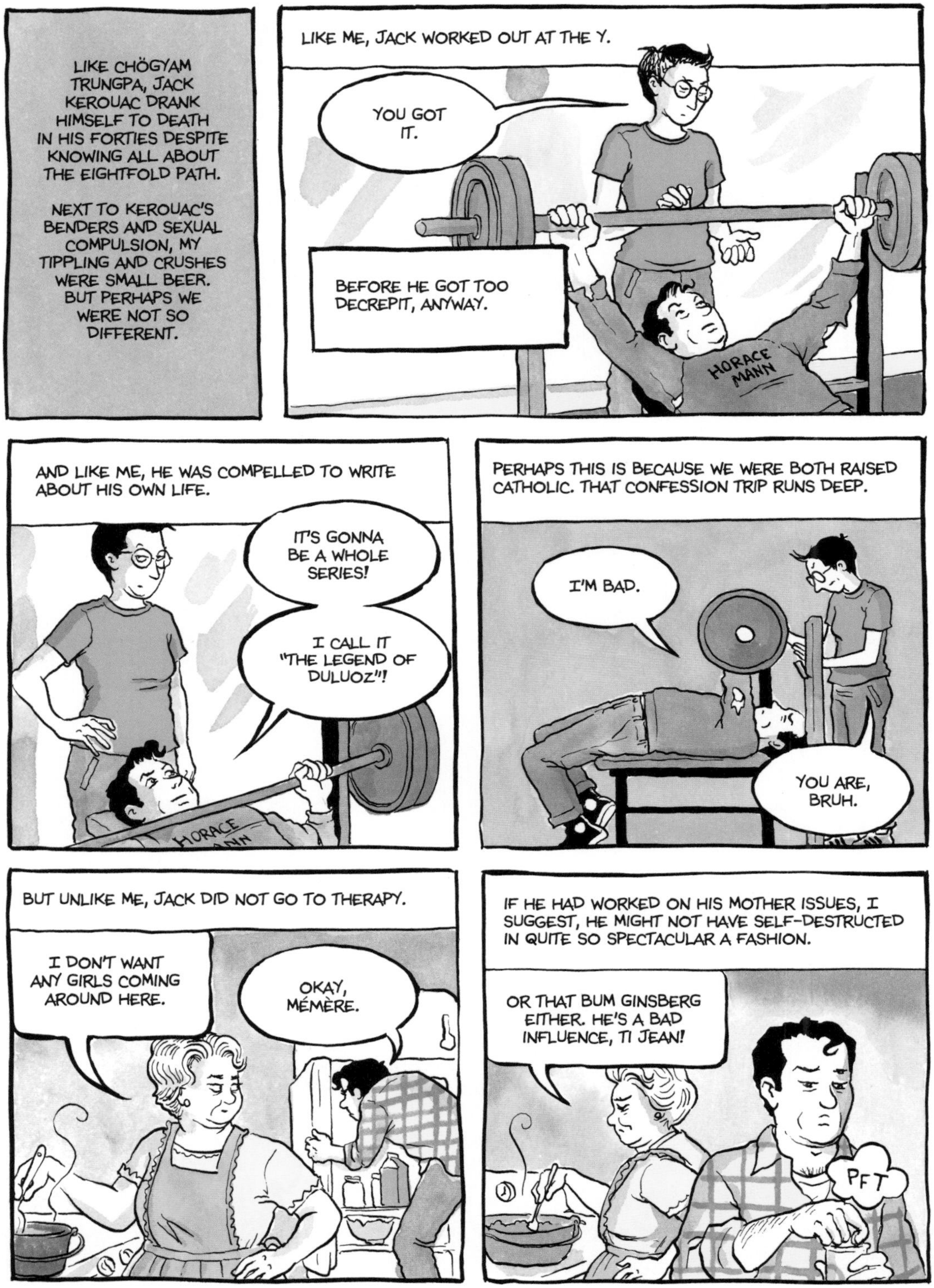

LIKE CHÖGYAM TRUNGPA, JACK KEROUAC DRANK HIMSELF TO DEATH IN HIS FORTIES DESPITE KNOWING ALL ABOUT THE EIGHTFOLD PATH.
NEXT TO KEROUAC'S BENDERS AND SEXUAL COMPULSION, MY TIPPLING AND CRUSHES WERE SMALL BEER. BUT PERHAPS WE WERE NOT SO DIFFERENT.
LIKE ME, JACK WORKED OUT AT THE Y.
YOU GOT IT.
BEFORE HE GOT TOO DECREPIT, ANYWAY.
HORACE MANN
AND LIKE ME, HE WAS COMPELLED TO WRITE ABOUT HIS OWN LIFE.
IT'S GONNA BE A WHOLE SERIES!
I CALL IT "THE LEGEND OF DULUOZ"!
HORACE MANN
PERHAPS THIS IS BECAUSE WE WERE BOTH RAISED CATHOLIC. THAT CONFESSION TRIP RUNS DEEP.
I'M BAD.
YOU ARE, BRUH.
BUT UNLIKE ME, JACK DID NOT GO TO THERAPY.
I DON'T WANT ANY GIRLS COMING AROUND HERE.
OKAY, MÉMÈRE.
IF HE HAD WORKED ON HIS MOTHER ISSUES, I SUGGEST, HE MIGHT NOT HAVE SELF-DESTRUCTED IN QUITE SO SPECTACULAR A FASHION.
OR THAT BUM GINSBERG EITHER. HE'S A BAD INFLUENCE, TI JEAN!
PFT

AS MOVINGLY AS KEROUAC WROTE ABOUT LIBERATION, HE WOULD NEVER ATTAIN IT IN REAL LIFE. DESPITE ALL HIS WANDERINGS, "GIRLS," AND BINGES, HE WOULD REMAIN A PSYCHIC PRISONER OF HIS MOTHER.

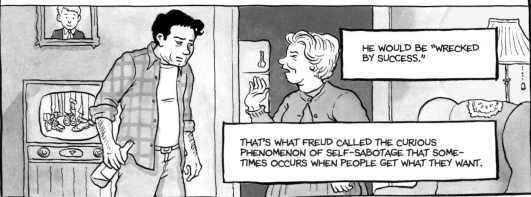

HE WOULD BE "WRECKED BY SUCCESS."

THAT'S WHAT FREUD CALLED THE CURIOUS PHENOMENON OF SELF-SABOTAGE THAT SOMETIMES OCCURS WHEN PEOPLE GET WHAT THEY WANT.

MOST PEOPLE DON'T EVEN TRY TO GET WHAT THEY WANT BECAUSE OF THE PAINFUL RECKONING WITH THEIR PARENTS IT ENTAILS.

I WOULD HAVE MY OWN STRUGGLES WITH "SUCCESS." I WAS STILL PLODDING ALONG ON THE DAD BOOK WHEN IT WAS BOUGHT BY A BIG PUBLISHER.

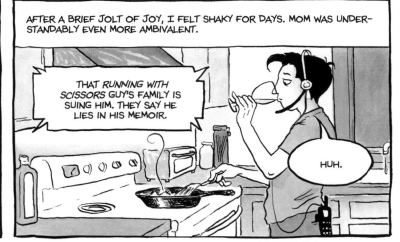

AFTER A BRIEF JOLT OF JOY, I FELT SHAKY FOR DAYS. MOM WAS UNDERSTANDABLY EVEN MORE AMBIVALENT.

THAT *RUNNING WITH SCISSORS* GUY'S FAMILY IS SUING HIM. THEY SAY HE LIES IN HIS MEMOIR.

HUH.

KEROUAC FAMOUSLY WROTE *ON THE ROAD* IN A FRENZIED THREE-WEEK BURST ON A LONG SCROLL OF TAPED-TOGETHER PAPER IN 1951. OVER THE NEXT FIVE YEARS, IT WAS REJECTED BY A BUNCH OF PUBLISHERS.

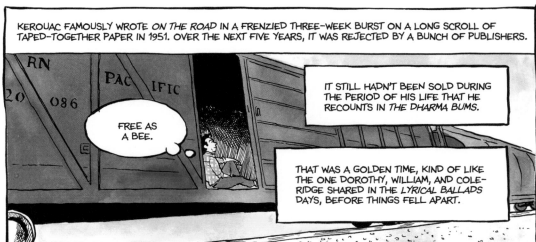

RN
20 086
PAC IFIC

FREE AS A BEE.

IT STILL HADN'T BEEN SOLD DURING THE PERIOD OF HIS LIFE THAT HE RECOUNTS IN *THE DHARMA BUMS*.

THAT WAS A GOLDEN TIME, KIND OF LIKE THE ONE DOROTHY, WILLIAM, AND COLERIDGE SHARED IN THE *LYRICAL BALLADS* DAYS, BEFORE THINGS FELL APART.

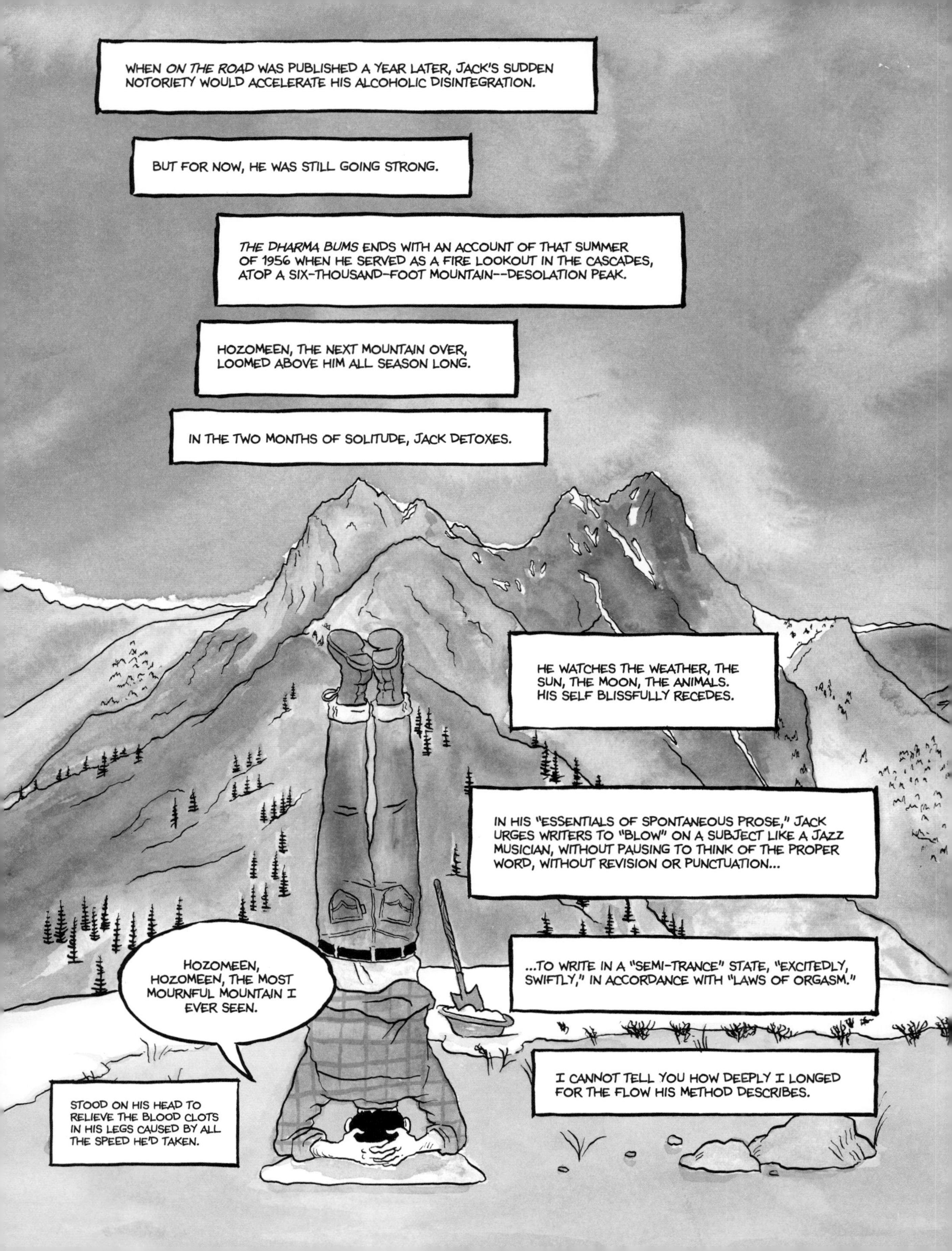
WHEN *ON THE ROAD* WAS PUBLISHED A YEAR LATER, JACK'S SUDDEN NOTORIETY WOULD ACCELERATE HIS ALCOHOLIC DISINTEGRATION.
BUT FOR NOW, HE WAS STILL GOING STRONG.
THE DHARMA BUMS ENDS WITH AN ACCOUNT OF THAT SUMMER OF 1956 WHEN HE SERVED AS A FIRE LOOKOUT IN THE CASCADES, ATOP A SIX-THOUSAND-FOOT MOUNTAIN--DESOLATION PEAK.
HOZOMEEN, THE NEXT MOUNTAIN OVER, LOOMED ABOVE HIM ALL SEASON LONG.
IN THE TWO MONTHS OF SOLITUDE, JACK DETOXES.
HE WATCHES THE WEATHER, THE SUN, THE MOON, THE ANIMALS. HIS SELF BLISSFULLY RECEDES.
IN HIS "ESSENTIALS OF SPONTANEOUS PROSE," JACK URGES WRITERS TO "BLOW" ON A SUBJECT LIKE A JAZZ MUSICIAN, WITHOUT PAUSING TO THINK OF THE PROPER WORD, WITHOUT REVISION OR PUNCTUATION...
...TO WRITE IN A "SEMI-TRANCE" STATE, "EXCITEDLY, SWIFTLY," IN ACCORDANCE WITH "LAWS OF ORGASM."
HOZOMEEN, HOZOMEEN, THE MOST MOURNFUL MOUNTAIN I EVER SEEN.
STOOD ON HIS HEAD TO RELIEVE THE BLOOD CLOTS IN HIS LEGS CAUSED BY ALL THE SPEED HE'D TAKEN.
I CANNOT TELL YOU HOW DEEPLY I LONGED FOR THE FLOW HIS METHOD DESCRIBES.

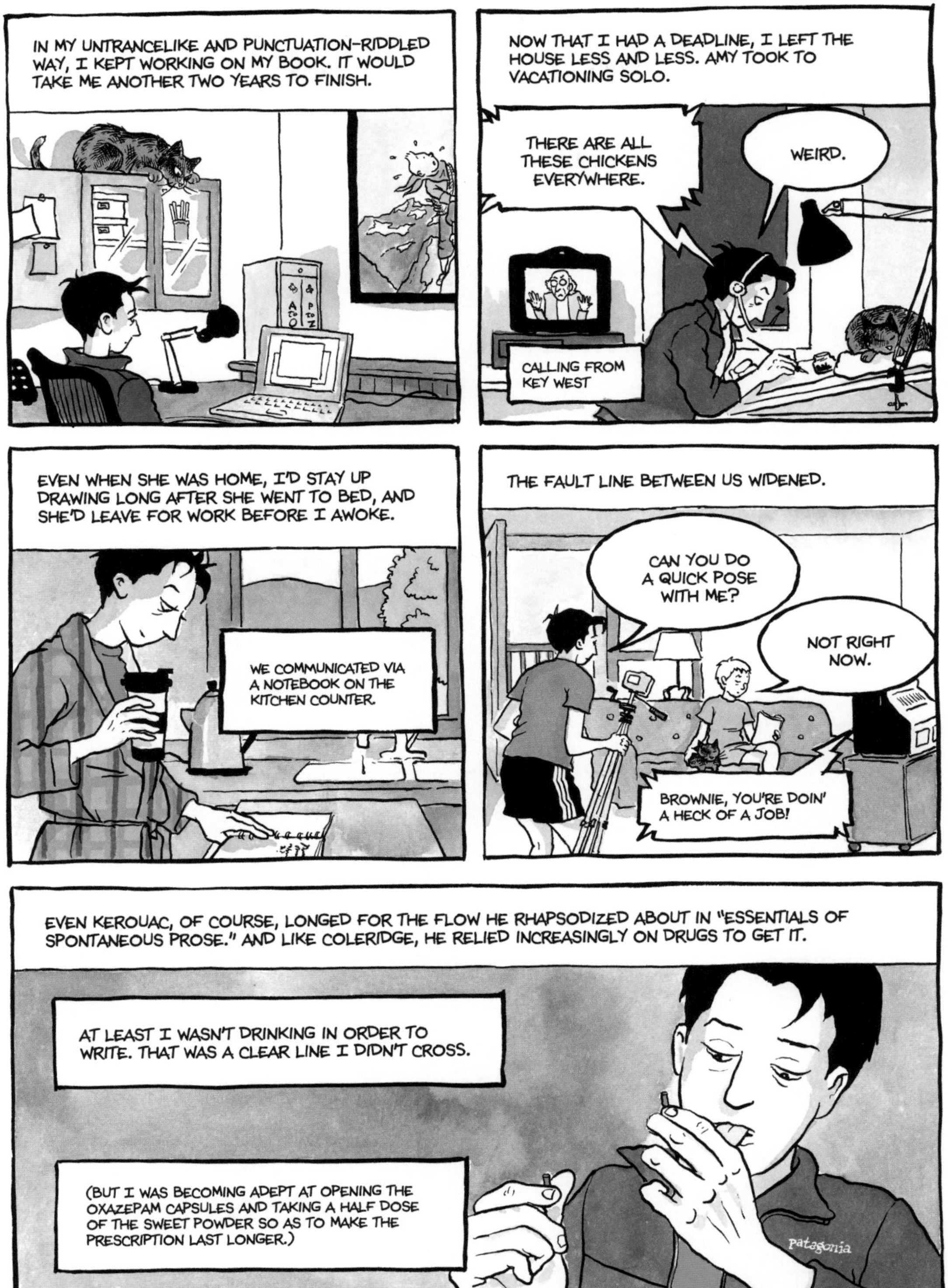
IN MY UNTRANCELIKE AND PUNCTUATION-RIDDLED WAY, I KEPT WORKING ON MY BOOK. IT WOULD TAKE ME ANOTHER TWO YEARS TO FINISH.
NOW THAT I HAD A DEADLINE, I LEFT THE HOUSE LESS AND LESS. AMY TOOK TO VACATIONING SOLO.
THERE ARE ALL THESE CHICKENS EVERYWHERE.
WEIRD.
CALLING FROM KEY WEST
EVEN WHEN SHE WAS HOME, I'D STAY UP DRAWING LONG AFTER SHE WENT TO BED, AND SHE'D LEAVE FOR WORK BEFORE I AWOKE.
WE COMMUNICATED VIA A NOTEBOOK ON THE KITCHEN COUNTER.
THE FAULT LINE BETWEEN US WIDENED.
CAN YOU DO A QUICK POSE WITH ME?
NOT RIGHT NOW.
BROWNIE, YOU'RE DOIN' A HECK OF A JOB!
EVEN KEROUAC, OF COURSE, LONGED FOR THE FLOW HE RHAPSODIZED ABOUT IN "ESSENTIALS OF SPONTANEOUS PROSE." AND LIKE COLERIDGE, HE RELIED INCREASINGLY ON DRUGS TO GET IT.
AT LEAST I WASN'T DRINKING IN ORDER TO WRITE. THAT WAS A CLEAR LINE I DIDN'T CROSS.
(BUT I WAS BECOMING ADEPT AT OPENING THE OXAZEPAM CAPSULES AND TAKING A HALF DOSE OF THE SWEET POWDER SO AS TO MAKE THE PRESCRIPTION LAST LONGER.)
patagonia

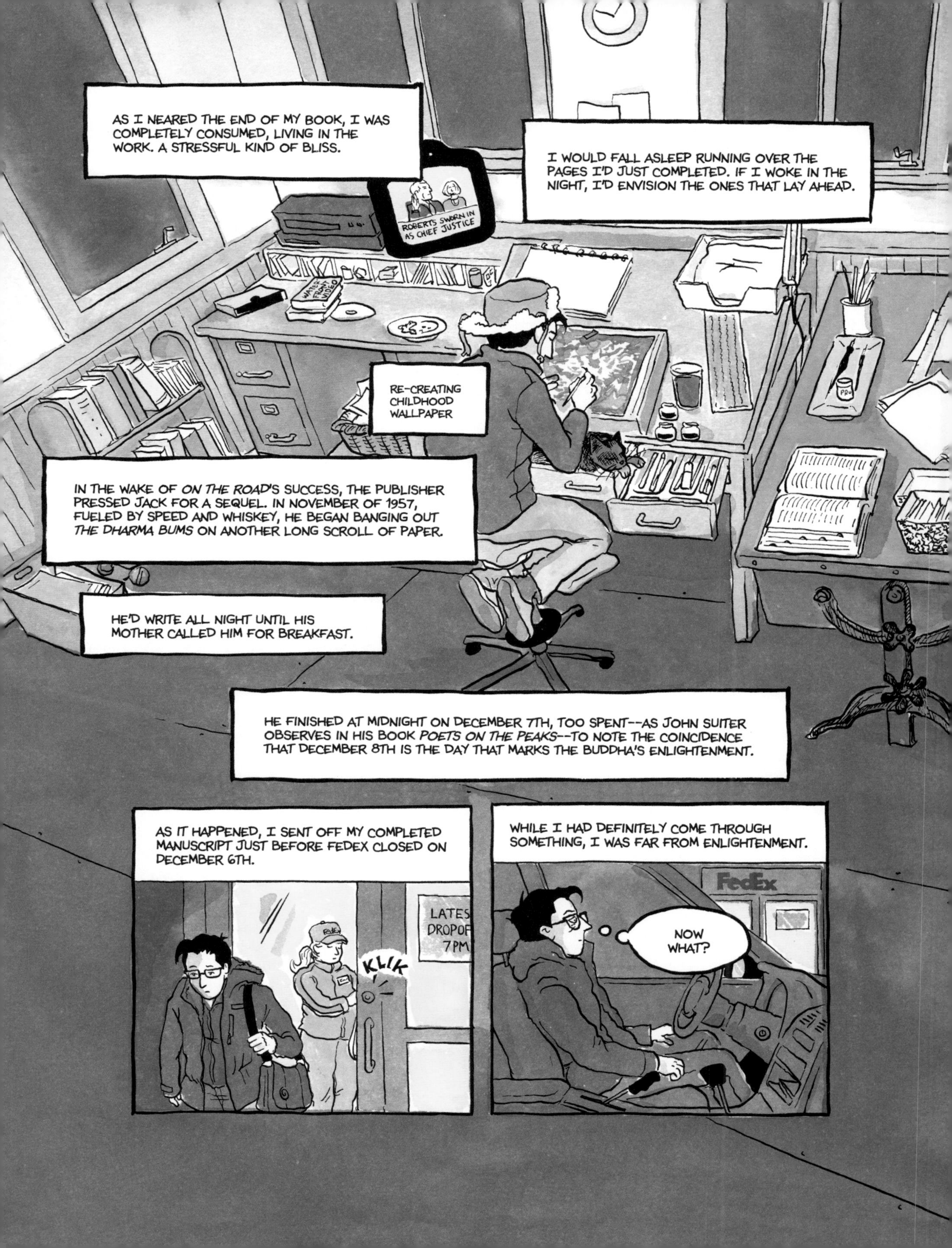
AS I NEARED THE END OF MY BOOK, I WAS COMPLETELY CONSUMED, LIVING IN THE WORK. A STRESSFUL KIND OF BLISS.
ROBERTS SWORN IN AS CHIEF JUSTICE
I WOULD FALL ASLEEP RUNNING OVER THE PAGES I'D JUST COMPLETED. IF I WOKE IN THE NIGHT, I'D ENVISION THE ONES THAT LAY AHEAD.
WATERFRONT VIDEO
RE-CREATING CHILDHOOD WALLPAPER
IN THE WAKE OF *ON THE ROAD*'S SUCCESS, THE PUBLISHER PRESSED JACK FOR A SEQUEL. IN NOVEMBER OF 1957, FUELED BY SPEED AND WHISKEY, HE BEGAN BANGING OUT *THE DHARMA BUMS* ON ANOTHER LONG SCROLL OF PAPER.
HE'D WRITE ALL NIGHT UNTIL HIS MOTHER CALLED HIM FOR BREAKFAST.
HE FINISHED AT MIDNIGHT ON DECEMBER 7TH, TOO SPENT--AS JOHN SUITER OBSERVES IN HIS BOOK *POETS ON THE PEAKS*--TO NOTE THE COINCIDENCE THAT DECEMBER 8TH IS THE DAY THAT MARKS THE BUDDHA'S ENLIGHTENMENT.
AS IT HAPPENED, I SENT OFF MY COMPLETED MANUSCRIPT JUST BEFORE FEDEX CLOSED ON DECEMBER 6TH.
LATES DROPOF 7PM
KLIK
WHILE I HAD DEFINITELY COME THROUGH SOMETHING, I WAS FAR FROM ENLIGHTENMENT.
FedEx
NOW WHAT?

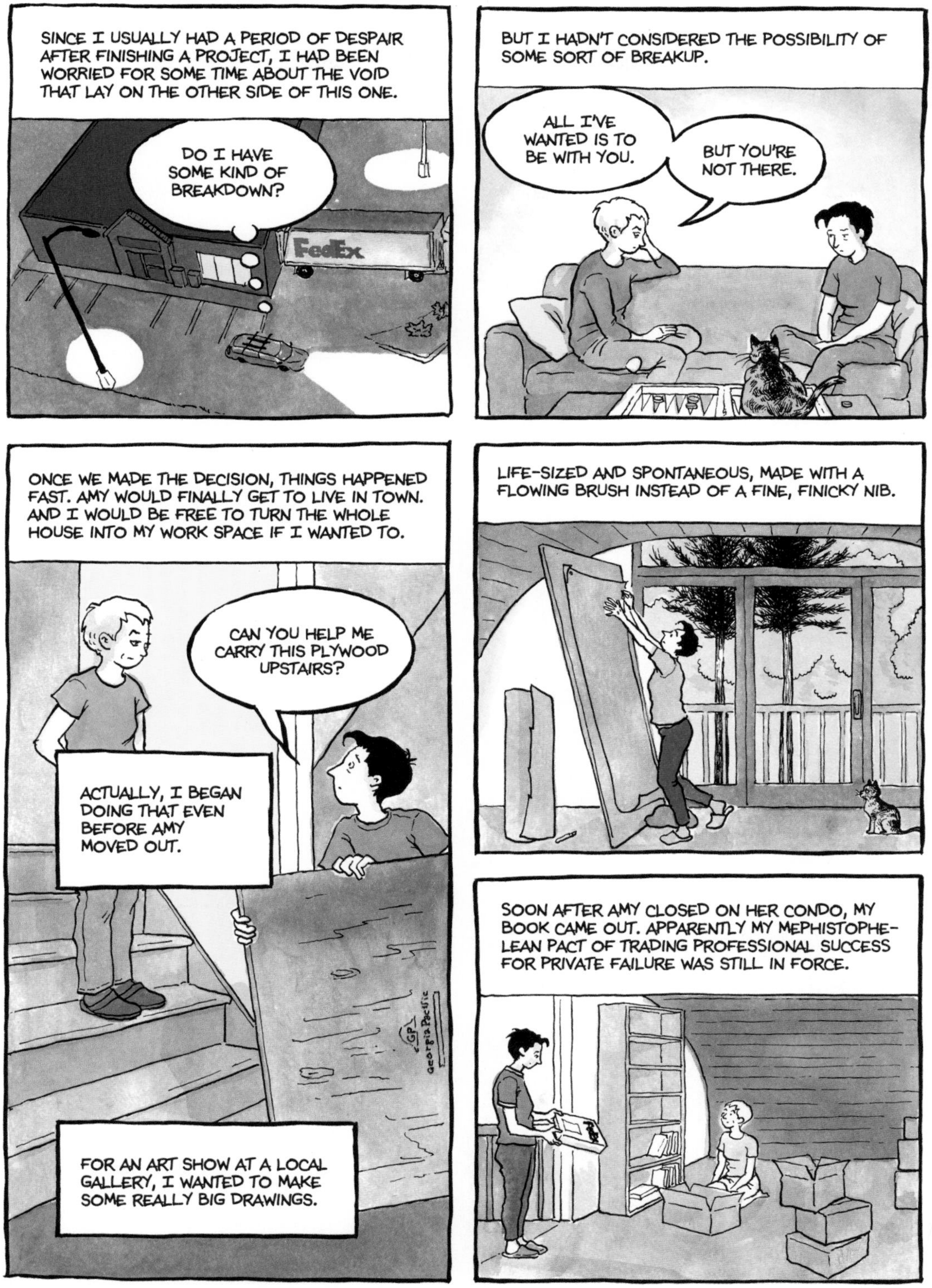
SINCE I USUALLY HAD A PERIOD OF DESPAIR AFTER FINISHING A PROJECT, I HAD BEEN WORRIED FOR SOME TIME ABOUT THE VOID THAT LAY ON THE OTHER SIDE OF THIS ONE.
DO I HAVE SOME KIND OF BREAKDOWN?
FedEx
BUT I HADN'T CONSIDERED THE POSSIBILITY OF SOME SORT OF BREAKUP.
ALL I'VE WANTED IS TO BE WITH YOU.
BUT YOU'RE NOT THERE.
ONCE WE MADE THE DECISION, THINGS HAPPENED FAST. AMY WOULD FINALLY GET TO LIVE IN TOWN. AND I WOULD BE FREE TO TURN THE WHOLE HOUSE INTO MY WORK SPACE IF I WANTED TO.
CAN YOU HELP ME CARRY THIS PLYWOOD UPSTAIRS?
ACTUALLY, I BEGAN DOING THAT EVEN BEFORE AMY MOVED OUT.
FOR AN ART SHOW AT A LOCAL GALLERY, I WANTED TO MAKE SOME REALLY BIG DRAWINGS.
LIFE-SIZED AND SPONTANEOUS, MADE WITH A FLOWING BRUSH INSTEAD OF A FINE, FINICKY NIB.
SOON AFTER AMY CLOSED ON HER CONDO, MY BOOK CAME OUT. APPARENTLY MY MEPHISTOPHE-LEAN PACT OF TRADING PROFESSIONAL SUCCESS FOR PRIVATE FAILURE WAS STILL IN FORCE.

MY THERAPIST WARNED ME THAT I'D HAVE TO TAKE BACK ALL THE UNWANTED ASPECTS OF MY OWN SELF I'D PROJECTED ONTO AMY.
YOU'LL HAVE TO FEEL YOUR SADNESS.
BUT I WAS TOO BUSY BEING SHOT OUT OF A CANNON TO FEEL SAD. AS WE DIVIDED OUR STUFF, THE PRESS CAMPAIGN FOR THE BOOK BEGAN.
GOD. THE PHOTOGRAPHER FROM *PEOPLE* IS COMING TOMORROW.
CUISINART?
TAKE IT.
MOM TOOK MY SPLIT WITH AMY IN STRIDE--INDEED, SHE SEEMED TO PREFER ME SINGLE. SHE ALSO SEEMED TO TAKE SOME VICARIOUS THOUGH NOT UNMIXED PLEASURE IN THE PUBLICITY BUZZ.
THEY'RE FLYING ME TO NEW YORK FOR A PHOTO SHOOT WITH *ENTERTAINMENT WEEKLY.*
ENTERTAINMENT WEEKLY?!
SHE'D JUST HAD A COLONOSCOPY THAT REVEALED A POLYP.
ENRON
SHE WOULD HAVE THIS SURGICALLY REMOVED WHILE I WAS ON MY BOOK TOUR.
OH, I DON'T NEED YOU. BOB* WILL TAKE ME.
OKAY, I'LL LET YOU GO. GOTTA GET MY LAPS IN.
SAVOY THEATER
kitchen stuff
*HER BOYFRIEND
I WASN'T TOO WORRIED. SHE WAS IN BETTER SHAPE THAN I WAS. BESIDES, I WAS OFF.
STAYED WITH THE CAT WHILE I WAS GONE

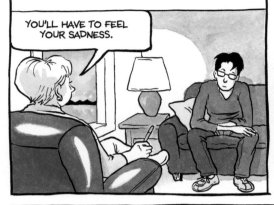

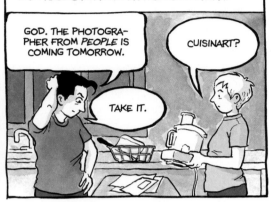

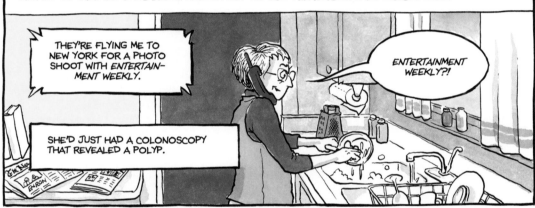

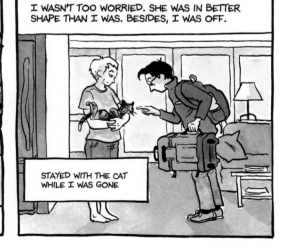

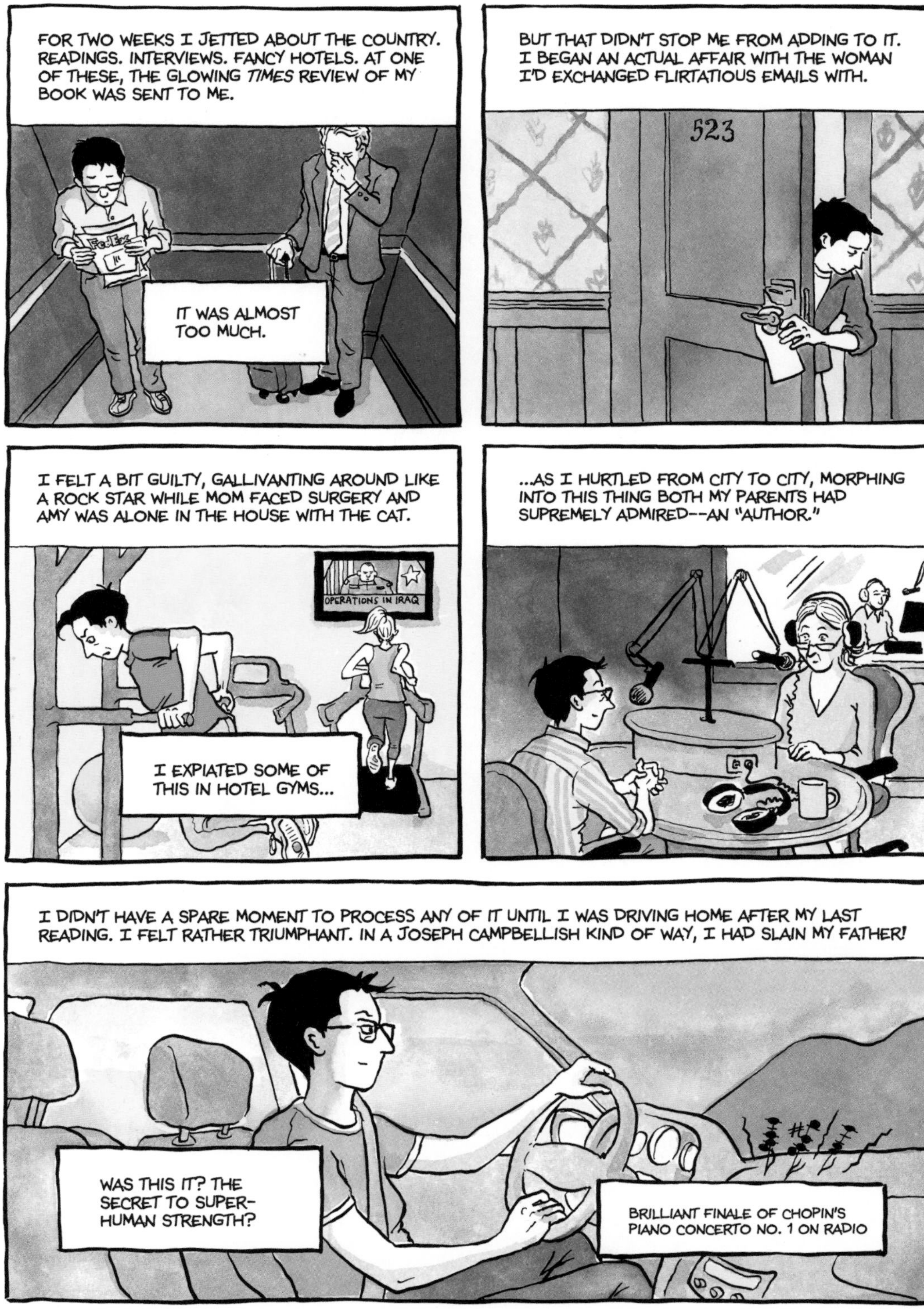

FOR TWO WEEKS I JETTED ABOUT THE COUNTRY. READINGS. INTERVIEWS. FANCY HOTELS. AT ONE OF THESE, THE GLOWING *TIMES* REVIEW OF MY BOOK WAS SENT TO ME.
FedEx
IT WAS ALMOST TOO MUCH.
BUT THAT DIDN'T STOP ME FROM ADDING TO IT. I BEGAN AN ACTUAL AFFAIR WITH THE WOMAN I'D EXCHANGED FLIRTATIOUS EMAILS WITH.
523
I FELT A BIT GUILTY, GALLIVANTING AROUND LIKE A ROCK STAR WHILE MOM FACED SURGERY AND AMY WAS ALONE IN THE HOUSE WITH THE CAT.
OPERATIONS IN IRAQ
I EXPIATED SOME OF THIS IN HOTEL GYMS...
...AS I HURTLED FROM CITY TO CITY, MORPHING INTO THIS THING BOTH MY PARENTS HAD SUPREMELY ADMIRED--AN "AUTHOR."
I DIDN'T HAVE A SPARE MOMENT TO PROCESS ANY OF IT UNTIL I WAS DRIVING HOME AFTER MY LAST READING. I FELT RATHER TRIUMPHANT. IN A JOSEPH CAMPBELLISH KIND OF WAY, I HAD SLAIN MY FATHER!
WAS THIS IT? THE SECRET TO SUPER-HUMAN STRENGTH?
BRILLIANT FINALE OF CHOPIN'S PIANO CONCERTO NO. 1 ON RADIO

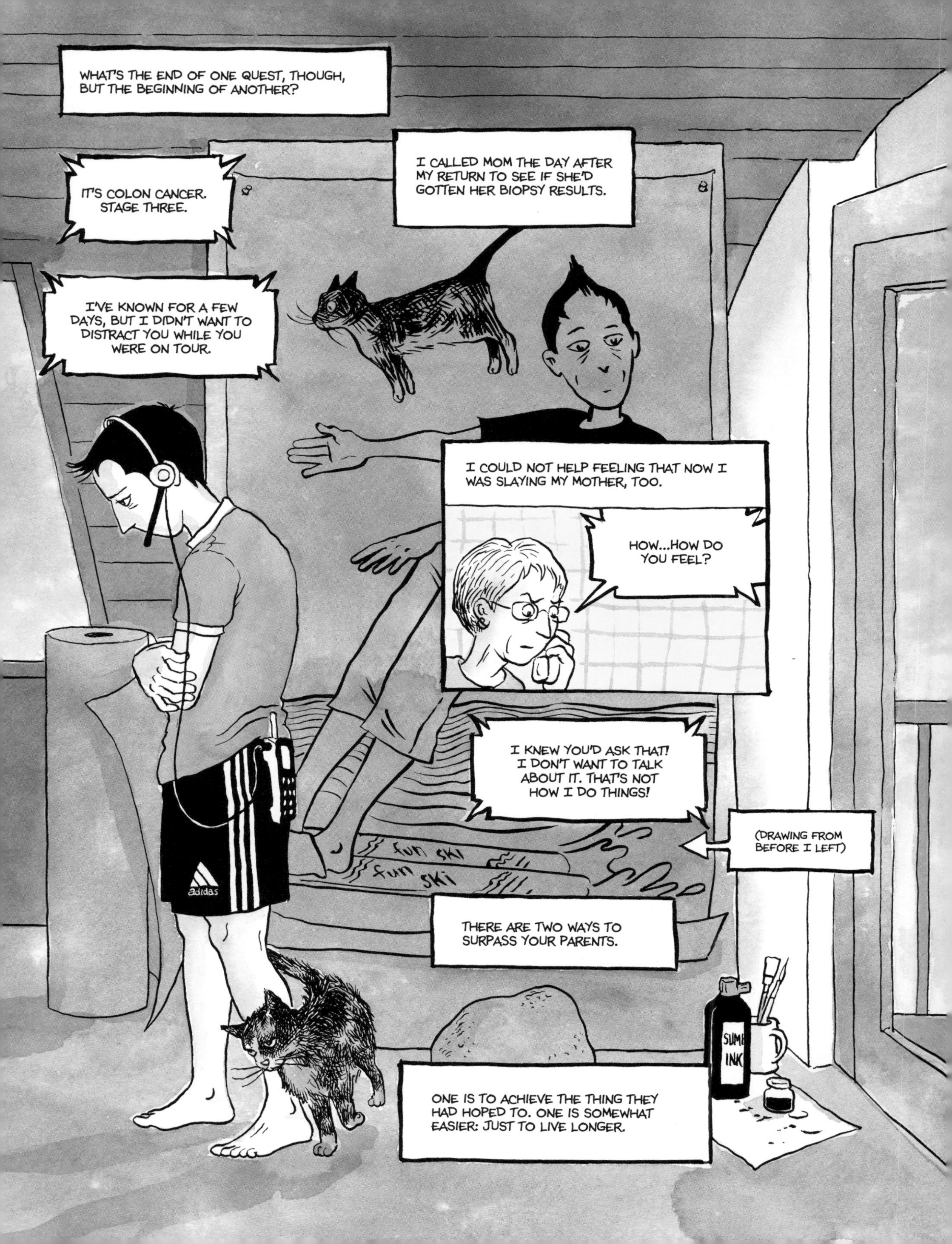
WHAT'S THE END OF ONE QUEST, THOUGH, BUT THE BEGINNING OF ANOTHER?
I CALLED MOM THE DAY AFTER MY RETURN TO SEE IF SHE'D GOTTEN HER BIOPSY RESULTS.
IT'S COLON CANCER. STAGE THREE.
I'VE KNOWN FOR A FEW DAYS, BUT I DIDN'T WANT TO DISTRACT YOU WHILE YOU WERE ON TOUR.
I COULD NOT HELP FEELING THAT NOW I WAS SLAYING MY MOTHER, TOO.
HOW...HOW DO YOU FEEL?
I KNEW YOU'D ASK THAT! I DON'T WANT TO TALK ABOUT IT. THAT'S NOT HOW I DO THINGS!
(DRAWING FROM BEFORE I LEFT)
fun ski
fun ski
adidas
THERE ARE TWO WAYS TO SURPASS YOUR PARENTS.
SUMI INK
ONE IS TO ACHIEVE THE THING THEY HAD HOPED TO. ONE IS SOMEWHAT EASIER: JUST TO LIVE LONGER.

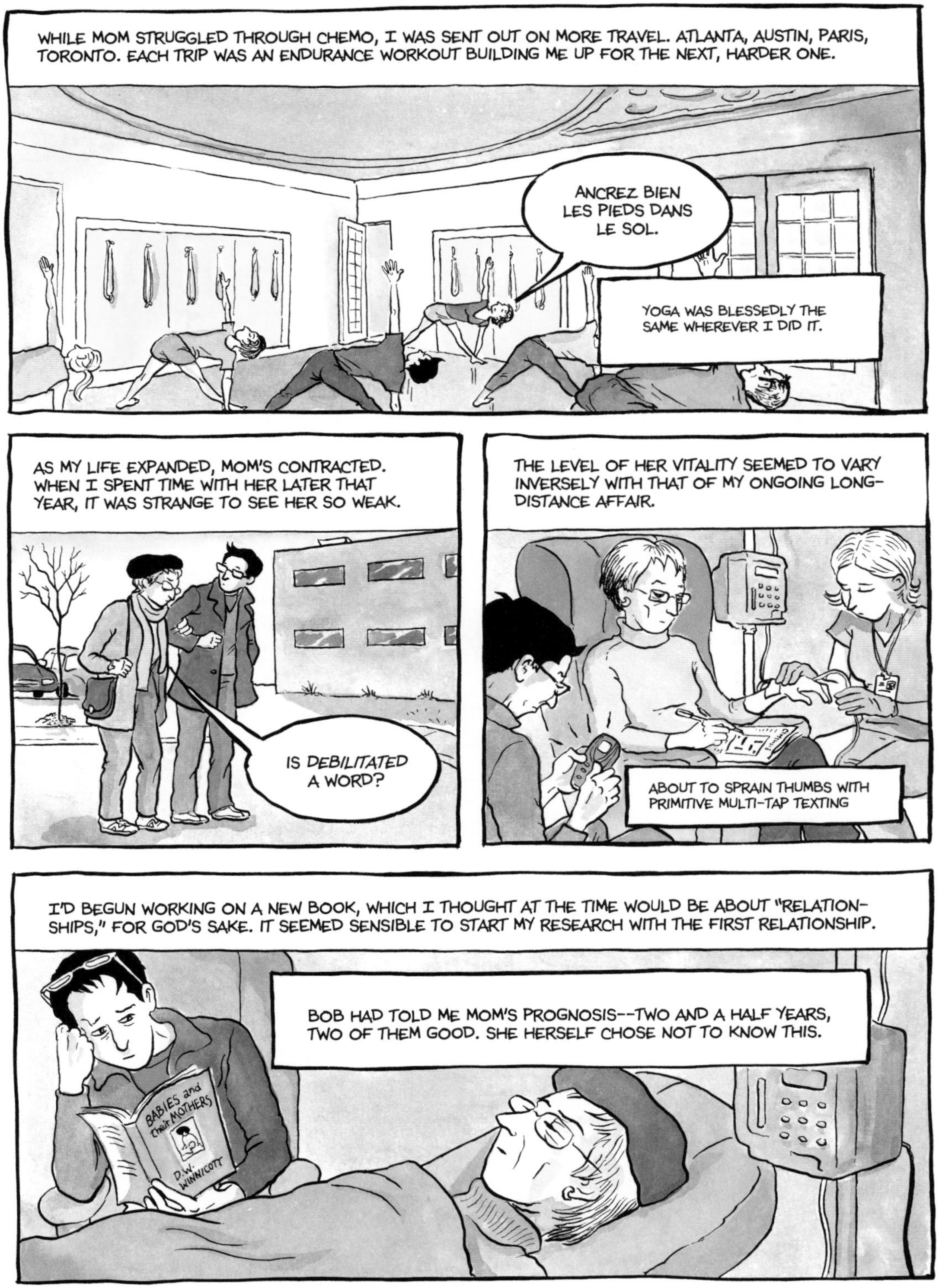
WHILE MOM STRUGGLED THROUGH CHEMO, I WAS SENT OUT ON MORE TRAVEL. ATLANTA, AUSTIN, PARIS, TORONTO. EACH TRIP WAS AN ENDURANCE WORKOUT BUILDING ME UP FOR THE NEXT, HARDER ONE.
ANCREZ BIEN LES PIEDS DANS LE SOL.
YOGA WAS BLESSEDLY THE SAME WHEREVER I DID IT.
AS MY LIFE EXPANDED, MOM'S CONTRACTED. WHEN I SPENT TIME WITH HER LATER THAT YEAR, IT WAS STRANGE TO SEE HER SO WEAK.
IS *DEBILITATED* A WORD?
THE LEVEL OF HER VITALITY SEEMED TO VARY INVERSELY WITH THAT OF MY ONGOING LONG-DISTANCE AFFAIR.
ABOUT TO SPRAIN THUMBS WITH PRIMITIVE MULTI-TAP TEXTING
I'D BEGUN WORKING ON A NEW BOOK, WHICH I THOUGHT AT THE TIME WOULD BE ABOUT "RELATIONSHIPS," FOR GOD'S SAKE. IT SEEMED SENSIBLE TO START MY RESEARCH WITH THE FIRST RELATIONSHIP.
BOB HAD TOLD ME MOM'S PROGNOSIS--TWO AND A HALF YEARS, TWO OF THEM GOOD. SHE HERSELF CHOSE NOT TO KNOW THIS.
BABIES and their MOTHERS
D.W. WINNICOTT

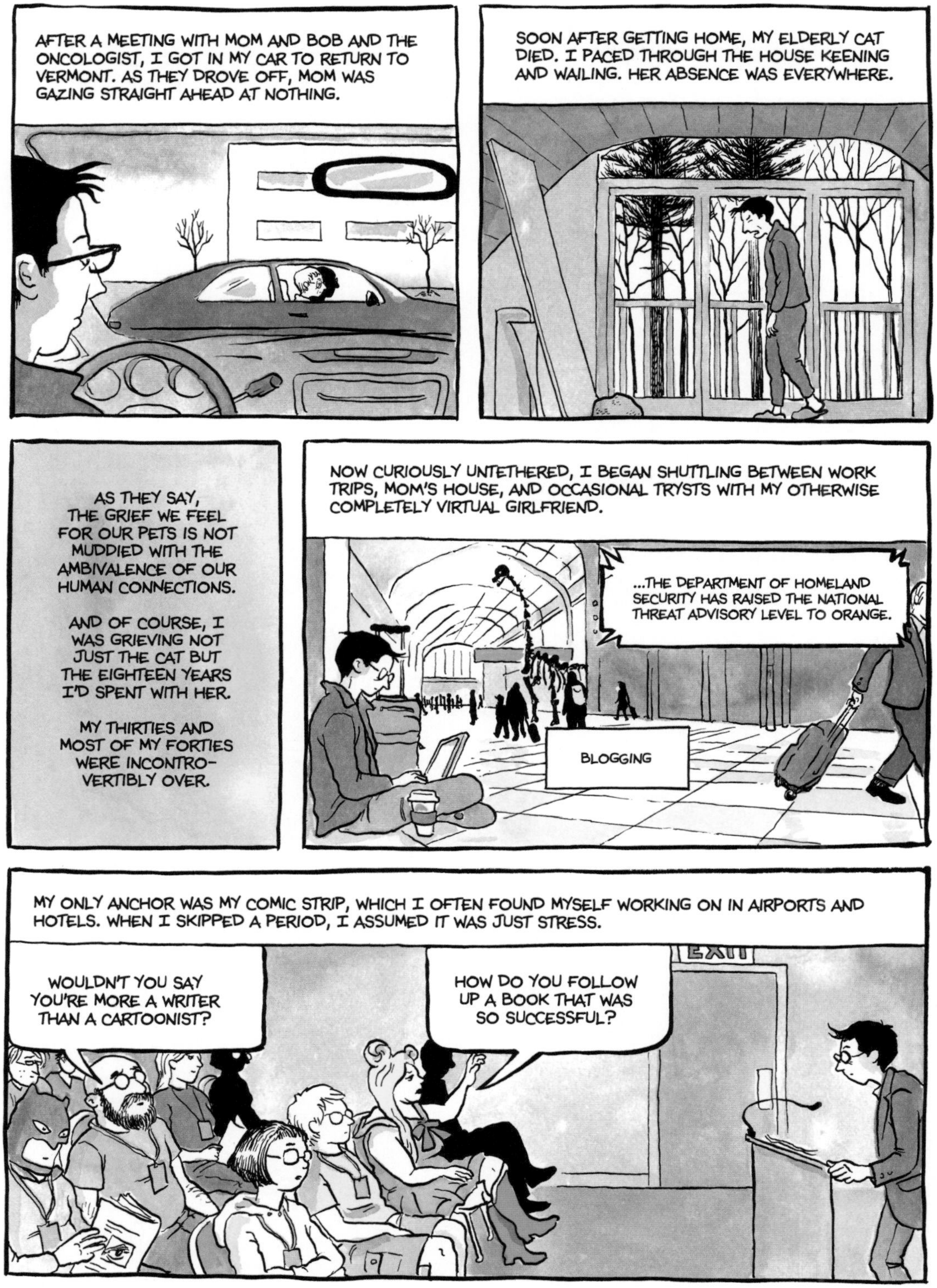
AFTER A MEETING WITH MOM AND BOB AND THE ONCOLOGIST, I GOT IN MY CAR TO RETURN TO VERMONT. AS THEY DROVE OFF, MOM WAS GAZING STRAIGHT AHEAD AT NOTHING.
SOON AFTER GETTING HOME, MY ELDERLY CAT DIED. I PACED THROUGH THE HOUSE KEENING AND WAILING. HER ABSENCE WAS EVERYWHERE.
AS THEY SAY, THE GRIEF WE FEEL FOR OUR PETS IS NOT MUDDIED WITH THE AMBIVALENCE OF OUR HUMAN CONNECTIONS.
AND OF COURSE, I WAS GRIEVING NOT JUST THE CAT BUT THE EIGHTEEN YEARS I'D SPENT WITH HER.
MY THIRTIES AND MOST OF MY FORTIES WERE INCONTRO-VERTIBLY OVER.
NOW CURIOUSLY UNTETHERED, I BEGAN SHUTTLING BETWEEN WORK TRIPS, MOM'S HOUSE, AND OCCASIONAL TRYSTS WITH MY OTHERWISE COMPLETELY VIRTUAL GIRLFRIEND.
...THE DEPARTMENT OF HOMELAND SECURITY HAS RAISED THE NATIONAL THREAT ADVISORY LEVEL TO ORANGE.
BLOGGING
MY ONLY ANCHOR WAS MY COMIC STRIP, WHICH I OFTEN FOUND MYSELF WORKING ON IN AIRPORTS AND HOTELS. WHEN I SKIPPED A PERIOD, I ASSUMED IT WAS JUST STRESS.
EXIT
WOULDN'T YOU SAY YOU'RE MORE A WRITER THAN A CARTOONIST?
HOW DO YOU FOLLOW UP A BOOK THAT WAS SO SUCCESSFUL?

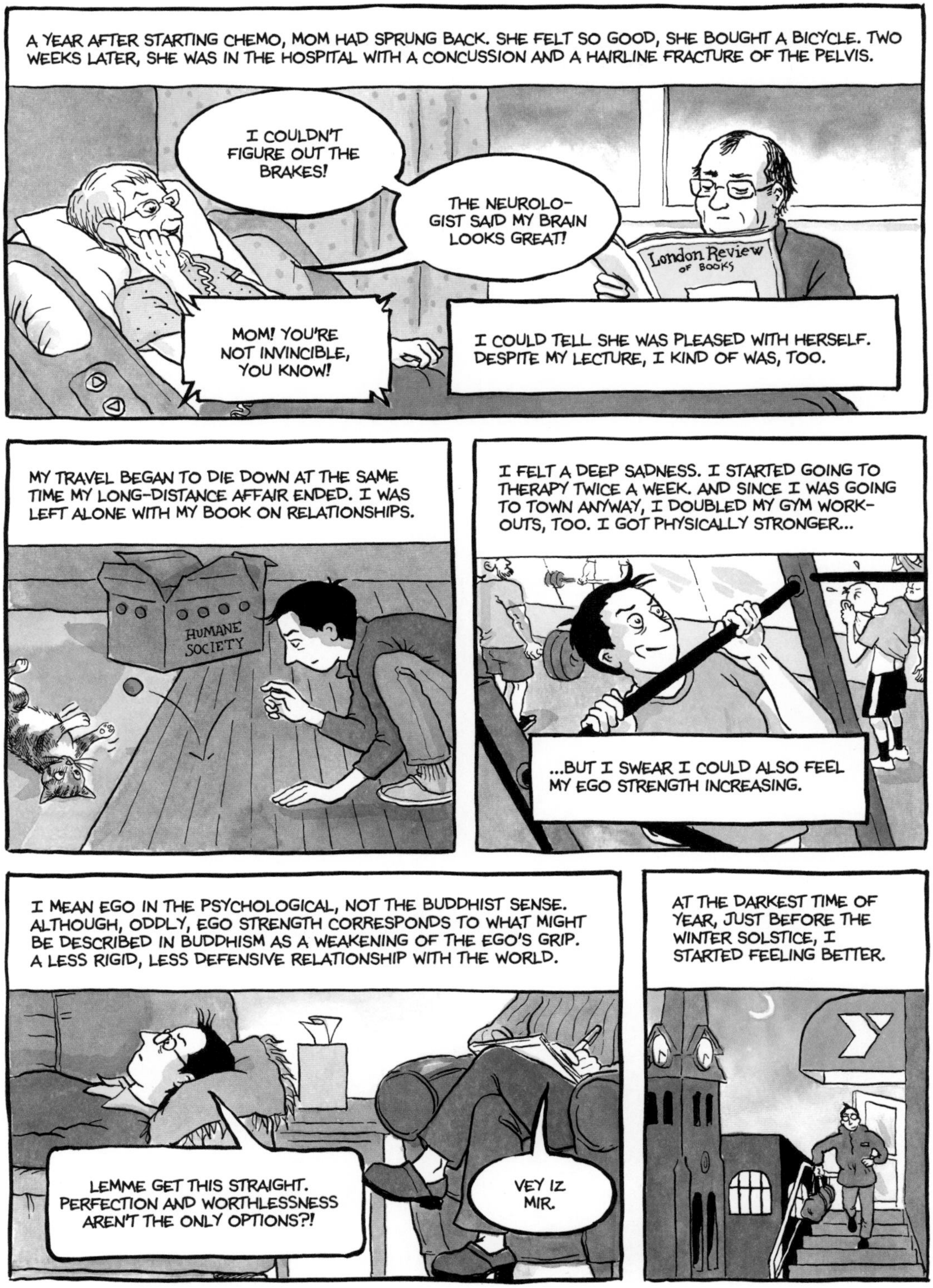
A YEAR AFTER STARTING CHEMO, MOM HAD SPRUNG BACK. SHE FELT SO GOOD, SHE BOUGHT A BICYCLE. TWO WEEKS LATER, SHE WAS IN THE HOSPITAL WITH A CONCUSSION AND A HAIRLINE FRACTURE OF THE PELVIS.
I COULDN'T FIGURE OUT THE BRAKES!
THE NEUROLOGIST SAID MY BRAIN LOOKS GREAT!
London Review OF BOOKS
MOM! YOU'RE NOT INVINCIBLE, YOU KNOW!
I COULD TELL SHE WAS PLEASED WITH HERSELF. DESPITE MY LECTURE, I KIND OF WAS, TOO.
MY TRAVEL BEGAN TO DIE DOWN AT THE SAME TIME MY LONG-DISTANCE AFFAIR ENDED. I WAS LEFT ALONE WITH MY BOOK ON RELATIONSHIPS.
HUMANE SOCIETY
I FELT A DEEP SADNESS. I STARTED GOING TO THERAPY TWICE A WEEK. AND SINCE I WAS GOING TO TOWN ANYWAY, I DOUBLED MY GYM WORKOUTS, TOO. I GOT PHYSICALLY STRONGER...
...BUT I SWEAR I COULD ALSO FEEL MY EGO STRENGTH INCREASING.
I MEAN EGO IN THE PSYCHOLOGICAL, NOT THE BUDDHIST SENSE. ALTHOUGH, ODDLY, EGO STRENGTH CORRESPONDS TO WHAT MIGHT BE DESCRIBED IN BUDDHISM AS A WEAKENING OF THE EGO'S GRIP. A LESS RIGID, LESS DEFENSIVE RELATIONSHIP WITH THE WORLD.
LEMME GET THIS STRAIGHT. PERFECTION AND WORTHLESSNESS AREN'T THE ONLY OPTIONS?!
VEY IZ MIR.
AT THE DARKEST TIME OF YEAR, JUST BEFORE THE WINTER SOLSTICE, I STARTED FEELING BETTER.

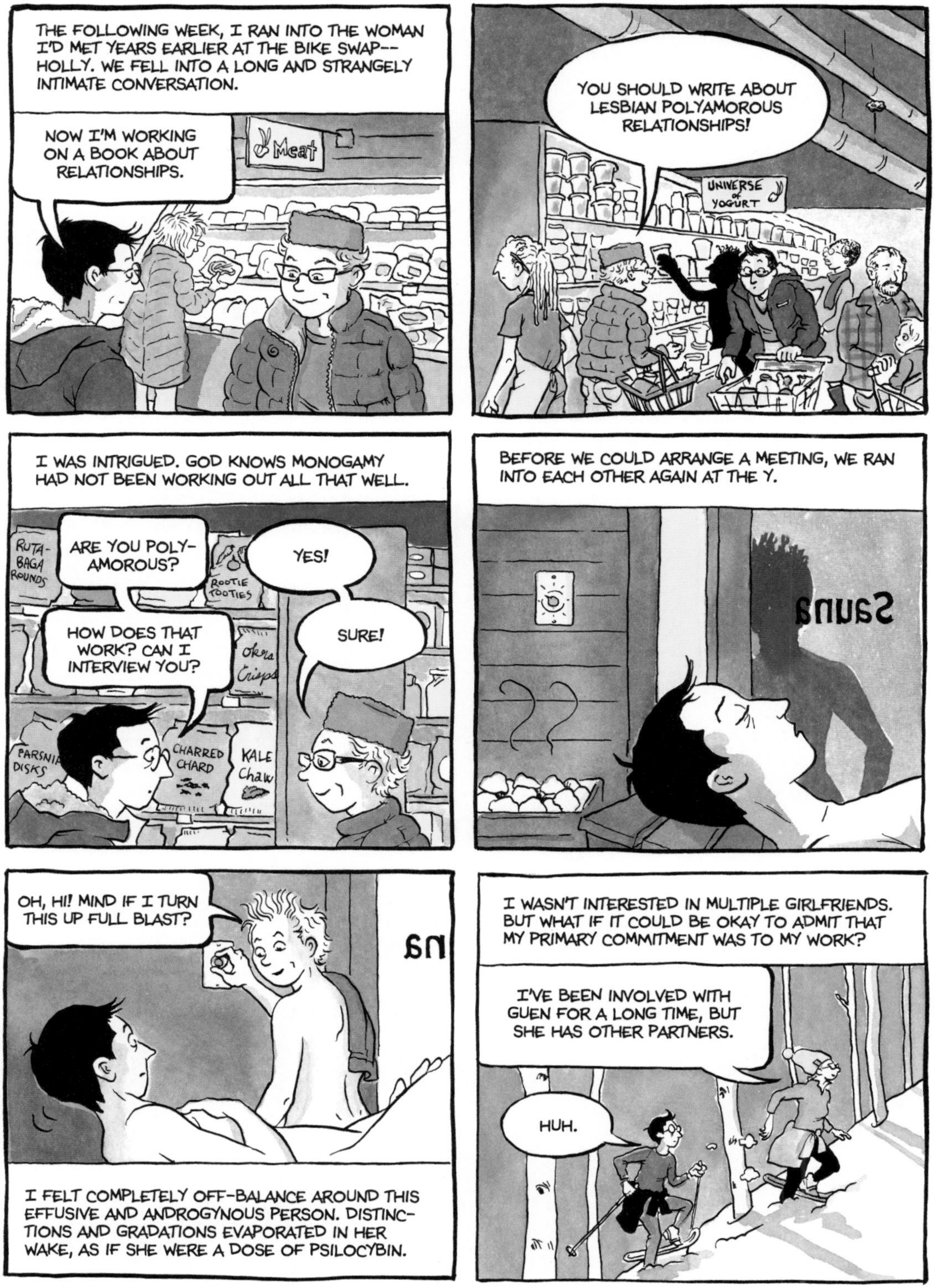

THE FOLLOWING WEEK, I RAN INTO THE WOMAN I'D MET YEARS EARLIER AT THE BIKE SWAP-- HOLLY. WE FELL INTO A LONG AND STRANGELY INTIMATE CONVERSATION.
NOW I'M WORKING ON A BOOK ABOUT RELATIONSHIPS.
Meat
YOU SHOULD WRITE ABOUT LESBIAN POLYAMOROUS RELATIONSHIPS!
UNIVERSE of YOGURT
I WAS INTRIGUED. GOD KNOWS MONOGAMY HAD NOT BEEN WORKING OUT ALL THAT WELL.
ARE YOU POLY-AMOROUS?
YES!
HOW DOES THAT WORK? CAN I INTERVIEW YOU?
SURE!
RUTA-BAGA ROUNDS
ROOTIE TOOTIES
Okra Crisps
CHARRED CHARD
KALE Chaw
BEFORE WE COULD ARRANGE A MEETING, WE RAN INTO EACH OTHER AGAIN AT THE Y.
OH, HI! MIND IF I TURN THIS UP FULL BLAST?
I FELT COMPLETELY OFF-BALANCE AROUND THIS EFFUSIVE AND ANDROGYNOUS PERSON. DISTINCTIONS AND GRADATIONS EVAPORATED IN HER WAKE, AS IF SHE WERE A DOSE OF PSILOCYBIN.
I WASN'T INTERESTED IN MULTIPLE GIRLFRIENDS. BUT WHAT IF IT COULD BE OKAY TO ADMIT THAT MY PRIMARY COMMITMENT WAS TO MY WORK?
I'VE BEEN INVOLVED WITH GUEN FOR A LONG TIME, BUT SHE HAS OTHER PARTNERS.
HUH.

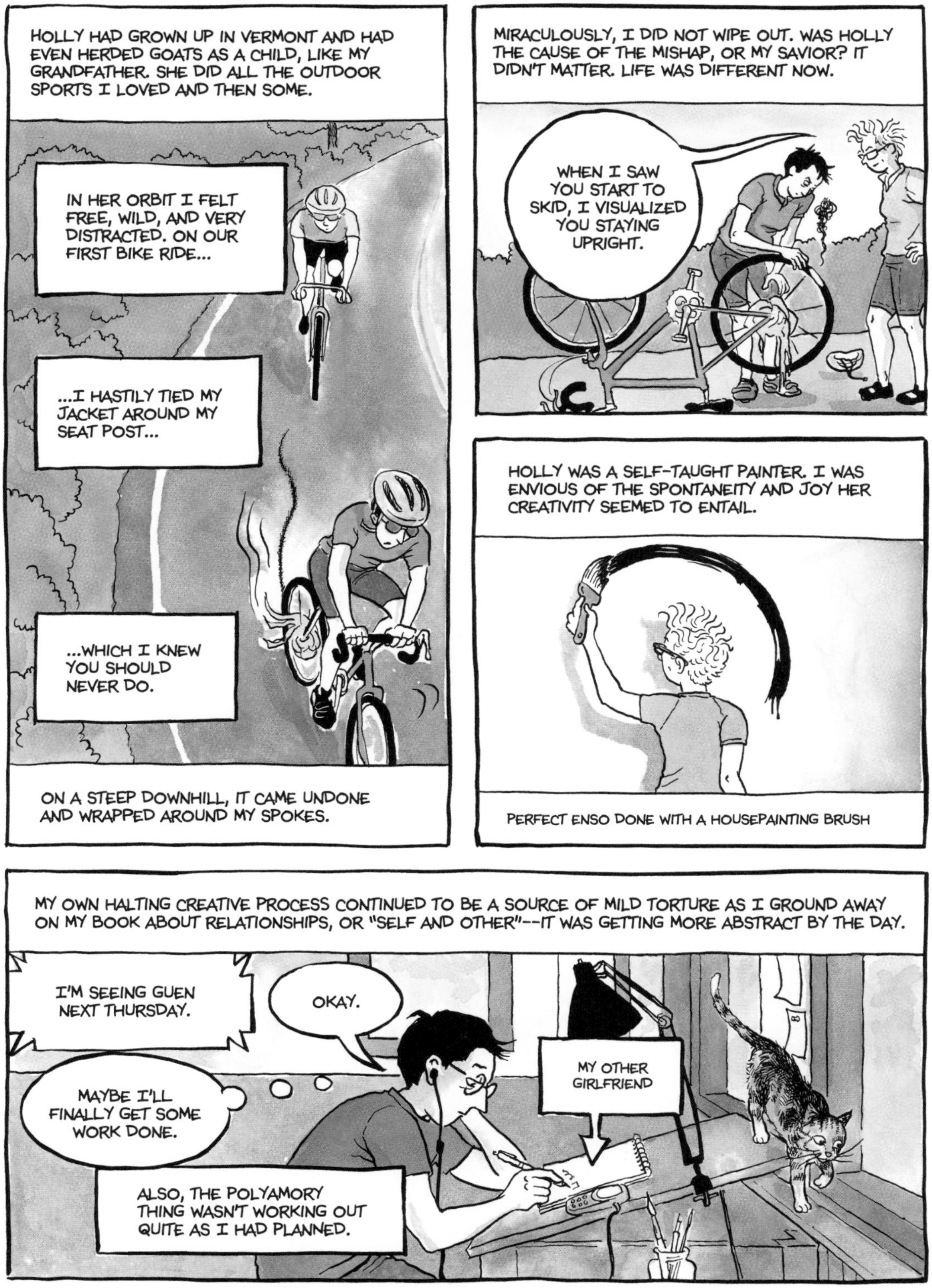
HOLLY HAD GROWN UP IN VERMONT AND HAD EVEN HERDED GOATS AS A CHILD, LIKE MY GRANDFATHER. SHE DID ALL THE OUTDOOR SPORTS I LOVED AND THEN SOME.
IN HER ORBIT I FELT FREE, WILD, AND VERY DISTRACTED. ON OUR FIRST BIKE RIDE...
...I HASTILY TIED MY JACKET AROUND MY SEAT POST...
...WHICH I KNEW YOU SHOULD NEVER DO.
ON A STEEP DOWNHILL, IT CAME UNDONE AND WRAPPED AROUND MY SPOKES.
MIRACULOUSLY, I DID NOT WIPE OUT. WAS HOLLY THE CAUSE OF THE MISHAP, OR MY SAVIOR? IT DIDN'T MATTER. LIFE WAS DIFFERENT NOW.
WHEN I SAW YOU START TO SKID, I VISUALIZED YOU STAYING UPRIGHT.
HOLLY WAS A SELF-TAUGHT PAINTER. I WAS ENVIOUS OF THE SPONTANEITY AND JOY HER CREATIVITY SEEMED TO ENTAIL.
PERFECT ENSO DONE WITH A HOUSEPAINTING BRUSH
MY OWN HALTING CREATIVE PROCESS CONTINUED TO BE A SOURCE OF MILD TORTURE AS I GROUND AWAY ON MY BOOK ABOUT RELATIONSHIPS, OR "SELF AND OTHER"--IT WAS GETTING MORE ABSTRACT BY THE DAY.
I'M SEEING GUEN NEXT THURSDAY.
OKAY.
MAYBE I'LL FINALLY GET SOME WORK DONE.
MY OTHER GIRLFRIEND
ALSO, THE POLYAMORY THING WASN'T WORKING OUT QUITE AS I HAD PLANNED.

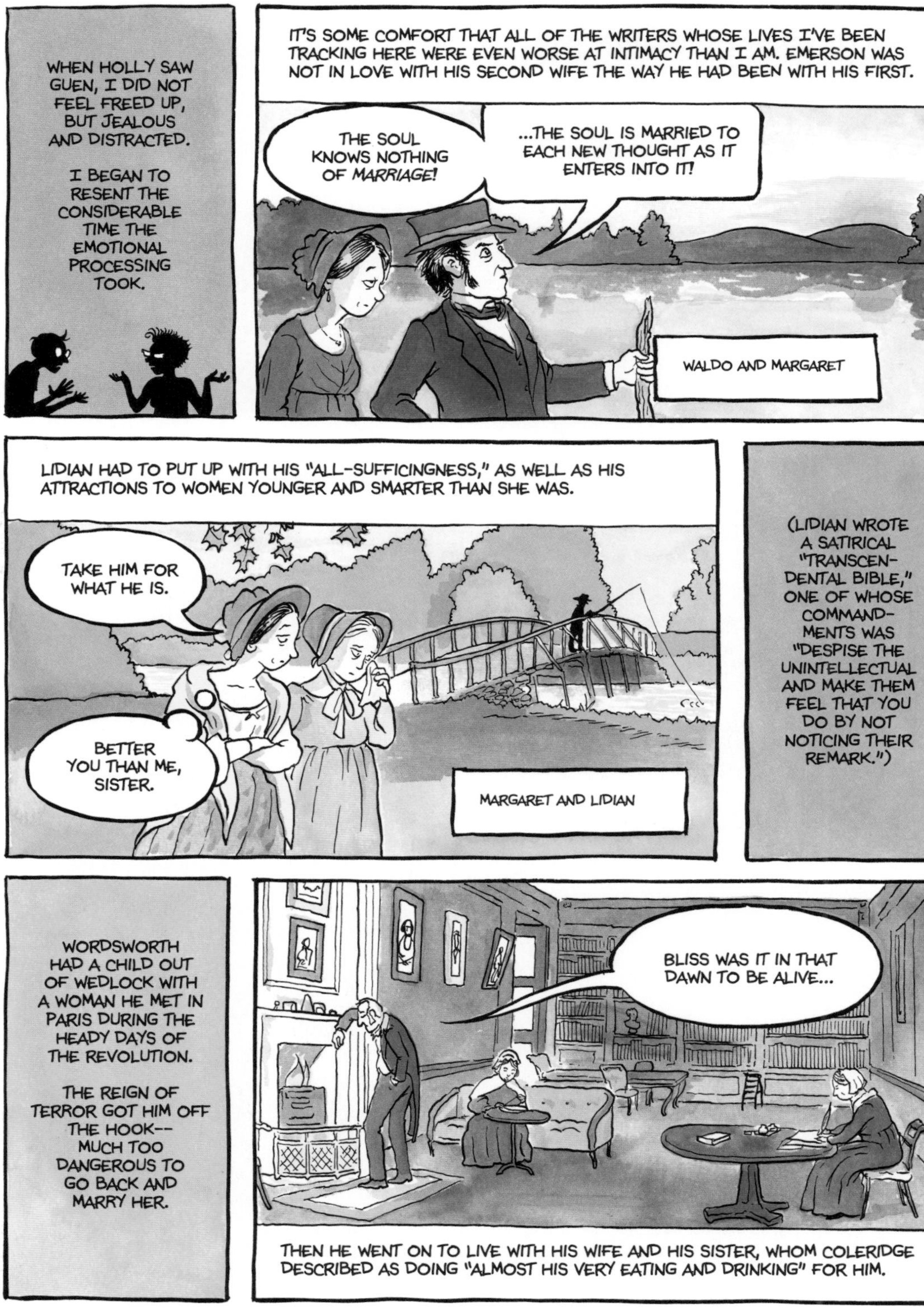
WHEN HOLLY SAW GUEN, I DID NOT FEEL FREED UP, BUT JEALOUS AND DISTRACTED.
I BEGAN TO RESENT THE CONSIDERABLE TIME THE EMOTIONAL PROCESSING TOOK.
IT'S SOME COMFORT THAT ALL OF THE WRITERS WHOSE LIVES I'VE BEEN TRACKING HERE WERE EVEN WORSE AT INTIMACY THAN I AM. EMERSON WAS NOT IN LOVE WITH HIS SECOND WIFE THE WAY HE HAD BEEN WITH HIS FIRST.
THE SOUL KNOWS NOTHING OF *MARRIAGE*!
...THE SOUL IS MARRIED TO EACH NEW THOUGHT AS IT ENTERS INTO IT!
WALDO AND MARGARET
LIDIAN HAD TO PUT UP WITH HIS "ALL-SUFFICINGNESS," AS WELL AS HIS ATTRACTIONS TO WOMEN YOUNGER AND SMARTER THAN SHE WAS.
TAKE HIM FOR WHAT HE IS.
BETTER YOU THAN ME, SISTER.
MARGARET AND LIDIAN
(LIDIAN WROTE A SATIRICAL "TRANSCEN-DENTAL BIBLE," ONE OF WHOSE COMMAND-MENTS WAS "DESPISE THE UNINTELLECTUAL AND MAKE THEM FEEL THAT YOU DO BY NOT NOTICING THEIR REMARK.")
WORDSWORTH HAD A CHILD OUT OF WEDLOCK WITH A WOMAN HE MET IN PARIS DURING THE HEADY DAYS OF THE REVOLUTION.
THE REIGN OF TERROR GOT HIM OFF THE HOOK-- MUCH TOO DANGEROUS TO GO BACK AND MARRY HER.
BLISS WAS IT IN THAT DAWN TO BE ALIVE...
THEN HE WENT ON TO LIVE WITH HIS WIFE AND HIS SISTER, WHOM COLERIDGE DESCRIBED AS DOING "ALMOST HIS VERY EATING AND DRINKING" FOR HIM.

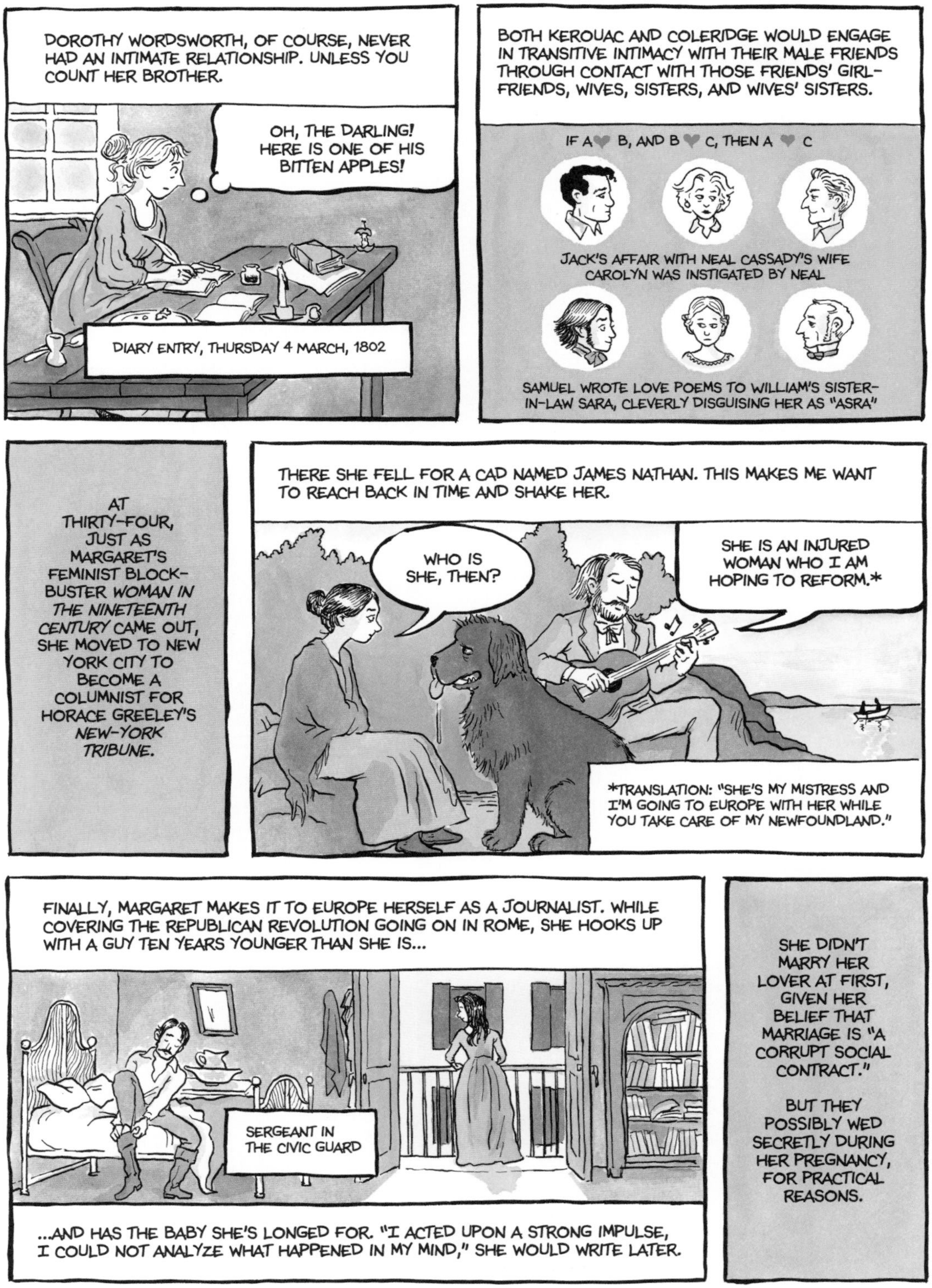

DOROTHY WORDSWORTH, OF COURSE, NEVER HAD AN INTIMATE RELATIONSHIP. UNLESS YOU COUNT HER BROTHER.
OH, THE DARLING! HERE IS ONE OF HIS BITTEN APPLES!
DIARY ENTRY, THURSDAY 4 MARCH, 1802
BOTH KEROUAC AND COLERIDGE WOULD ENGAGE IN TRANSITIVE INTIMACY WITH THEIR MALE FRIENDS THROUGH CONTACT WITH THOSE FRIENDS' GIRLFRIENDS, WIVES, SISTERS, AND WIVES' SISTERS.
IF A ♥ B, AND B ♥ C, THEN A ♥ C
JACK'S AFFAIR WITH NEAL CASSADY'S WIFE CAROLYN WAS INSTIGATED BY NEAL
SAMUEL WROTE LOVE POEMS TO WILLIAM'S SISTER-IN-LAW SARA, CLEVERLY DISGUISING HER AS "ASRA"
AT THIRTY-FOUR, JUST AS MARGARET'S FEMINIST BLOCKBUSTER *WOMAN IN THE NINETEENTH CENTURY* CAME OUT, SHE MOVED TO NEW YORK CITY TO BECOME A COLUMNIST FOR HORACE GREELEY'S *NEW-YORK TRIBUNE*.
THERE SHE FELL FOR A CAD NAMED JAMES NATHAN. THIS MAKES ME WANT TO REACH BACK IN TIME AND SHAKE HER.
WHO IS SHE, THEN?
SHE IS AN INJURED WOMAN WHO I AM HOPING TO REFORM.*
*TRANSLATION: "SHE'S MY MISTRESS AND I'M GOING TO EUROPE WITH HER WHILE YOU TAKE CARE OF MY NEWFOUNDLAND."
FINALLY, MARGARET MAKES IT TO EUROPE HERSELF AS A JOURNALIST. WHILE COVERING THE REPUBLICAN REVOLUTION GOING ON IN ROME, SHE HOOKS UP WITH A GUY TEN YEARS YOUNGER THAN SHE IS...
SERGEANT IN THE CIVIC GUARD
...AND HAS THE BABY SHE'S LONGED FOR. "I ACTED UPON A STRONG IMPULSE, I COULD NOT ANALYZE WHAT HAPPENED IN MY MIND," SHE WOULD WRITE LATER.
SHE DIDN'T MARRY HER LOVER AT FIRST, GIVEN HER BELIEF THAT MARRIAGE IS "A CORRUPT SOCIAL CONTRACT."
BUT THEY POSSIBLY WED SECRETLY DURING HER PREGNANCY, FOR PRACTICAL REASONS.

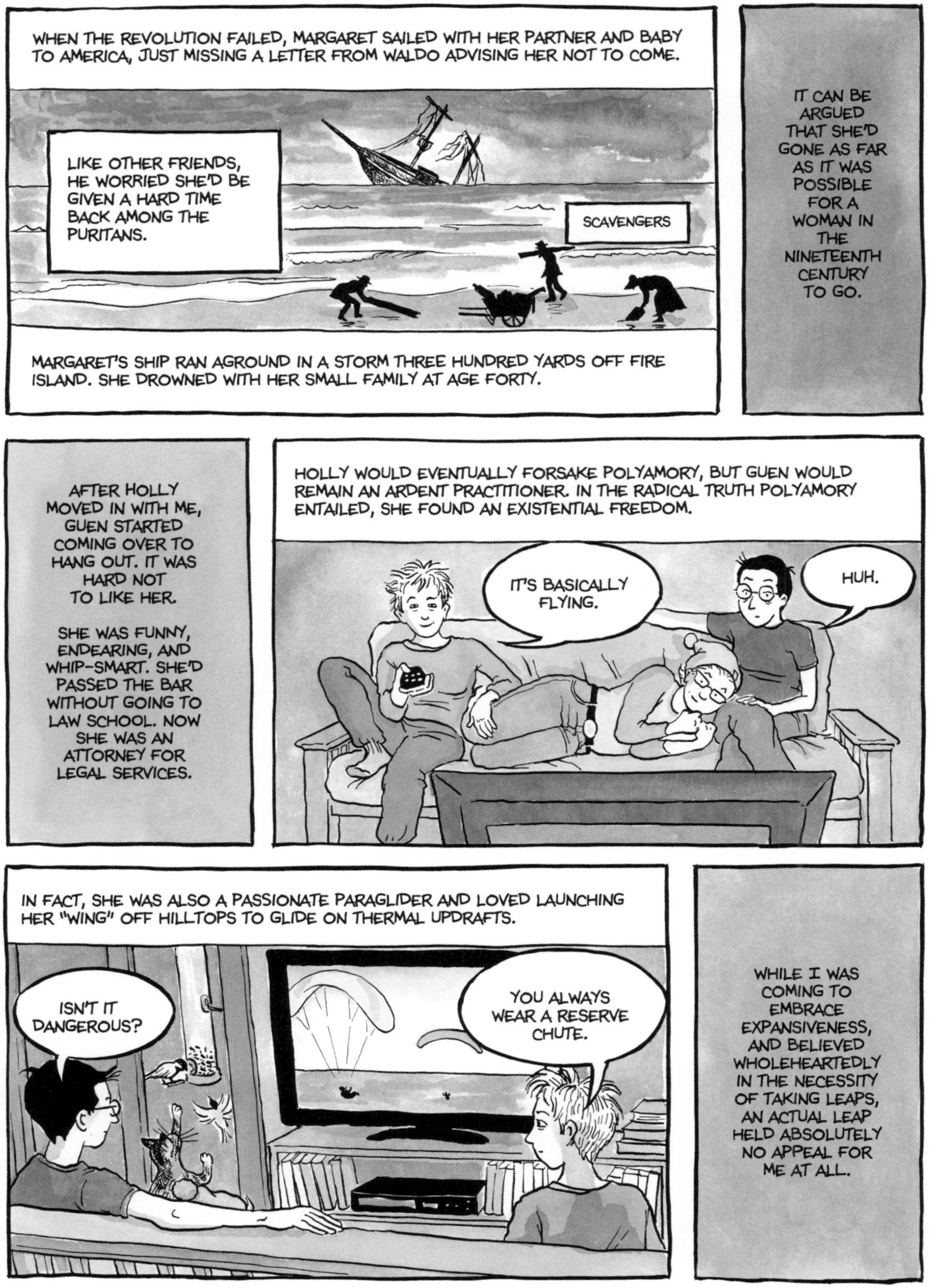
WHEN THE REVOLUTION FAILED, MARGARET SAILED WITH HER PARTNER AND BABY TO AMERICA, JUST MISSING A LETTER FROM WALDO ADVISING HER NOT TO COME.
LIKE OTHER FRIENDS, HE WORRIED SHE'D BE GIVEN A HARD TIME BACK AMONG THE PURITANS.
SCAVENGERS
MARGARET'S SHIP RAN AGROUND IN A STORM THREE HUNDRED YARDS OFF FIRE ISLAND. SHE DROWNED WITH HER SMALL FAMILY AT AGE FORTY.
IT CAN BE ARGUED THAT SHE'D GONE AS FAR AS IT WAS POSSIBLE FOR A WOMAN IN THE NINETEENTH CENTURY TO GO.
AFTER HOLLY MOVED IN WITH ME, GUEN STARTED COMING OVER TO HANG OUT. IT WAS HARD NOT TO LIKE HER.
SHE WAS FUNNY, ENDEARING, AND WHIP-SMART. SHE'D PASSED THE BAR WITHOUT GOING TO LAW SCHOOL. NOW SHE WAS AN ATTORNEY FOR LEGAL SERVICES.
HOLLY WOULD EVENTUALLY FORSAKE POLYAMORY, BUT GUEN WOULD REMAIN AN ARDENT PRACTITIONER. IN THE RADICAL TRUTH POLYAMORY ENTAILED, SHE FOUND AN EXISTENTIAL FREEDOM.
IT'S BASICALLY FLYING.
HUH.
IN FACT, SHE WAS ALSO A PASSIONATE PARAGLIDER AND LOVED LAUNCHING HER "WING" OFF HILLTOPS TO GLIDE ON THERMAL UPDRAFTS.
ISN'T IT DANGEROUS?
YOU ALWAYS WEAR A RESERVE CHUTE.
WHILE I WAS COMING TO EMBRACE EXPANSIVENESS, AND BELIEVED WHOLEHEARTEDLY IN THE NECESSITY OF TAKING LEAPS, AN ACTUAL LEAP HELD ABSOLUTELY NO APPEAL FOR ME AT ALL.

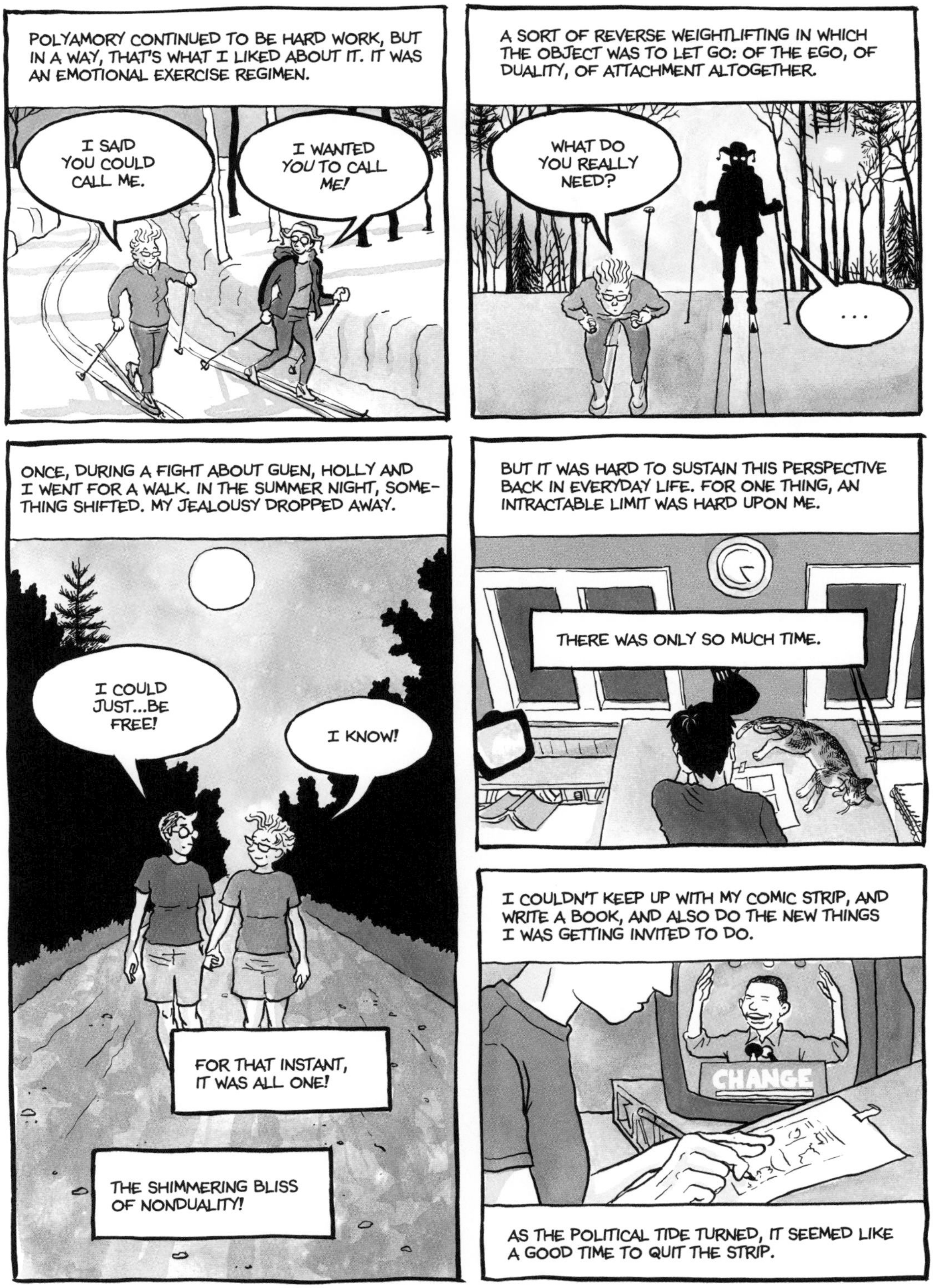
POLYAMORY CONTINUED TO BE HARD WORK, BUT IN A WAY, THAT'S WHAT I LIKED ABOUT IT. IT WAS AN EMOTIONAL EXERCISE REGIMEN.
I SAID YOU COULD CALL ME.
I WANTED YOU TO CALL ME!
A SORT OF REVERSE WEIGHTLIFTING IN WHICH THE OBJECT WAS TO LET GO: OF THE EGO, OF DUALITY, OF ATTACHMENT ALTOGETHER.
WHAT DO YOU REALLY NEED?
...
ONCE, DURING A FIGHT ABOUT GUEN, HOLLY AND I WENT FOR A WALK. IN THE SUMMER NIGHT, SOMETHING SHIFTED. MY JEALOUSY DROPPED AWAY.
I COULD JUST...BE FREE!
I KNOW!
FOR THAT INSTANT, IT WAS ALL ONE!
THE SHIMMERING BLISS OF NONDUALITY!
BUT IT WAS HARD TO SUSTAIN THIS PERSPECTIVE BACK IN EVERYDAY LIFE. FOR ONE THING, AN INTRACTABLE LIMIT WAS HARD UPON ME.
THERE WAS ONLY SO MUCH TIME.
I COULDN'T KEEP UP WITH MY COMIC STRIP, AND WRITE A BOOK, AND ALSO DO THE NEW THINGS I WAS GETTING INVITED TO DO.
CHANGE
AS THE POLITICAL TIDE TURNED, IT SEEMED LIKE A GOOD TIME TO QUIT THE STRIP.

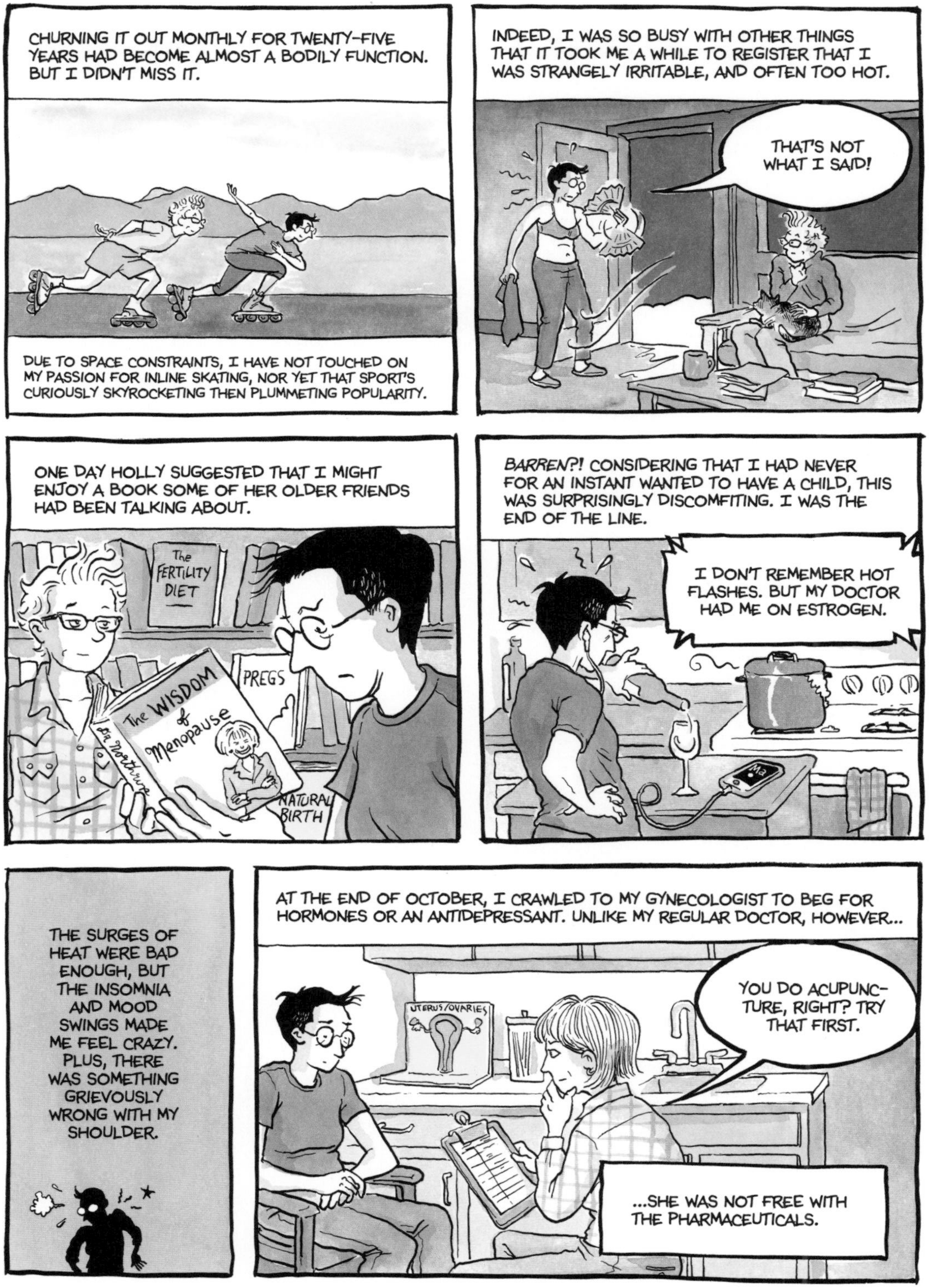
CHURNING IT OUT MONTHLY FOR TWENTY-FIVE YEARS HAD BECOME ALMOST A BODILY FUNCTION. BUT I DIDN'T MISS IT.
DUE TO SPACE CONSTRAINTS, I HAVE NOT TOUCHED ON MY PASSION FOR INLINE SKATING, NOR YET THAT SPORT'S CURIOUSLY SKYROCKETING THEN PLUMMETING POPULARITY.
INDEED, I WAS SO BUSY WITH OTHER THINGS THAT IT TOOK ME A WHILE TO REGISTER THAT I WAS STRANGELY IRRITABLE, AND OFTEN TOO HOT.
THAT'S NOT WHAT I SAID!
ONE DAY HOLLY SUGGESTED THAT I MIGHT ENJOY A BOOK SOME OF HER OLDER FRIENDS HAD BEEN TALKING ABOUT.
The FERTILITY DIET
PREGS
The WISDOM of Menopause
Dr. Northrup
NATURAL BIRTH
BARREN?! CONSIDERING THAT I HAD NEVER FOR AN INSTANT WANTED TO HAVE A CHILD, THIS WAS SURPRISINGLY DISCOMFITING. I WAS THE END OF THE LINE.
I DON'T REMEMBER HOT FLASHES. BUT MY DOCTOR HAD ME ON ESTROGEN.
Ma
THE SURGES OF HEAT WERE BAD ENOUGH, BUT THE INSOMNIA AND MOOD SWINGS MADE ME FEEL CRAZY. PLUS, THERE WAS SOMETHING GRIEVOUSLY WRONG WITH MY SHOULDER.
AT THE END OF OCTOBER, I CRAWLED TO MY GYNECOLOGIST TO BEG FOR HORMONES OR AN ANTIDEPRESSANT. UNLIKE MY REGULAR DOCTOR, HOWEVER...
UTERUS/OVARIES
YOU DO ACUPUNCTURE, RIGHT? TRY THAT FIRST.
...SHE WAS NOT FREE WITH THE PHARMACEUTICALS.

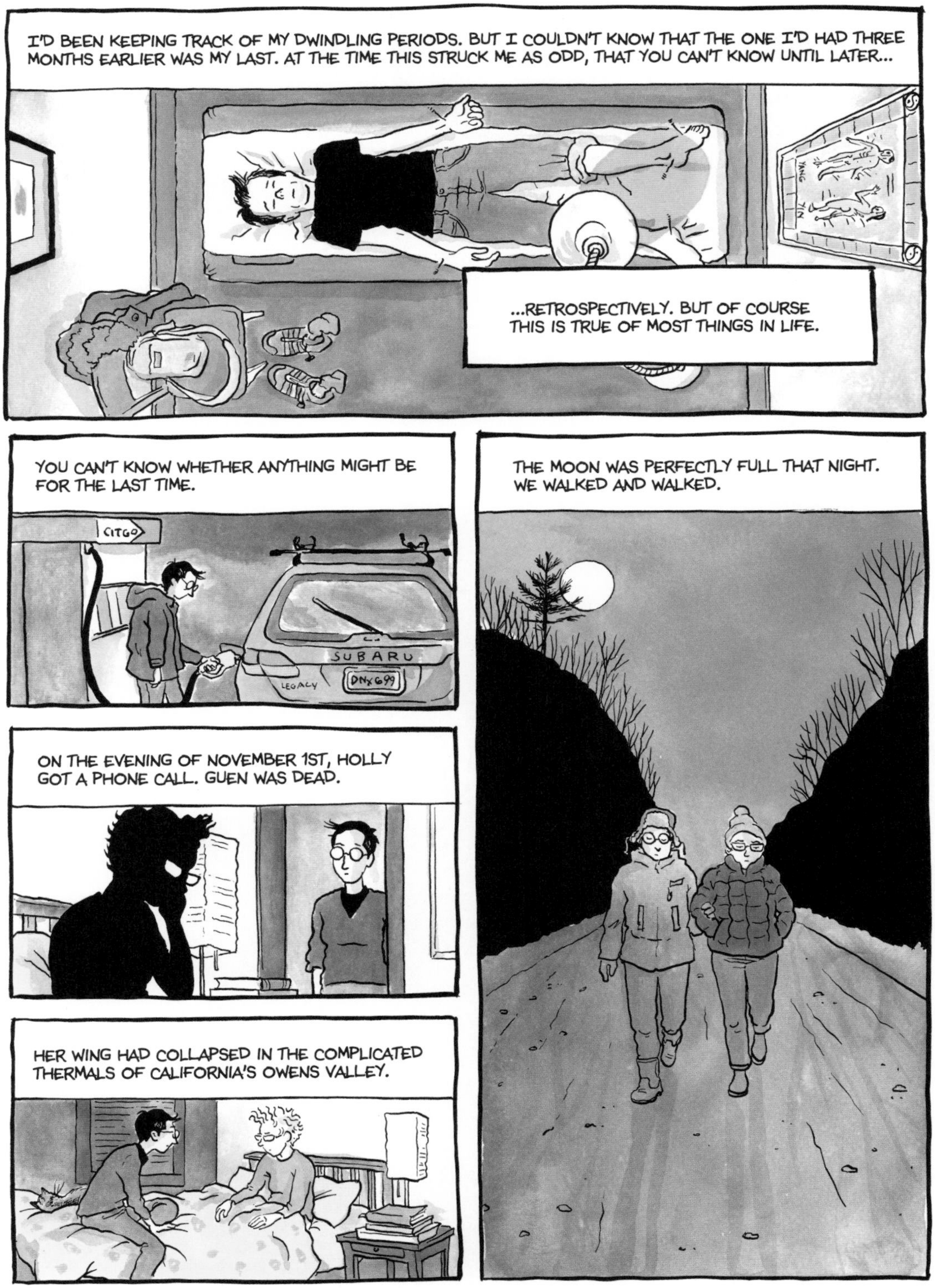
I'D BEEN KEEPING TRACK OF MY DWINDLING PERIODS. BUT I COULDN'T KNOW THAT THE ONE I'D HAD THREE MONTHS EARLIER WAS MY LAST. AT THE TIME THIS STRUCK ME AS ODD, THAT YOU CAN'T KNOW UNTIL LATER...
YANG
YIN
...RETROSPECTIVELY. BUT OF COURSE THIS IS TRUE OF MOST THINGS IN LIFE.
YOU CAN'T KNOW WHETHER ANYTHING MIGHT BE FOR THE LAST TIME.
CITGO
SUBARU
LEGACY
DNX699
ON THE EVENING OF NOVEMBER 1ST, HOLLY GOT A PHONE CALL. GUEN WAS DEAD.
HER WING HAD COLLAPSED IN THE COMPLICATED THERMALS OF CALIFORNIA'S OWENS VALLEY.
THE MOON WAS PERFECTLY FULL THAT NIGHT. WE WALKED AND WALKED.

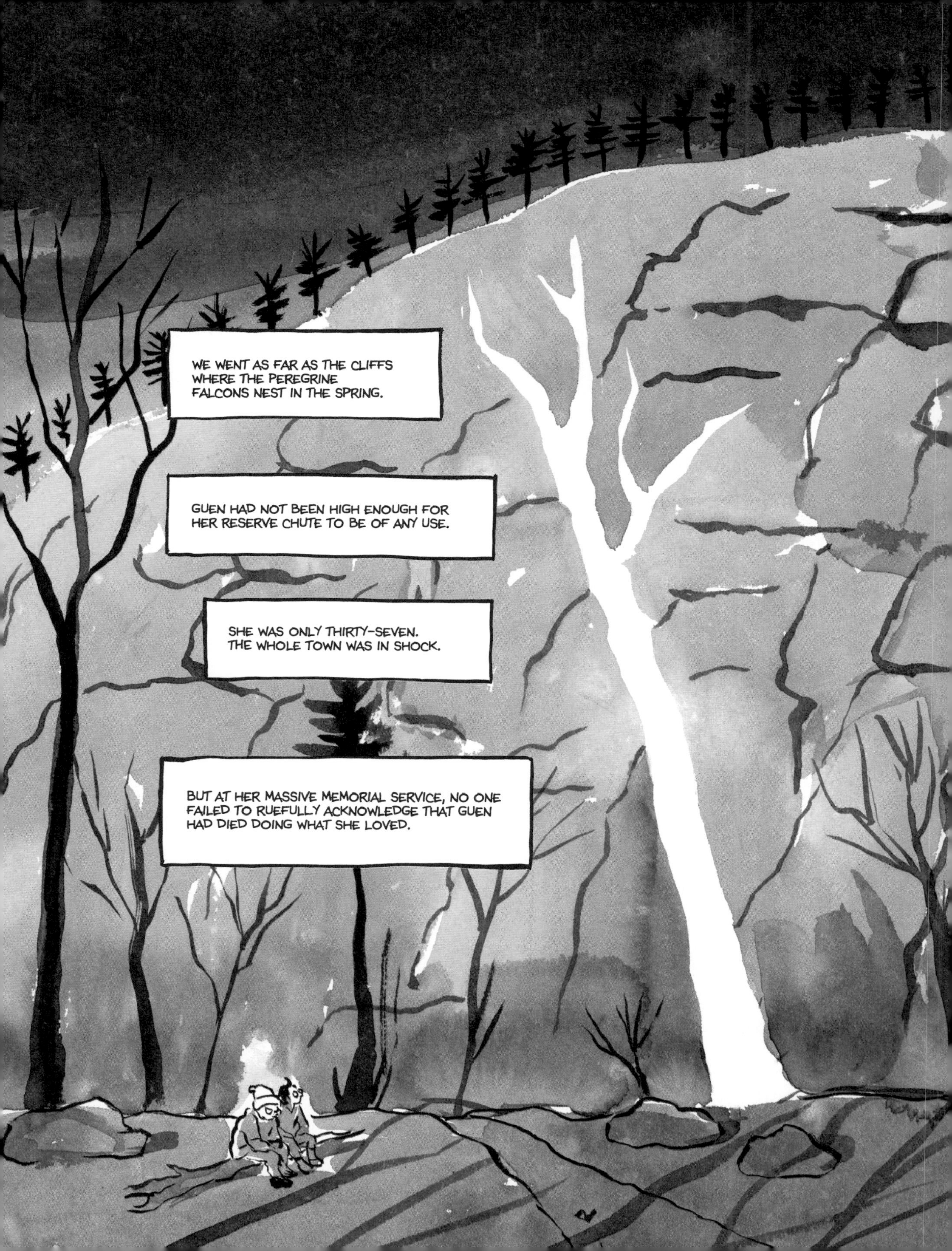
WE WENT AS FAR AS THE CLIFFS WHERE THE PEREGRINE FALCONS NEST IN THE SPRING.
GUEN HAD NOT BEEN HIGH ENOUGH FOR HER RESERVE CHUTE TO BE OF ANY USE.
SHE WAS ONLY THIRTY-SEVEN. THE WHOLE TOWN WAS IN SHOCK.
BUT AT HER MASSIVE MEMORIAL SERVICE, NO ONE FAILED TO RUEFULLY ACKNOWLEDGE THAT GUEN HAD DIED DOING WHAT SHE LOVED.

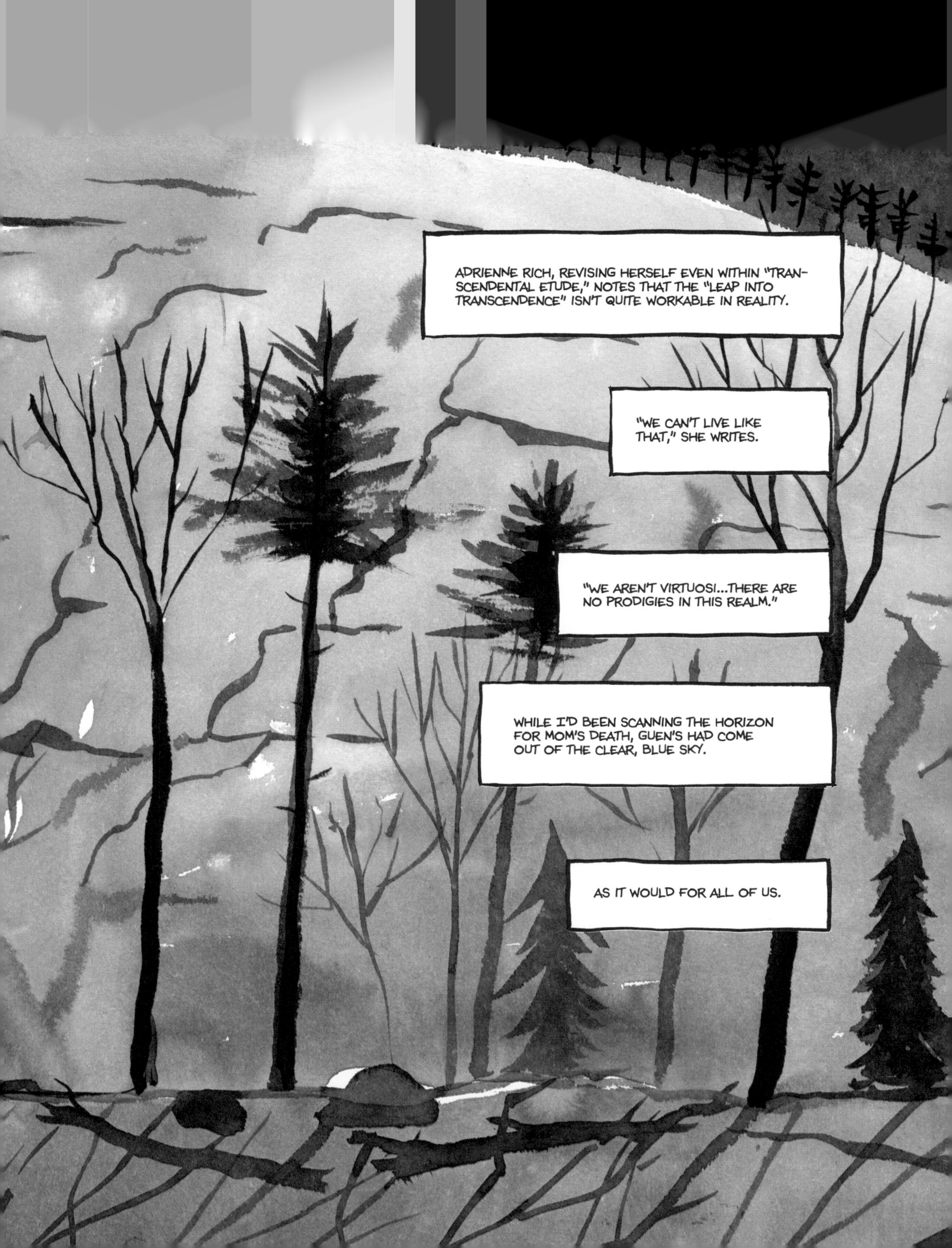
ADRIENNE RICH, REVISING HERSELF EVEN WITHIN "TRANSCENDENTAL ETUDE," NOTES THAT THE "LEAP INTO TRANSCENDENCE" ISN'T QUITE WORKABLE IN REALITY.
"WE CAN'T LIVE LIKE THAT," SHE WRITES.
"WE AREN'T VIRTUOSI...THERE ARE NO PRODIGIES IN THIS REALM."
WHILE I'D BEEN SCANNING THE HORIZON FOR MOM'S DEATH, GUEN'S HAD COME OUT OF THE CLEAR, BLUE SKY.
AS IT WOULD FOR ALL OF US.

2010s

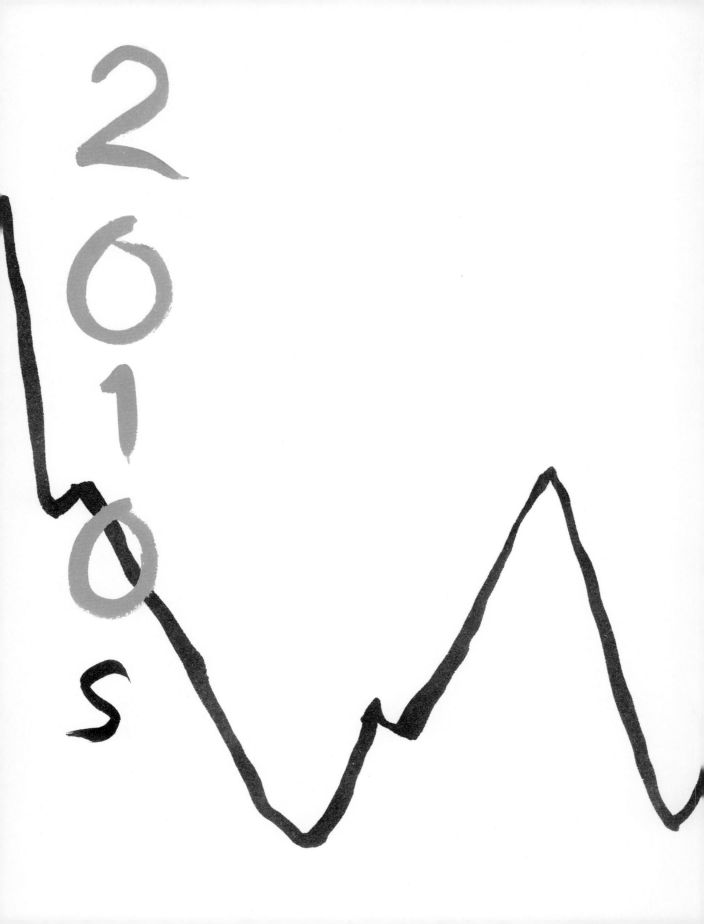

5
0
5

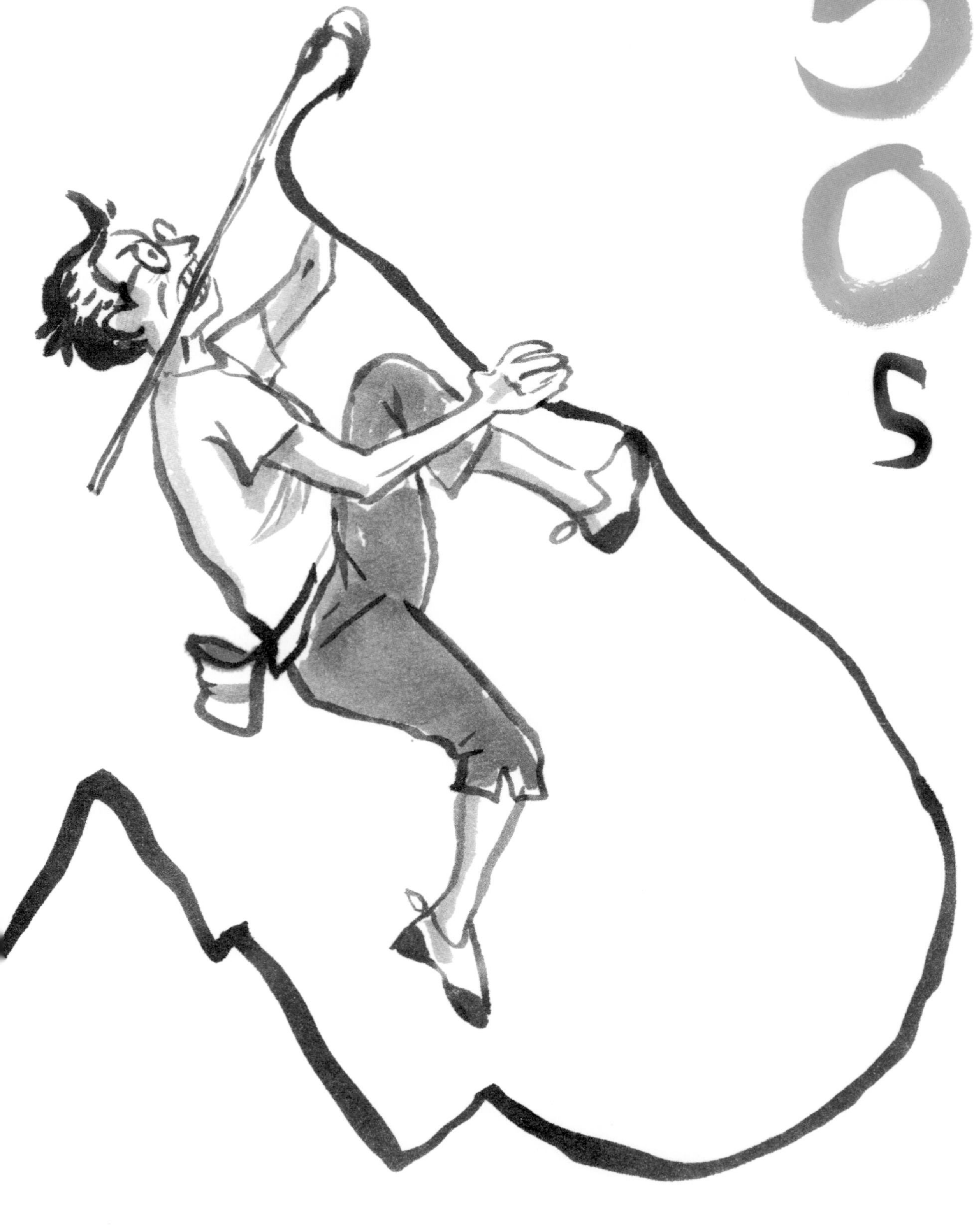

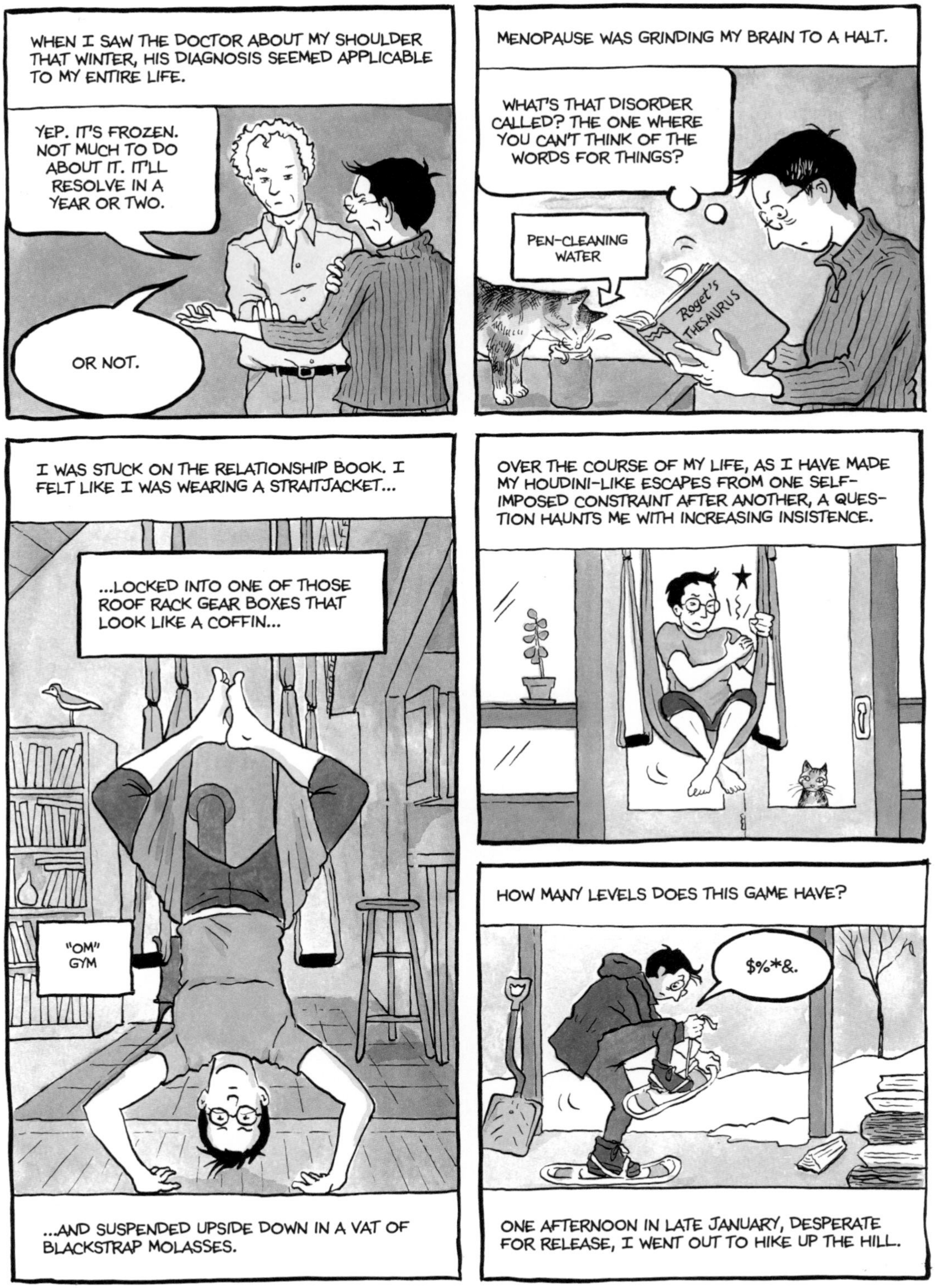
WHEN I SAW THE DOCTOR ABOUT MY SHOULDER THAT WINTER, HIS DIAGNOSIS SEEMED APPLICABLE TO MY ENTIRE LIFE.
YEP. IT'S FROZEN. NOT MUCH TO DO ABOUT IT. IT'LL RESOLVE IN A YEAR OR TWO.
OR NOT.
MENOPAUSE WAS GRINDING MY BRAIN TO A HALT.
WHAT'S THAT DISORDER CALLED? THE ONE WHERE YOU CAN'T THINK OF THE WORDS FOR THINGS?
PEN-CLEANING WATER
Roget's THESAURUS
I WAS STUCK ON THE RELATIONSHIP BOOK. I FELT LIKE I WAS WEARING A STRAITJACKET...
...LOCKED INTO ONE OF THOSE ROOF RACK GEAR BOXES THAT LOOK LIKE A COFFIN...
"OM" GYM
...AND SUSPENDED UPSIDE DOWN IN A VAT OF BLACKSTRAP MOLASSES.
OVER THE COURSE OF MY LIFE, AS I HAVE MADE MY HOUDINI-LIKE ESCAPES FROM ONE SELF-IMPOSED CONSTRAINT AFTER ANOTHER, A QUESTION HAUNTS ME WITH INCREASING INSISTENCE.
HOW MANY LEVELS DOES THIS GAME HAVE?
$%*&.
ONE AFTERNOON IN LATE JANUARY, DESPERATE FOR RELEASE, I WENT OUT TO HIKE UP THE HILL.

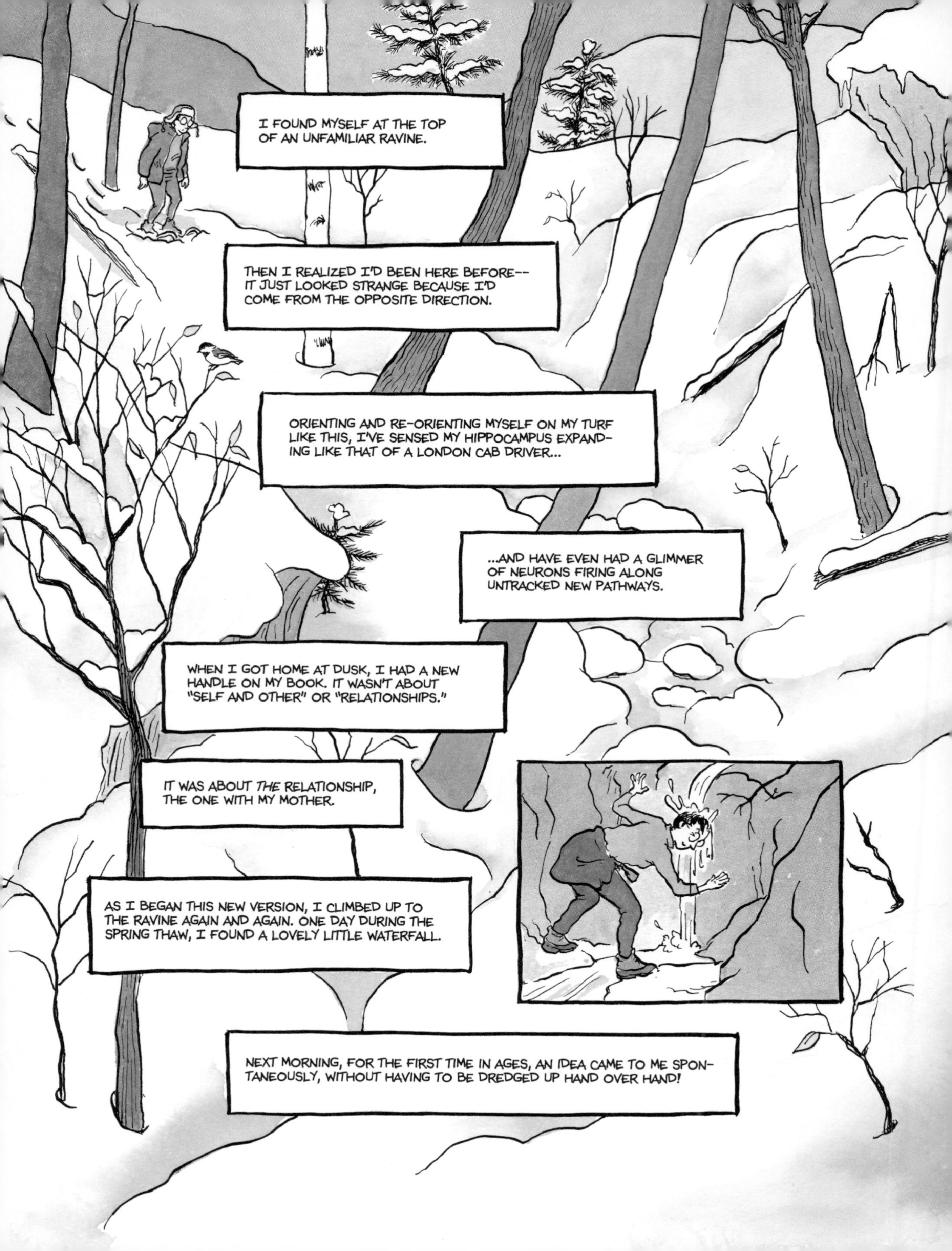
I FOUND MYSELF AT THE TOP OF AN UNFAMILIAR RAVINE.
THEN I REALIZED I'D BEEN HERE BEFORE-- IT JUST LOOKED STRANGE BECAUSE I'D COME FROM THE OPPOSITE DIRECTION.
ORIENTING AND RE-ORIENTING MYSELF ON MY TURF LIKE THIS, I'VE SENSED MY HIPPOCAMPUS EXPANDING LIKE THAT OF A LONDON CAB DRIVER...
...AND HAVE EVEN HAD A GLIMMER OF NEURONS FIRING ALONG UNTRACKED NEW PATHWAYS.
WHEN I GOT HOME AT DUSK, I HAD A NEW HANDLE ON MY BOOK. IT WASN'T ABOUT "SELF AND OTHER" OR "RELATIONSHIPS."
IT WAS ABOUT *THE* RELATIONSHIP, THE ONE WITH MY MOTHER.
AS I BEGAN THIS NEW VERSION, I CLIMBED UP TO THE RAVINE AGAIN AND AGAIN. ONE DAY DURING THE SPRING THAW, I FOUND A LOVELY LITTLE WATERFALL.
NEXT MORNING, FOR THE FIRST TIME IN AGES, AN IDEA CAME TO ME SPONTANEOUSLY, WITHOUT HAVING TO BE DREDGED UP HAND OVER HAND!

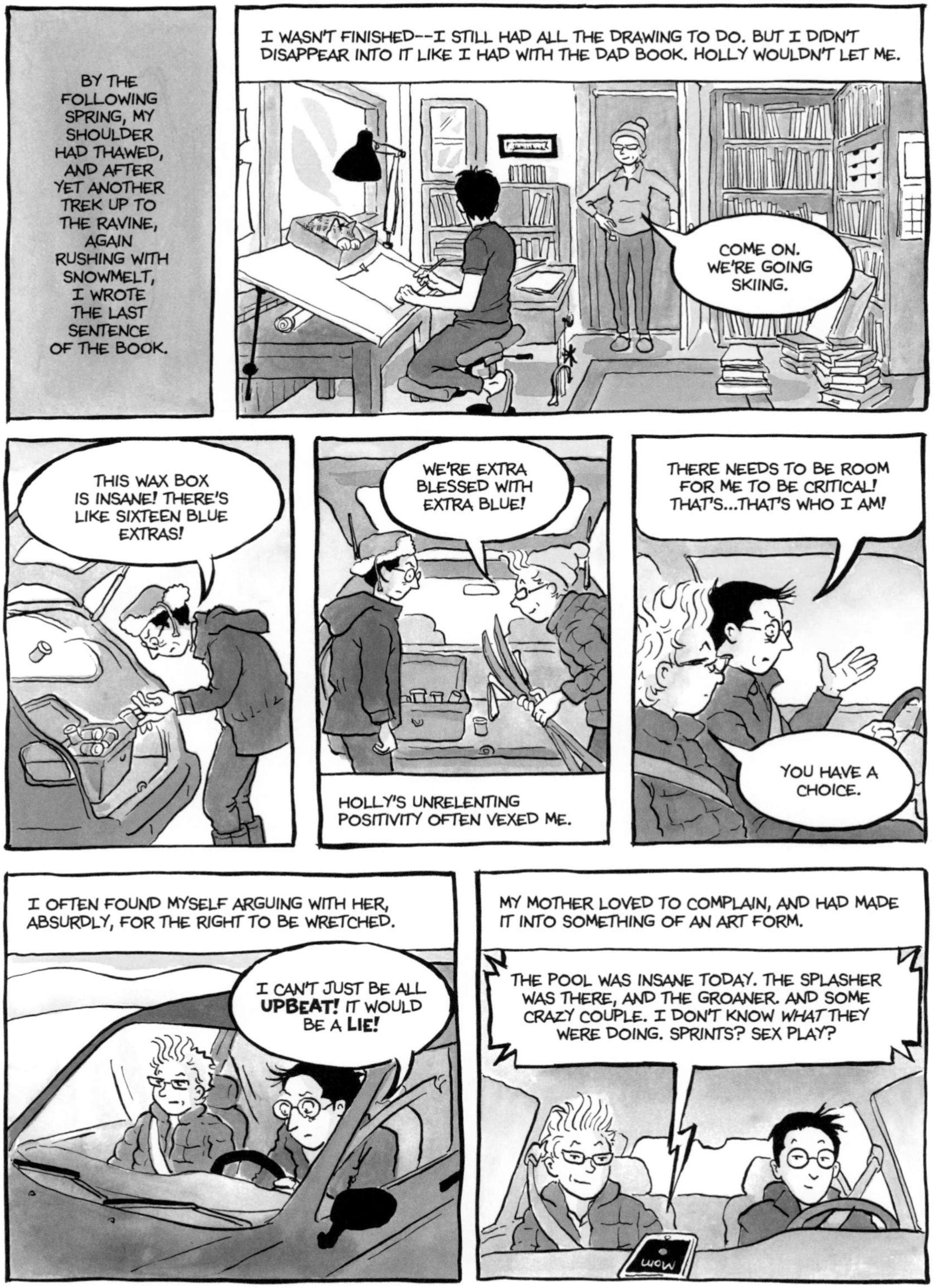
BY THE FOLLOWING SPRING, MY SHOULDER HAD THAWED, AND AFTER YET ANOTHER TREK UP TO THE RAVINE, AGAIN RUSHING WITH SNOWMELT, I WROTE THE LAST SENTENCE OF THE BOOK.
I WASN'T FINISHED--I STILL HAD ALL THE DRAWING TO DO. BUT I DIDN'T DISAPPEAR INTO IT LIKE I HAD WITH THE DAD BOOK. HOLLY WOULDN'T LET ME.
COME ON. WE'RE GOING SKIING.
THIS WAX BOX IS INSANE! THERE'S LIKE SIXTEEN BLUE EXTRAS!
WE'RE EXTRA BLESSED WITH EXTRA BLUE!
HOLLY'S UNRELENTING POSITIVITY OFTEN VEXED ME.
THERE NEEDS TO BE ROOM FOR ME TO BE CRITICAL! THAT'S...THAT'S WHO I AM!
YOU HAVE A CHOICE.
I OFTEN FOUND MYSELF ARGUING WITH HER, ABSURDLY, FOR THE RIGHT TO BE WRETCHED.
I CAN'T JUST BE ALL UPBEAT! IT WOULD BE A LIE!
MY MOTHER LOVED TO COMPLAIN, AND HAD MADE IT INTO SOMETHING OF AN ART FORM.
THE POOL WAS INSANE TODAY. THE SPLASHER WAS THERE, AND THE GROANER. AND SOME CRAZY COUPLE. I DON'T KNOW WHAT THEY WERE DOING. SPRINTS? SEX PLAY?
Mom

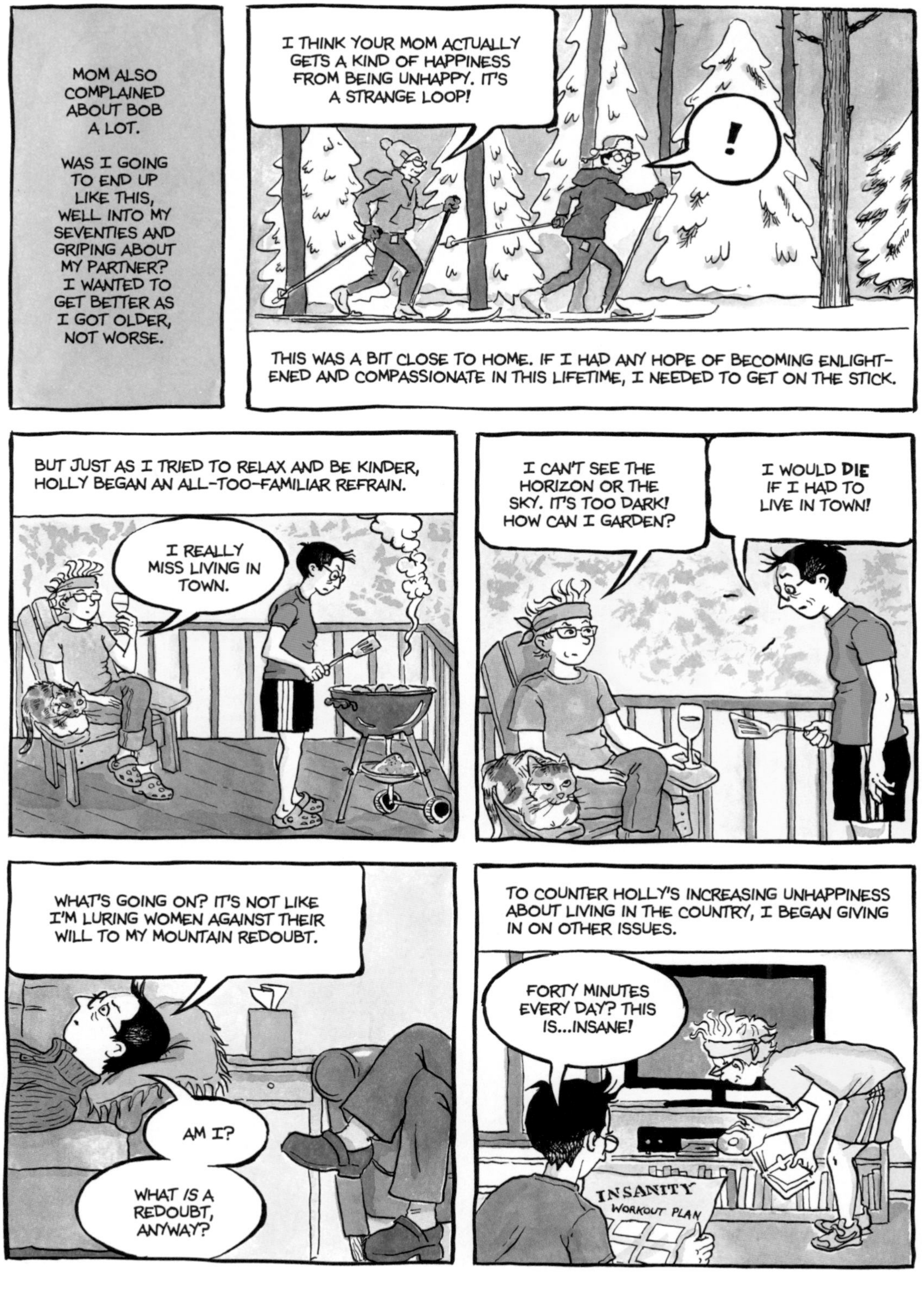

MOM ALSO COMPLAINED ABOUT BOB A LOT.
WAS I GOING TO END UP LIKE THIS, WELL INTO MY SEVENTIES AND GRIPING ABOUT MY PARTNER? I WANTED TO GET BETTER AS I GOT OLDER, NOT WORSE.
I THINK YOUR MOM ACTUALLY GETS A KIND OF HAPPINESS FROM BEING UNHAPPY. IT'S A STRANGE LOOP!
!
THIS WAS A BIT CLOSE TO HOME. IF I HAD ANY HOPE OF BECOMING ENLIGHTENED AND COMPASSIONATE IN THIS LIFETIME, I NEEDED TO GET ON THE STICK.
BUT JUST AS I TRIED TO RELAX AND BE KINDER, HOLLY BEGAN AN ALL-TOO-FAMILIAR REFRAIN.
I REALLY MISS LIVING IN TOWN.
I CAN'T SEE THE HORIZON OR THE SKY. IT'S TOO DARK! HOW CAN I GARDEN?
I WOULD **DIE** IF I HAD TO LIVE IN TOWN!
WHAT'S GOING ON? IT'S NOT LIKE I'M LURING WOMEN AGAINST THEIR WILL TO MY MOUNTAIN REDOUBT.
AM I?
WHAT *IS* A REDOUBT, ANYWAY?
TO COUNTER HOLLY'S INCREASING UNHAPPINESS ABOUT LIVING IN THE COUNTRY, I BEGAN GIVING IN ON OTHER ISSUES.
FORTY MINUTES EVERY DAY? THIS IS...INSANE!
INSANITY
WORKOUT PLAN

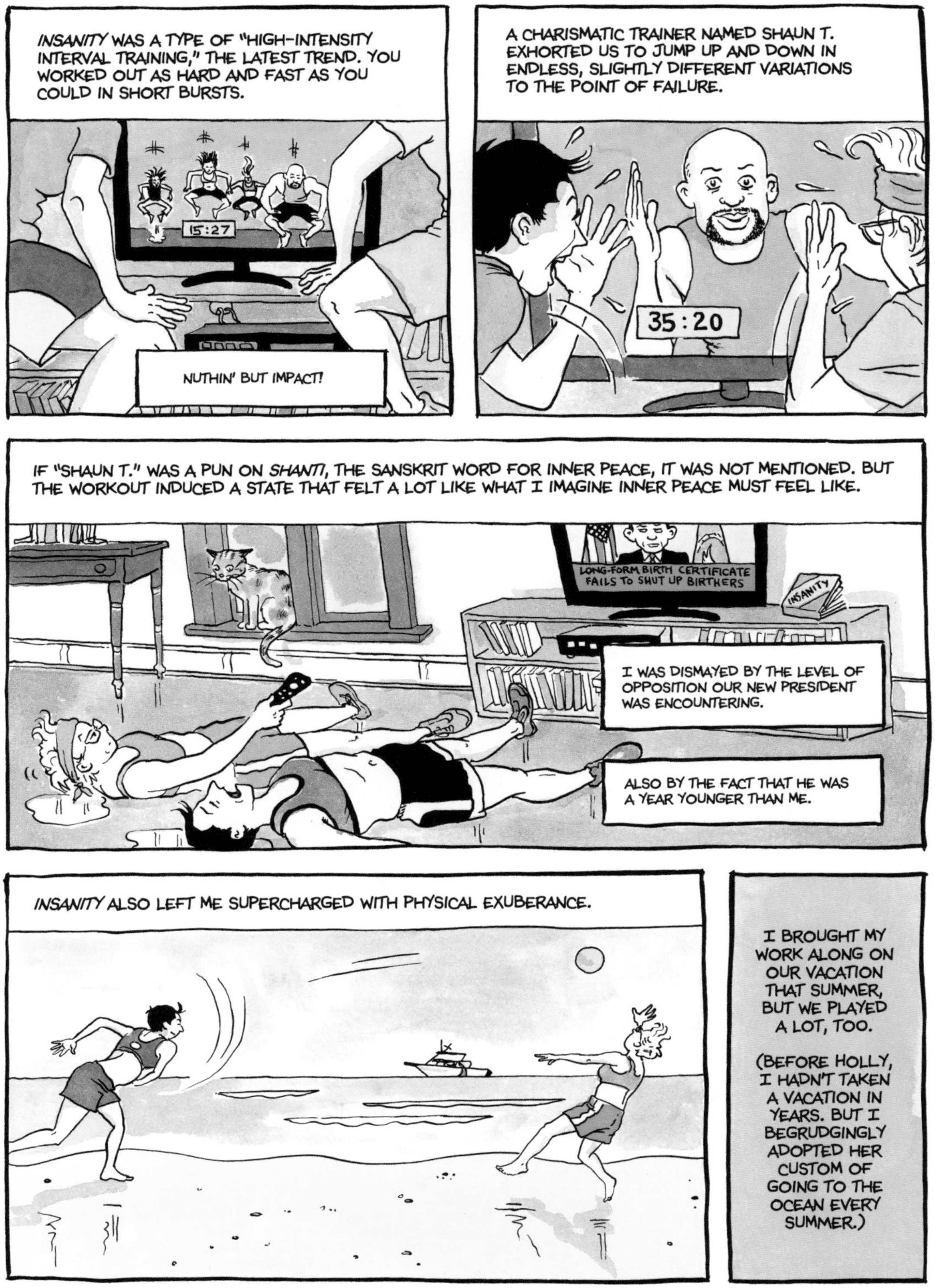

INSANITY WAS A TYPE OF "HIGH-INTENSITY INTERVAL TRAINING," THE LATEST TREND. YOU WORKED OUT AS HARD AND FAST AS YOU COULD IN SHORT BURSTS.
15:27
NUTHIN' BUT IMPACT!
A CHARISMATIC TRAINER NAMED SHAUN T. EXHORTED US TO JUMP UP AND DOWN IN ENDLESS, SLIGHTLY DIFFERENT VARIATIONS TO THE POINT OF FAILURE.
35:20
IF "SHAUN T." WAS A PUN ON SHANTI, THE SANSKRIT WORD FOR INNER PEACE, IT WAS NOT MENTIONED. BUT THE WORKOUT INDUCED A STATE THAT FELT A LOT LIKE WHAT I IMAGINE INNER PEACE MUST FEEL LIKE.
LONG-FORM BIRTH CERTIFICATE FAILS TO SHUT UP BIRTHERS
INSANITY
I WAS DISMAYED BY THE LEVEL OF OPPOSITION OUR NEW PRESIDENT WAS ENCOUNTERING.
ALSO BY THE FACT THAT HE WAS A YEAR YOUNGER THAN ME.
INSANITY ALSO LEFT ME SUPERCHARGED WITH PHYSICAL EXUBERANCE.
I BROUGHT MY WORK ALONG ON OUR VACATION THAT SUMMER, BUT WE PLAYED A LOT, TOO.
(BEFORE HOLLY, I HADN'T TAKEN A VACATION IN YEARS. BUT I BEGRUDGINGLY ADOPTED HER CUSTOM OF GOING TO THE OCEAN EVERY SUMMER.)

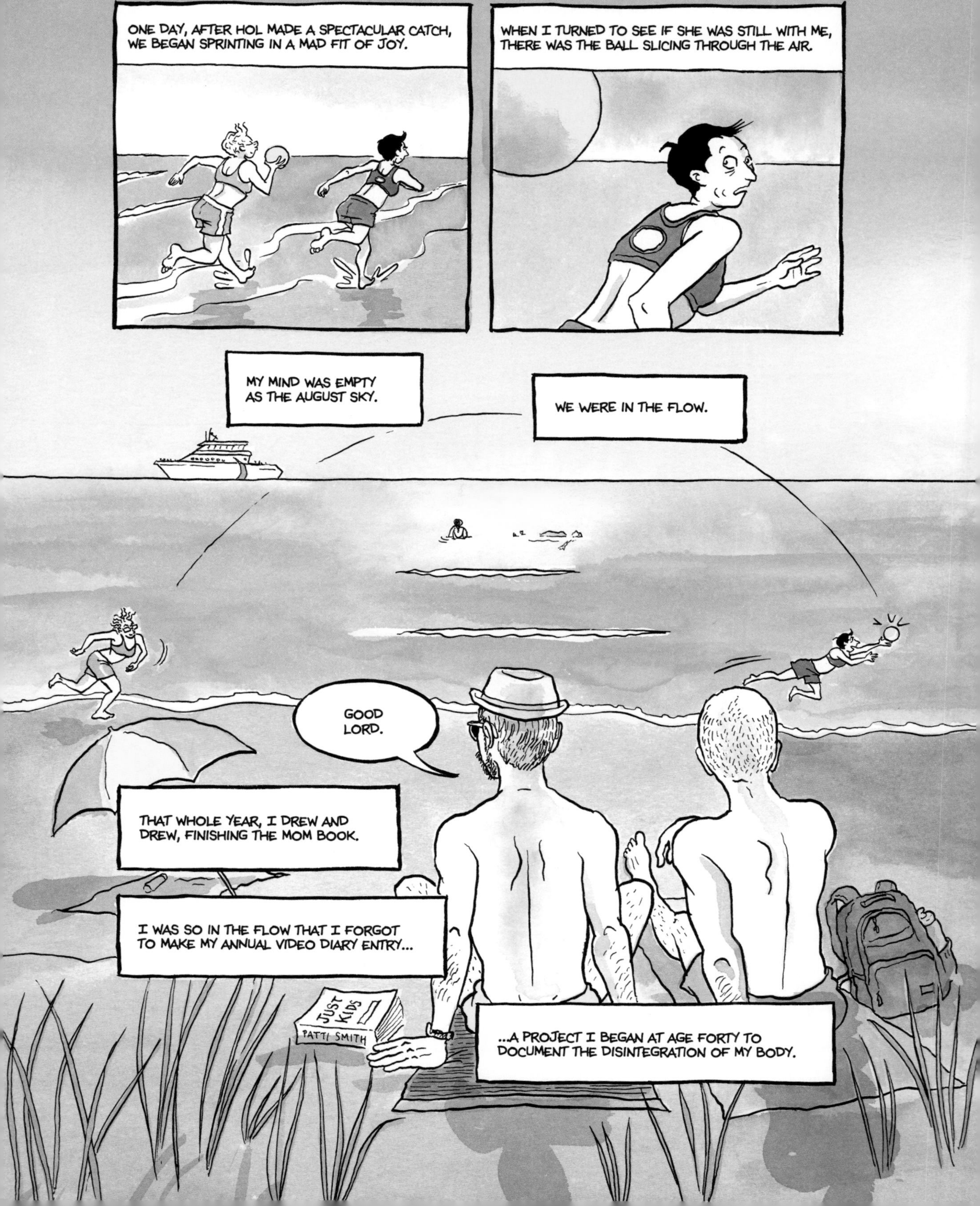
ONE DAY, AFTER HOL MADE A SPECTACULAR CATCH, WE BEGAN SPRINTING IN A MAD FIT OF JOY.
WHEN I TURNED TO SEE IF SHE WAS STILL WITH ME, THERE WAS THE BALL SLICING THROUGH THE AIR.
MY MIND WAS EMPTY AS THE AUGUST SKY.
WE WERE IN THE FLOW.
GOOD LORD.
THAT WHOLE YEAR, I DREW AND DREW, FINISHING THE MOM BOOK.
I WAS SO IN THE FLOW THAT I FORGOT TO MAKE MY ANNUAL VIDEO DIARY ENTRY...
JUST KIDS
PATTI SMITH
...A PROJECT I BEGAN AT AGE FORTY TO DOCUMENT THE DISINTEGRATION OF MY BODY.

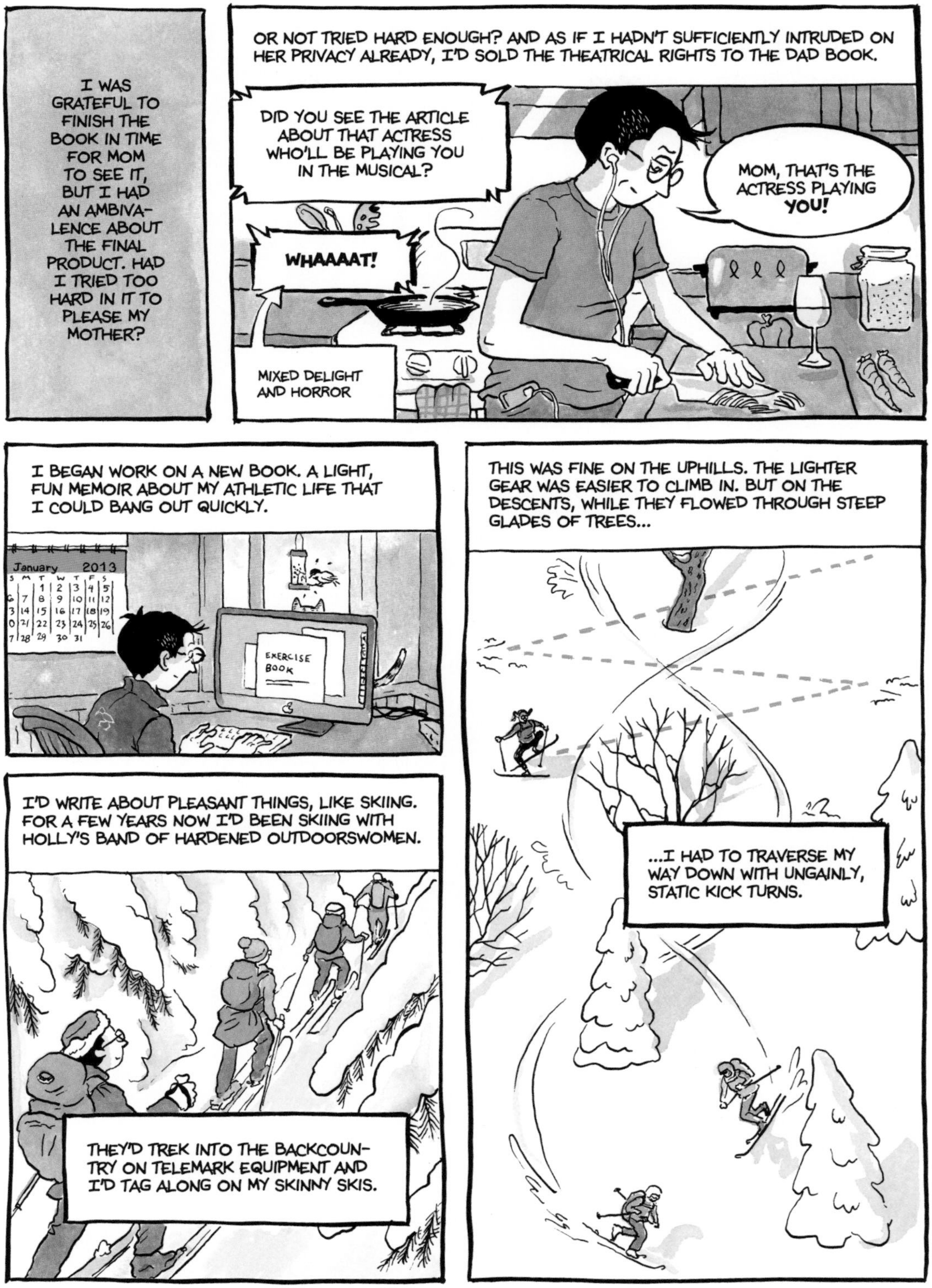
I WAS GRATEFUL TO FINISH THE BOOK IN TIME FOR MOM TO SEE IT, BUT I HAD AN AMBIVALENCE ABOUT THE FINAL PRODUCT. HAD I TRIED TOO HARD IN IT TO PLEASE MY MOTHER?
OR NOT TRIED HARD ENOUGH? AND AS IF I HADN'T SUFFICIENTLY INTRUDED ON HER PRIVACY ALREADY, I'D SOLD THE THEATRICAL RIGHTS TO THE DAD BOOK.
DID YOU SEE THE ARTICLE ABOUT THAT ACTRESS WHO'LL BE PLAYING YOU IN THE MUSICAL?
MOM, THAT'S THE ACTRESS PLAYING **YOU!**
WHAAAAT!
MIXED DELIGHT AND HORROR
I BEGAN WORK ON A NEW BOOK. A LIGHT, FUN MEMOIR ABOUT MY ATHLETIC LIFE THAT I COULD BANG OUT QUICKLY.
January 2013
EXERCISE BOOK
I'D WRITE ABOUT PLEASANT THINGS, LIKE SKIING. FOR A FEW YEARS NOW I'D BEEN SKIING WITH HOLLY'S BAND OF HARDENED OUTDOORSWOMEN.
THEY'D TREK INTO THE BACKCOUNTRY ON TELEMARK EQUIPMENT AND I'D TAG ALONG ON MY SKINNY SKIS.
THIS WAS FINE ON THE UPHILLS. THE LIGHTER GEAR WAS EASIER TO CLIMB IN. BUT ON THE DESCENTS, WHILE THEY FLOWED THROUGH STEEP GLADES OF TREES...
...I HAD TO TRAVERSE MY WAY DOWN WITH UNGAINLY, STATIC KICK TURNS.

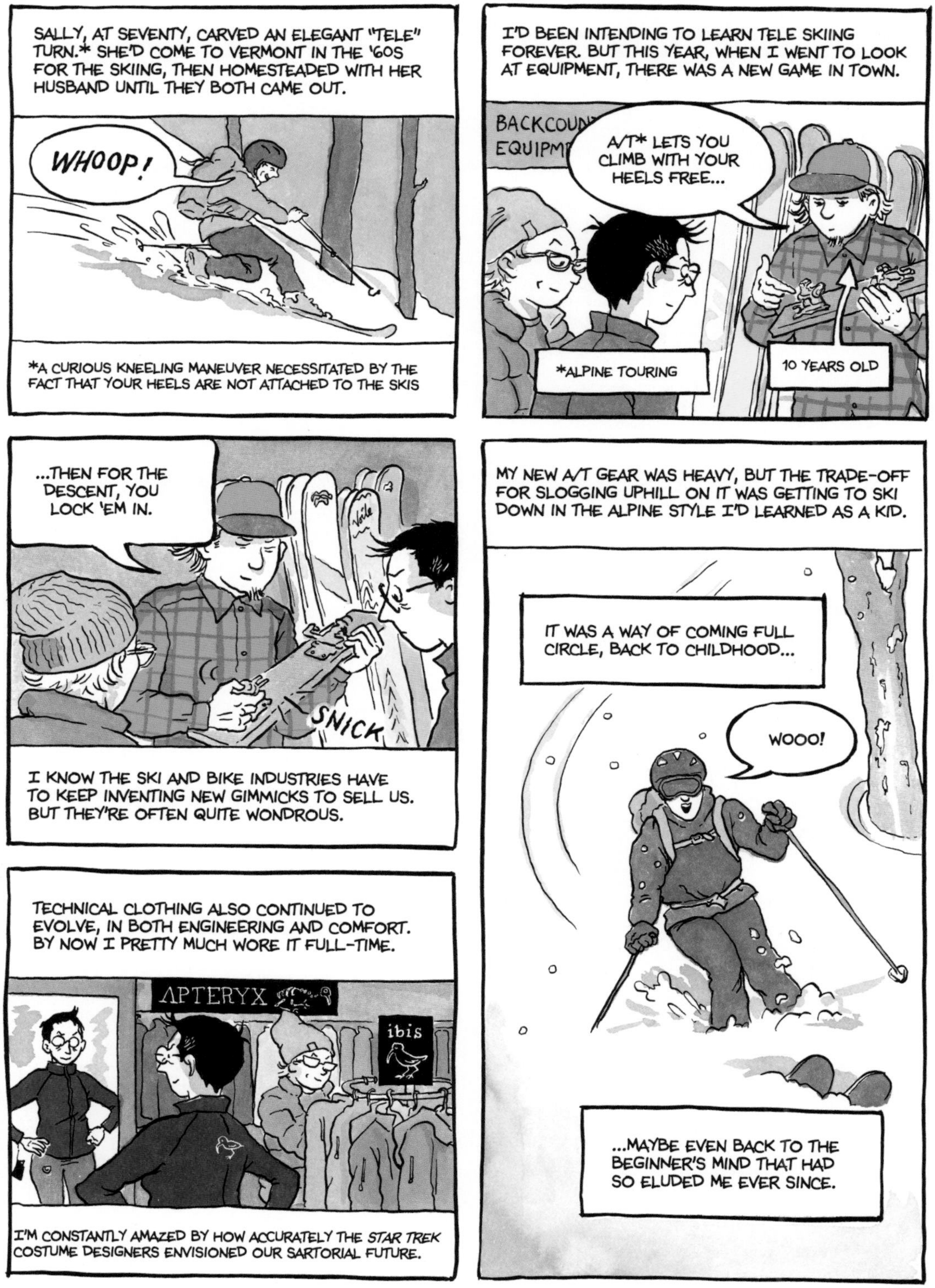

SALLY, AT SEVENTY, CARVED AN ELEGANT "TELE" TURN.* SHE'D COME TO VERMONT IN THE '60S FOR THE SKIING, THEN HOMESTEADED WITH HER HUSBAND UNTIL THEY BOTH CAME OUT.
WHOOP!
*A CURIOUS KNEELING MANEUVER NECESSITATED BY THE FACT THAT YOUR HEELS ARE NOT ATTACHED TO THE SKIS
I'D BEEN INTENDING TO LEARN TELE SKIING FOREVER. BUT THIS YEAR, WHEN I WENT TO LOOK AT EQUIPMENT, THERE WAS A NEW GAME IN TOWN.
A/T* LETS YOU CLIMB WITH YOUR HEELS FREE...
*ALPINE TOURING
10 YEARS OLD
...THEN FOR THE DESCENT, YOU LOCK 'EM IN.
SNICK
I KNOW THE SKI AND BIKE INDUSTRIES HAVE TO KEEP INVENTING NEW GIMMICKS TO SELL US. BUT THEY'RE OFTEN QUITE WONDROUS.
TECHNICAL CLOTHING ALSO CONTINUED TO EVOLVE, IN BOTH ENGINEERING AND COMFORT. BY NOW I PRETTY MUCH WORE IT FULL-TIME.
APTERYX
ibis
I'M CONSTANTLY AMAZED BY HOW ACCURATELY THE STAR TREK COSTUME DESIGNERS ENVISIONED OUR SARTORIAL FUTURE.
MY NEW A/T GEAR WAS HEAVY, BUT THE TRADE-OFF FOR SLOGGING UPHILL ON IT WAS GETTING TO SKI DOWN IN THE ALPINE STYLE I'D LEARNED AS A KID.
IT WAS A WAY OF COMING FULL CIRCLE, BACK TO CHILDHOOD...
WOOO!
...MAYBE EVEN BACK TO THE BEGINNER'S MIND THAT HAD SO ELUDED ME EVER SINCE.

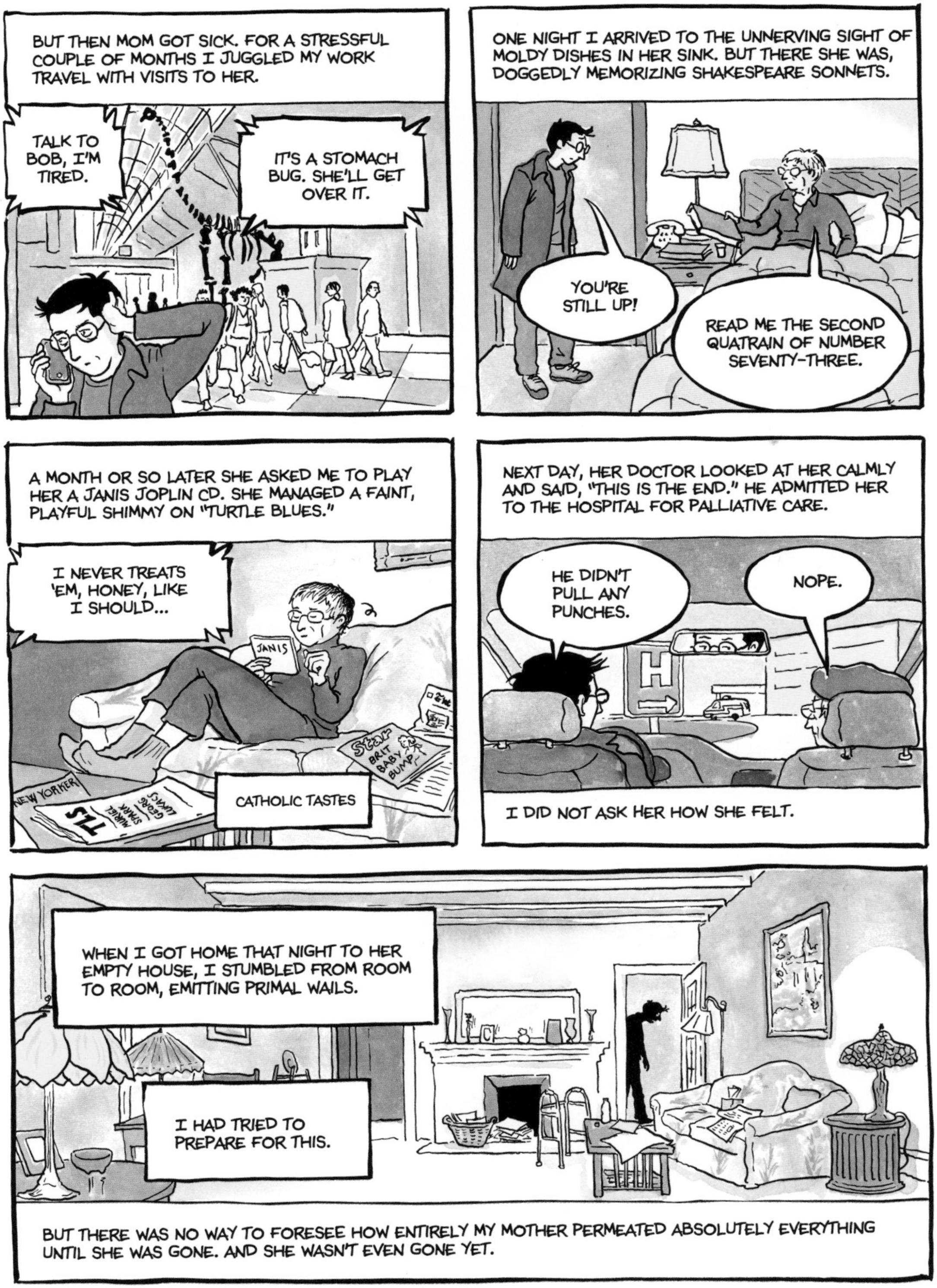
BUT THEN MOM GOT SICK. FOR A STRESSFUL COUPLE OF MONTHS I JUGGLED MY WORK TRAVEL WITH VISITS TO HER.
TALK TO BOB, I'M TIRED.
IT'S A STOMACH BUG. SHE'LL GET OVER IT.
ONE NIGHT I ARRIVED TO THE UNNERVING SIGHT OF MOLDY DISHES IN HER SINK. BUT THERE SHE WAS, DOGGEDLY MEMORIZING SHAKESPEARE SONNETS.
YOU'RE STILL UP!
READ ME THE SECOND QUATRAIN OF NUMBER SEVENTY-THREE.
A MONTH OR SO LATER SHE ASKED ME TO PLAY HER A JANIS JOPLIN CD. SHE MANAGED A FAINT, PLAYFUL SHIMMY ON "TURTLE BLUES."
I NEVER TREATS 'EM, HONEY, LIKE I SHOULD...
JANIS
Star
BRIT BABY BUMP
NEW YORKER
TLS
CATHOLIC TASTES
NEXT DAY, HER DOCTOR LOOKED AT HER CALMLY AND SAID, "THIS IS THE END." HE ADMITTED HER TO THE HOSPITAL FOR PALLIATIVE CARE.
HE DIDN'T PULL ANY PUNCHES.
NOPE.
H
I DID NOT ASK HER HOW SHE FELT.
WHEN I GOT HOME THAT NIGHT TO HER EMPTY HOUSE, I STUMBLED FROM ROOM TO ROOM, EMITTING PRIMAL WAILS.
I HAD TRIED TO PREPARE FOR THIS.
BUT THERE WAS NO WAY TO FORESEE HOW ENTIRELY MY MOTHER PERMEATED ABSOLUTELY EVERYTHING UNTIL SHE WAS GONE. AND SHE WASN'T EVEN GONE YET.

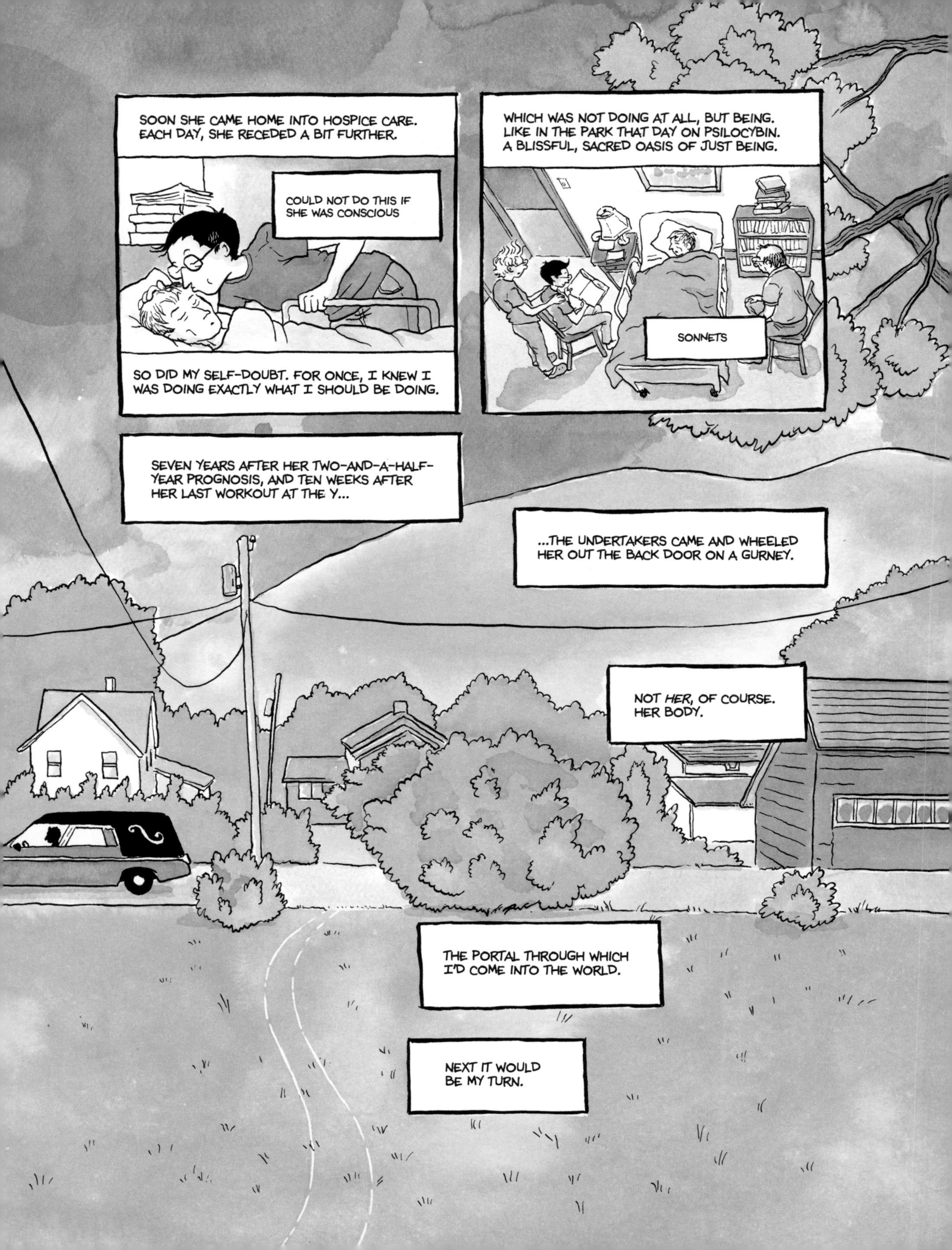
SOON SHE CAME HOME INTO HOSPICE CARE. EACH DAY, SHE RECEDED A BIT FURTHER.
COULD NOT DO THIS IF SHE WAS CONSCIOUS
SO DID MY SELF-DOUBT. FOR ONCE, I KNEW I WAS DOING EXACTLY WHAT I SHOULD BE DOING.
WHICH WAS NOT DOING AT ALL, BUT BEING. LIKE IN THE PARK THAT DAY ON PSILOCYBIN. A BLISSFUL, SACRED OASIS OF JUST BEING.
SONNETS
SEVEN YEARS AFTER HER TWO-AND-A-HALF-YEAR PROGNOSIS, AND TEN WEEKS AFTER HER LAST WORKOUT AT THE Y...
...THE UNDERTAKERS CAME AND WHEELED HER OUT THE BACK DOOR ON A GURNEY.
NOT *HER*, OF COURSE. HER BODY.
THE PORTAL THROUGH WHICH I'D COME INTO THE WORLD.
NEXT IT WOULD BE MY TURN.

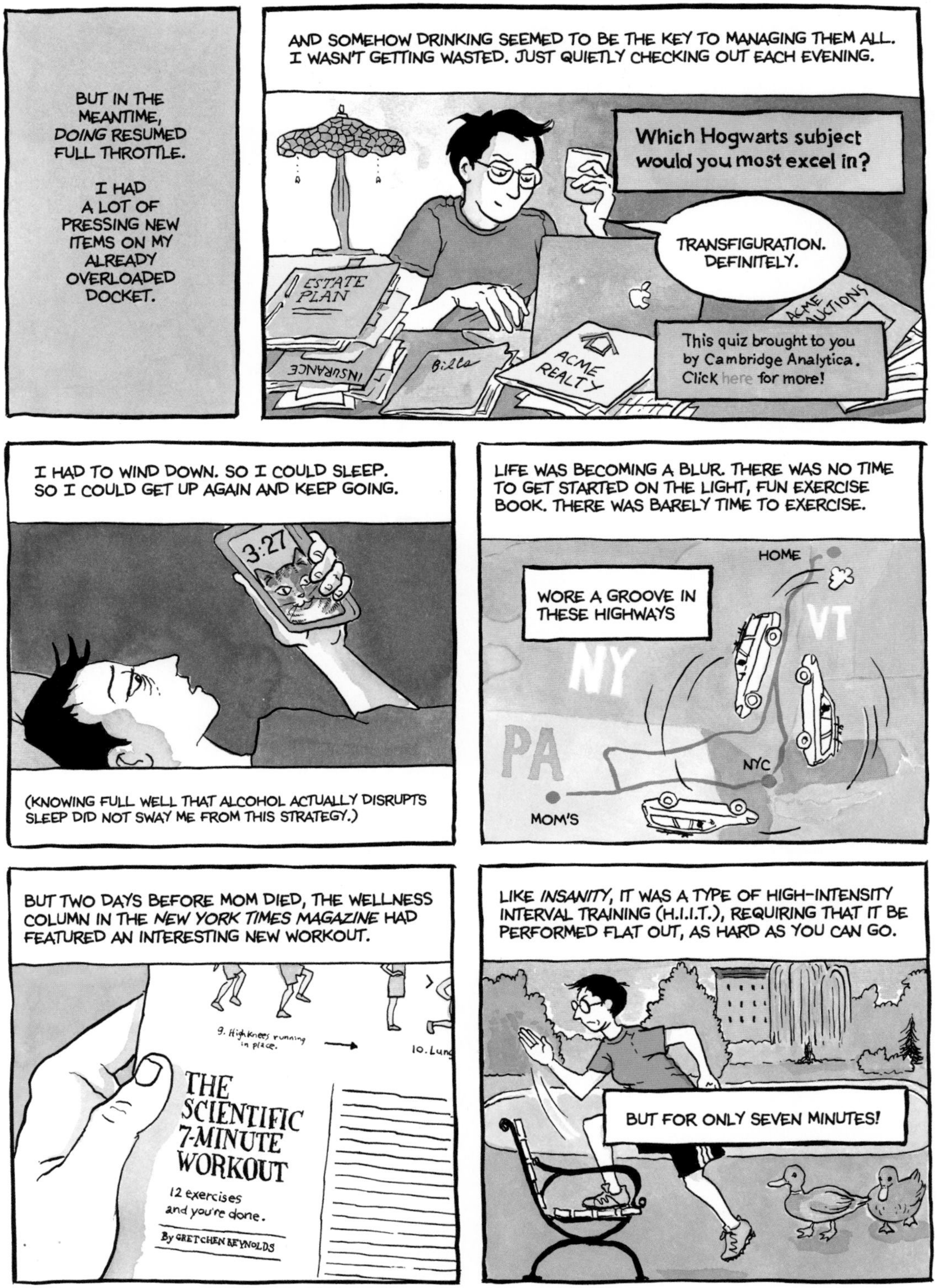
BUT IN THE MEANTIME, *DOING* RESUMED FULL THROTTLE.
I HAD A LOT OF PRESSING NEW ITEMS ON MY ALREADY OVERLOADED DOCKET.
AND SOMEHOW DRINKING SEEMED TO BE THE KEY TO MANAGING THEM ALL. I WASN'T GETTING WASTED. JUST QUIETLY CHECKING OUT EACH EVENING.
Which Hogwarts subject would you most excel in?
TRANSFIGURATION. DEFINITELY.
ESTATE PLAN
INSURANCE
Bills
ACME REALTY
ACME AUCTIONS
This quiz brought to you by Cambridge Analytica. Click here for more!
I HAD TO WIND DOWN. SO I COULD SLEEP. SO I COULD GET UP AGAIN AND KEEP GOING.
3:27
(KNOWING FULL WELL THAT ALCOHOL ACTUALLY DISRUPTS SLEEP DID NOT SWAY ME FROM THIS STRATEGY.)
LIFE WAS BECOMING A BLUR. THERE WAS NO TIME TO GET STARTED ON THE LIGHT, FUN EXERCISE BOOK. THERE WAS BARELY TIME TO EXERCISE.
WORE A GROOVE IN THESE HIGHWAYS
HOME
VT
NY
PA
NYC
MOM'S
BUT TWO DAYS BEFORE MOM DIED, THE WELLNESS COLUMN IN THE *NEW YORK TIMES MAGAZINE* HAD FEATURED AN INTERESTING NEW WORKOUT.
9. High knees running in place.
10. Lung
THE SCIENTIFIC 7-MINUTE WORKOUT
12 exercises and you're done.
By GRETCHEN REYNOLDS
LIKE *INSANITY*, IT WAS A TYPE OF HIGH-INTENSITY INTERVAL TRAINING (H.I.I.T.), REQUIRING THAT IT BE PERFORMED FLAT OUT, AS HARD AS YOU CAN GO.
BUT FOR ONLY SEVEN MINUTES!

THE SEMI-SADISTIC 7-MINUTE WORKOUT

12 exercises, and you're done for.

AS MY LIFE ITSELF BECAME A KIND OF HIGH-INTENSITY INTERVAL TRAINING, THIS WORKOUT WOULD BE MY SALVATION. I WOULD DO IT ON THREE CONTINENTS, AND MORE CITIES THAN I CAN COUNT, FIRST THING IN THE MORNING BEFORE I COULD THINK BETTER OF IT. IT RESTORED ELASTICITY TO MY BODY, CLARITY TO MY MIND, AND BUOYANCY TO MY SOUL--THOUGH I WAS STILL UNSURE WHAT A SOUL WAS.

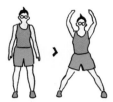

1. Rent a dumpster and, in a grief-stricken daze, fill it with the contents of your dead mother's house.

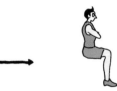

2. Rush to your dead mother's partner's deathbed when he, also grief-stricken, decides to stop treatment for his multiple illnesses.

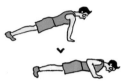

3. Rush off again in order to attend Off-Broadway musical based on your family memoir.

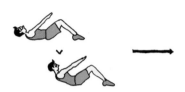

4. Round up wayward family members in logistically and emotionally complex operation for matinée of same.

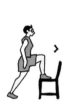

5. On grueling round of speaking engagements, realize you are performing some kind of version of yourself. Wonder if this is what it's like to be a sex worker.

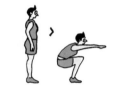

6. Fly to comics festival in France, give talk in English about your lesbian comic strip and gay dad to bewildered immigrant high school students.

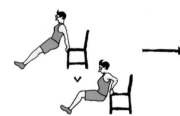

7. Travel to antipodes for a month of public appearances. Note incremental but inexorable ebb of life force with each one.

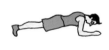

8. While struggling to feel that you deserve to be at an artist's residency in Italy, learn that you have won a MacArthur "genius" grant, and that the musical is moving to Broadway.

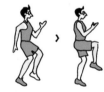

9. Become seized with a sense of profound fraudulence, made worse by knowledge that this is actually quite narcissistic and self-indulgent.

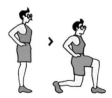

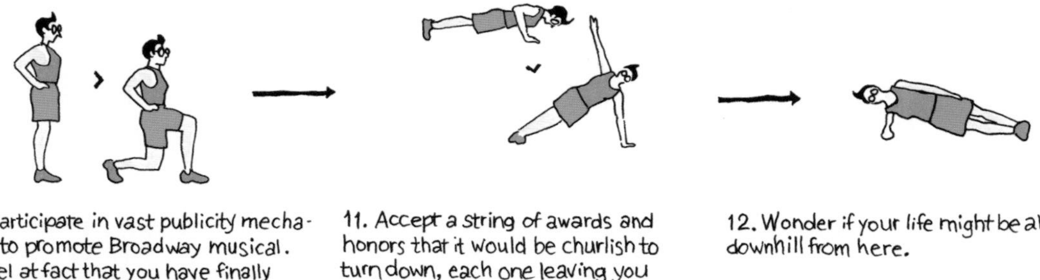

10. Participate in vast publicity mechanism to promote Broadway musical. Marvel at fact that you have finally become sick of talking about yourself.

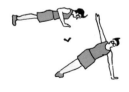

11. Accept a string of awards and honors that it would be churlish to turn down, each one leaving you feeling more depleted and foolish than the last.

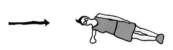

12. Wonder if your life might be all downhill from here.

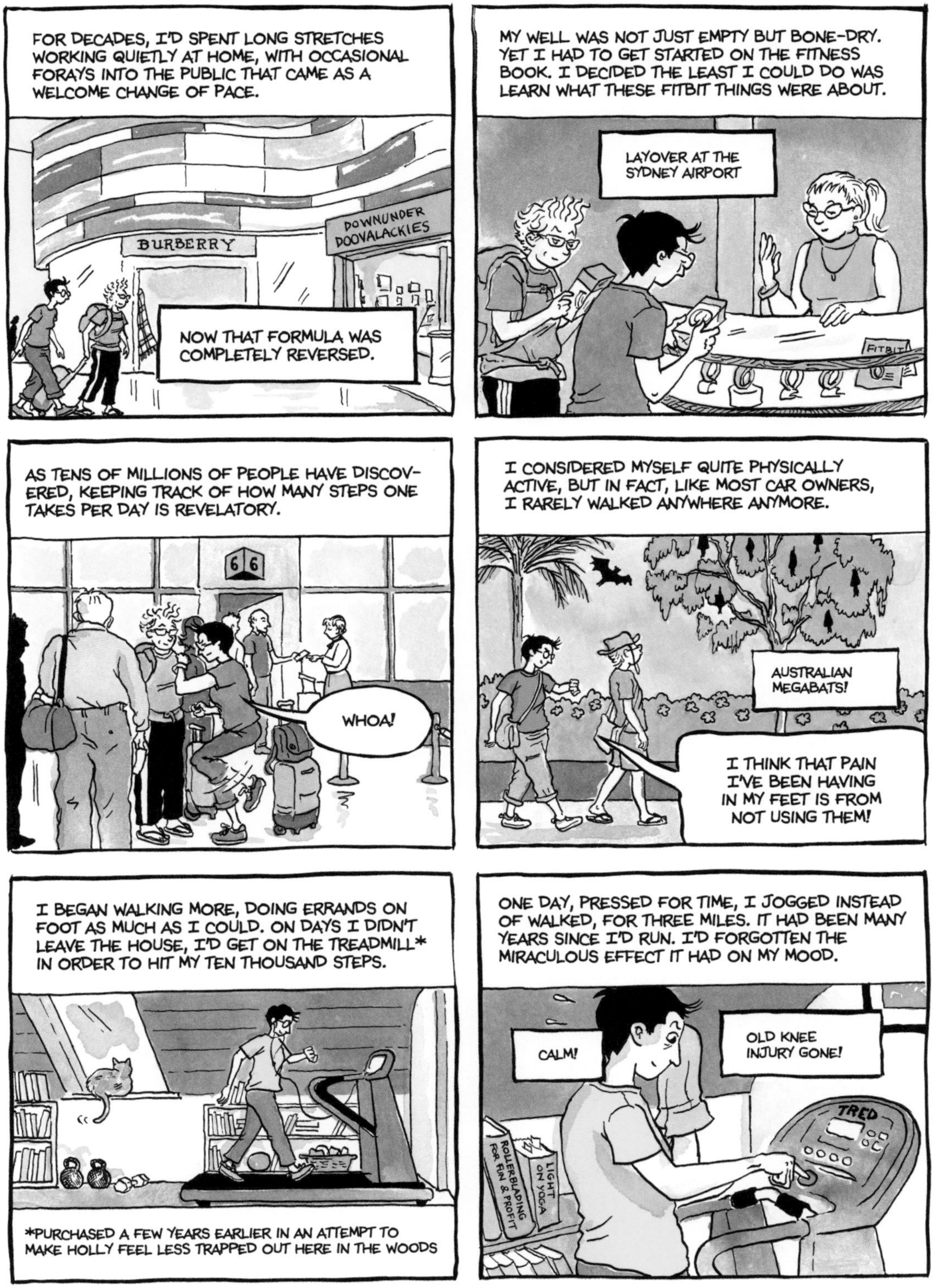
FOR DECADES, I'D SPENT LONG STRETCHES WORKING QUIETLY AT HOME, WITH OCCASIONAL FORAYS INTO THE PUBLIC THAT CAME AS A WELCOME CHANGE OF PACE.
BURBERRY
DOWNUNDER DOOVALACKIES
NOW THAT FORMULA WAS COMPLETELY REVERSED.
MY WELL WAS NOT JUST EMPTY BUT BONE-DRY. YET I HAD TO GET STARTED ON THE FITNESS BOOK. I DECIDED THE LEAST I COULD DO WAS LEARN WHAT THESE FITBIT THINGS WERE ABOUT.
LAYOVER AT THE SYDNEY AIRPORT
FITBIT
AS TENS OF MILLIONS OF PEOPLE HAVE DISCOVERED, KEEPING TRACK OF HOW MANY STEPS ONE TAKES PER DAY IS REVELATORY.
66
WHOA!
I CONSIDERED MYSELF QUITE PHYSICALLY ACTIVE, BUT IN FACT, LIKE MOST CAR OWNERS, I RARELY WALKED ANYWHERE ANYMORE.
AUSTRALIAN MEGABATS!
I THINK THAT PAIN I'VE BEEN HAVING IN MY FEET IS FROM NOT USING THEM!
I BEGAN WALKING MORE, DOING ERRANDS ON FOOT AS MUCH AS I COULD. ON DAYS I DIDN'T LEAVE THE HOUSE, I'D GET ON THE TREADMILL* IN ORDER TO HIT MY TEN THOUSAND STEPS.
*PURCHASED A FEW YEARS EARLIER IN AN ATTEMPT TO MAKE HOLLY FEEL LESS TRAPPED OUT HERE IN THE WOODS
ONE DAY, PRESSED FOR TIME, I JOGGED INSTEAD OF WALKED, FOR THREE MILES. IT HAD BEEN MANY YEARS SINCE I'D RUN. I'D FORGOTTEN THE MIRACULOUS EFFECT IT HAD ON MY MOOD.
CALM!
OLD KNEE INJURY GONE!
TRED
ROLLERBLADING FOR FUN & PROFIT
LIGHT ON YOGA

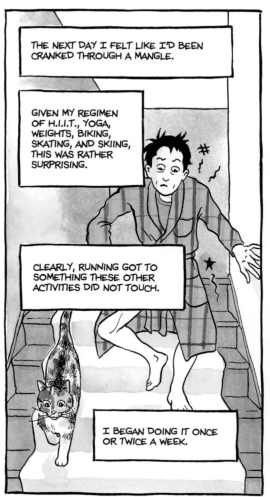

THE NEXT DAY I FELT LIKE I'D BEEN CRANKED THROUGH A MANGLE.

GIVEN MY REGIMEN OF H.I.I.T., YOGA, WEIGHTS, BIKING, SKATING, AND SKIING, THIS WAS RATHER SURPRISING.

CLEARLY, RUNNING GOT TO SOMETHING THESE OTHER ACTIVITIES DID NOT TOUCH.

I BEGAN DOING IT ONCE OR TWICE A WEEK.

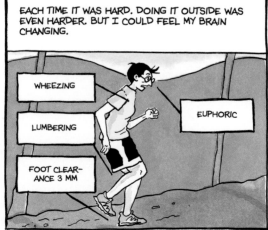

EACH TIME IT WAS HARD. DOING IT OUTSIDE WAS EVEN HARDER. BUT I COULD FEEL MY BRAIN CHANGING.

WHEEZING

LUMBERING

FOOT CLEAR-ANCE 3 MM

EUPHORIC

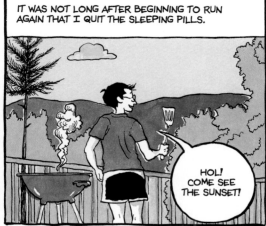

IT WAS NOT LONG AFTER BEGINNING TO RUN AGAIN THAT I QUIT THE SLEEPING PILLS.

HOL! COME SEE THE SUNSET!

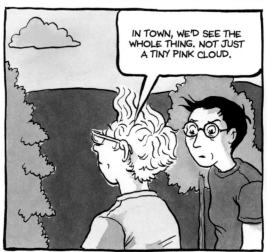

IN TOWN, WE'D SEE THE WHOLE THING. NOT JUST A TINY PINK CLOUD.

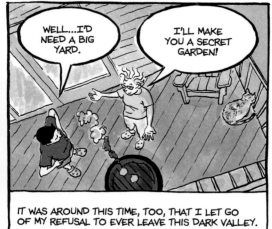

WELL...I'D NEED A BIG YARD.

I'LL MAKE YOU A SECRET GARDEN!

IT WAS AROUND THIS TIME, TOO, THAT I LET GO OF MY REFUSAL TO EVER LEAVE THIS DARK VALLEY.

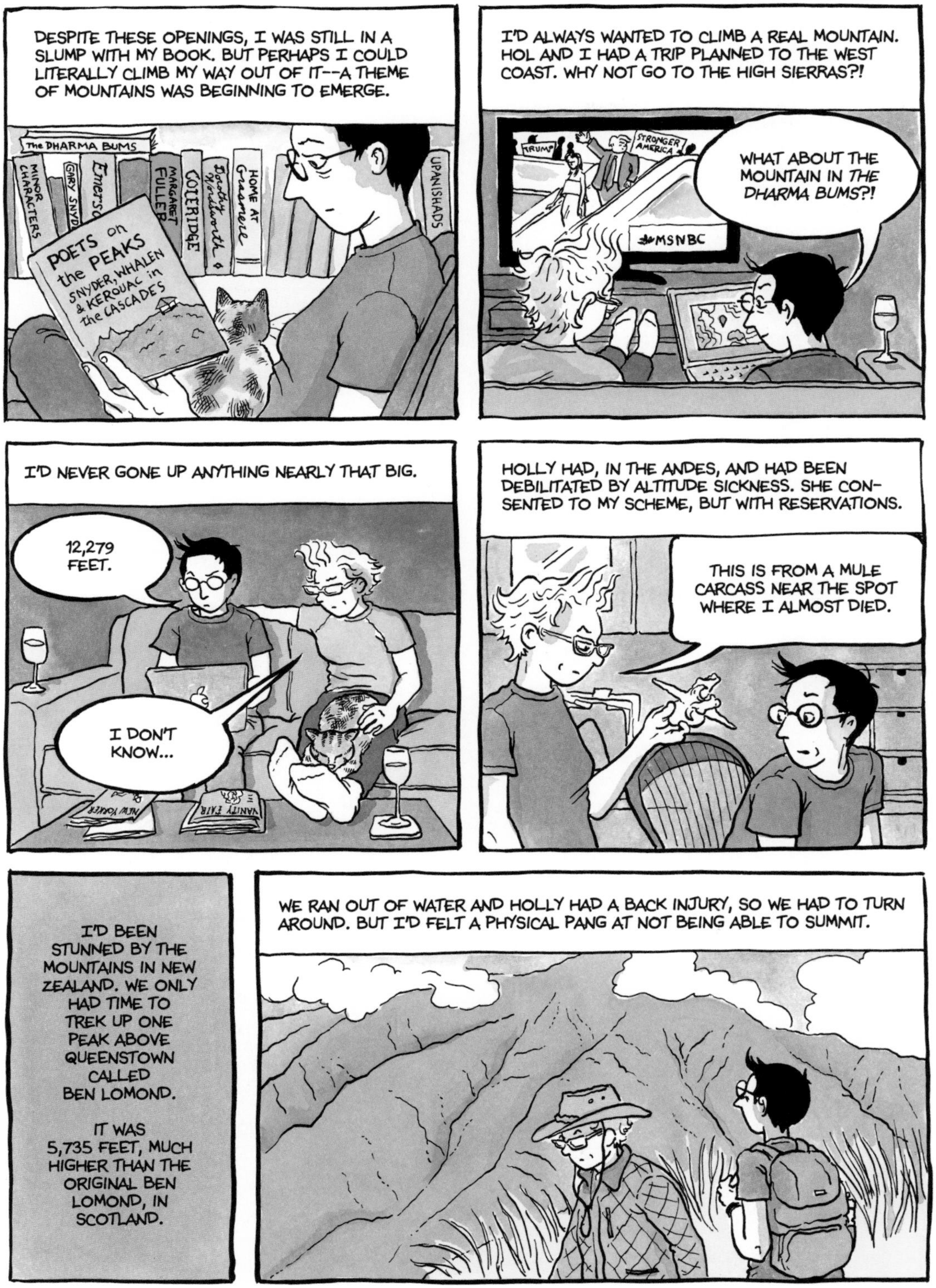
DESPITE THESE OPENINGS, I WAS STILL IN A SLUMP WITH MY BOOK. BUT PERHAPS I COULD LITERALLY CLIMB MY WAY OUT OF IT--A THEME OF MOUNTAINS WAS BEGINNING TO EMERGE.
The DHARMA BUMS
MINOR CHARACTERS
GARY SNYD
Emerso
MARGARET FULLER
COLERIDGE
Dorothy Wordsworth
HOME AT Grasmere
UPANISHADS
POETS on the PEAKS SNYDER, WHALEN & KEROUAC in the CASCADES
I'D ALWAYS WANTED TO CLIMB A REAL MOUNTAIN. HOL AND I HAD A TRIP PLANNED TO THE WEST COAST. WHY NOT GO TO THE HIGH SIERRAS?!
TRUMP
STRONGER AMERICA
MSNBC
WHAT ABOUT THE MOUNTAIN IN *THE DHARMA BUMS*?!
I'D NEVER GONE UP ANYTHING NEARLY THAT BIG.
12,279 FEET.
I DON'T KNOW...
NEW YORKER
VANITY FAIR
HOLLY HAD, IN THE ANDES, AND HAD BEEN DEBILITATED BY ALTITUDE SICKNESS. SHE CONSENTED TO MY SCHEME, BUT WITH RESERVATIONS.
THIS IS FROM A MULE CARCASS NEAR THE SPOT WHERE I ALMOST DIED.
I'D BEEN STUNNED BY THE MOUNTAINS IN NEW ZEALAND. WE ONLY HAD TIME TO TREK UP ONE PEAK ABOVE QUEENSTOWN CALLED BEN LOMOND.
IT WAS 5,735 FEET, MUCH HIGHER THAN THE ORIGINAL BEN LOMOND, IN SCOTLAND.
WE RAN OUT OF WATER AND HOLLY HAD A BACK INJURY, SO WE HAD TO TURN AROUND. BUT I'D FELT A PHYSICAL PANG AT NOT BEING ABLE TO SUMMIT.

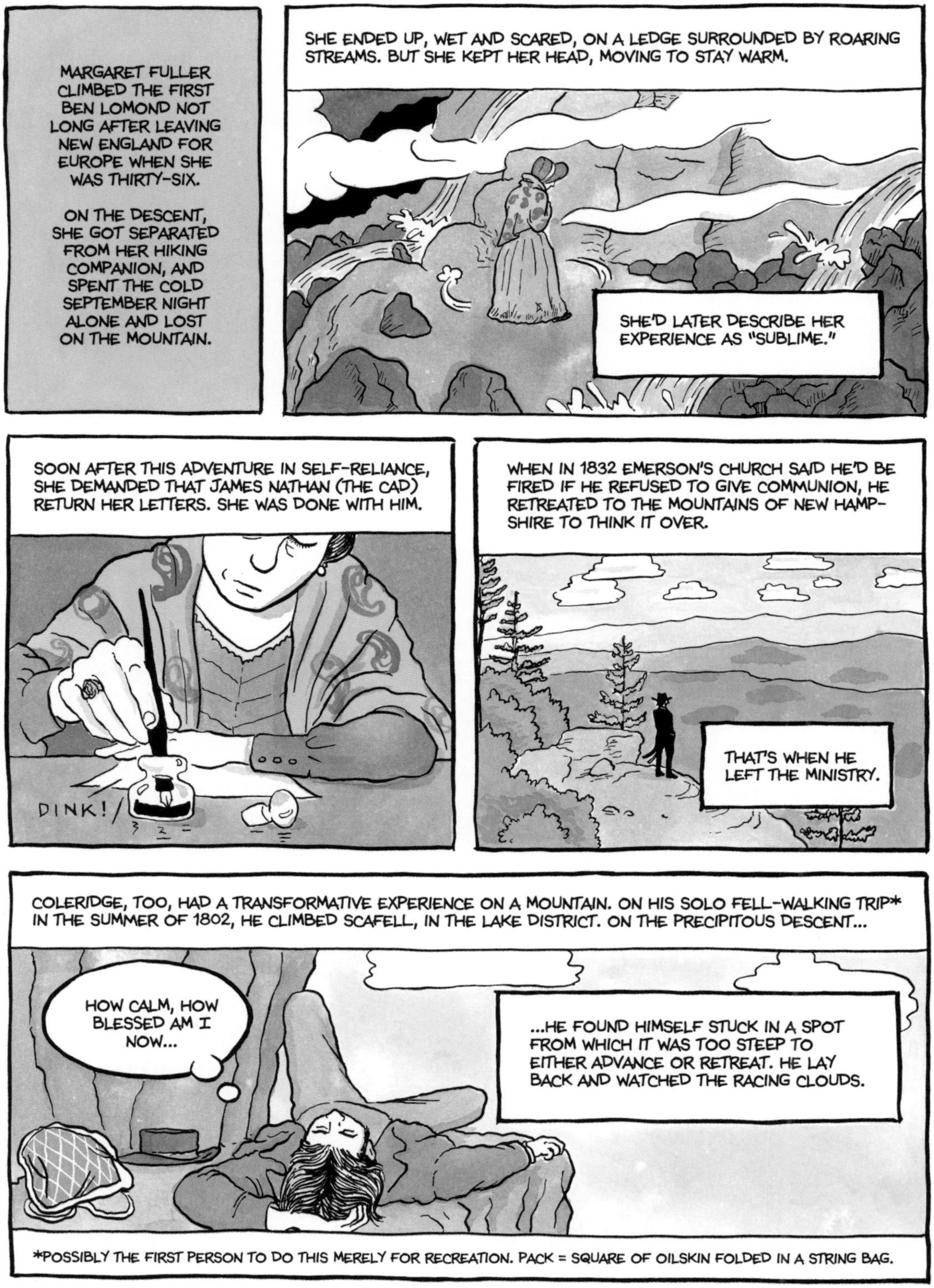
MARGARET FULLER CLIMBED THE FIRST BEN LOMOND NOT LONG AFTER LEAVING NEW ENGLAND FOR EUROPE WHEN SHE WAS THIRTY-SIX.
ON THE DESCENT, SHE GOT SEPARATED FROM HER HIKING COMPANION, AND SPENT THE COLD SEPTEMBER NIGHT ALONE AND LOST ON THE MOUNTAIN.
SHE ENDED UP, WET AND SCARED, ON A LEDGE SURROUNDED BY ROARING STREAMS. BUT SHE KEPT HER HEAD, MOVING TO STAY WARM.
SHE'D LATER DESCRIBE HER EXPERIENCE AS "SUBLIME."
SOON AFTER THIS ADVENTURE IN SELF-RELIANCE, SHE DEMANDED THAT JAMES NATHAN (THE CAD) RETURN HER LETTERS. SHE WAS DONE WITH HIM.
DINK!
WHEN IN 1832 EMERSON'S CHURCH SAID HE'D BE FIRED IF HE REFUSED TO GIVE COMMUNION, HE RETREATED TO THE MOUNTAINS OF NEW HAMP-SHIRE TO THINK IT OVER.
THAT'S WHEN HE LEFT THE MINISTRY.
COLERIDGE, TOO, HAD A TRANSFORMATIVE EXPERIENCE ON A MOUNTAIN. ON HIS SOLO FELL-WALKING TRIP* IN THE SUMMER OF 1802, HE CLIMBED SCAFELL, IN THE LAKE DISTRICT. ON THE PRECIPITOUS DESCENT...
HOW CALM, HOW BLESSED AM I NOW...
...HE FOUND HIMSELF STUCK IN A SPOT FROM WHICH IT WAS TOO STEEP TO EITHER ADVANCE OR RETREAT. HE LAY BACK AND WATCHED THE RACING CLOUDS.
*POSSIBLY THE FIRST PERSON TO DO THIS MERELY FOR RECREATION. PACK = SQUARE OF OILSKIN FOLDED IN A STRING BAG.

HE'D MADE THE TREK, IN PART, TO STAVE OFF HIS GROWING OPIUM HABIT.

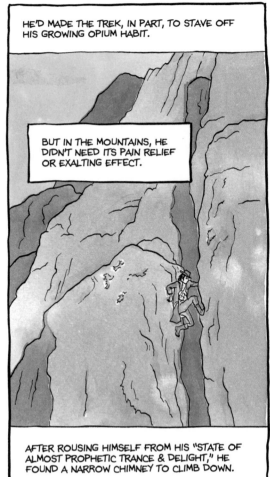

BUT IN THE MOUNTAINS, HE DIDN'T NEED ITS PAIN RELIEF OR EXALTING EFFECT.

AFTER ROUSING HIMSELF FROM HIS "STATE OF ALMOST PROPHETIC TRANCE & DELIGHT," HE FOUND A NARROW CHIMNEY TO CLIMB DOWN.

IN 1818, DOROTHY WOULD CLIMB NEIGHBORING SCAFELL PIKE, THE HIGHEST PEAK IN ENGLAND, WITH A SMALL PARTY. SHE WAS FORTY-SIX.

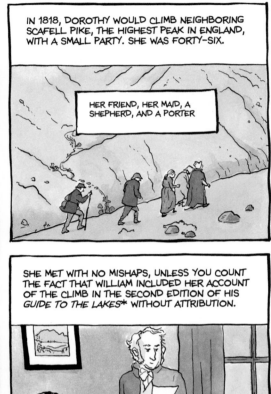

HER FRIEND, HER MAID, A SHEPHERD, AND A PORTER

SHE MET WITH NO MISHAPS, UNLESS YOU COUNT THE FACT THAT WILLIAM INCLUDED HER ACCOUNT OF THE CLIMB IN THE SECOND EDITION OF HIS *GUIDE TO THE LAKES** WITHOUT ATTRIBUTION.

*AT THE TIME, HE WAS ALMOST BETTER KNOWN FOR THIS GUIDEBOOK THAN FOR HIS POETRY.

AT AGE FIFTY-SEVEN, DOROTHY WENT INTO A DECLINE UNDERSTOOD AT THE TIME AS "PREMATURE DOTAGE."

BUT SOMETIMES SHE'D SNAP OUT OF IT AND SEEM FINE. AND SHE LIVED TO BE EIGHTY-THREE.

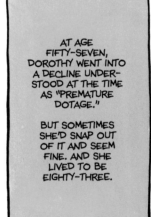

HER BIOGRAPHER FRANCES WILSON DIAGNOSES HER WITH "DEPRESSIVE PSEUDO-DEMENTIA," A PROFOUND DEPRESSION THAT MIMICS DEMENTIA...

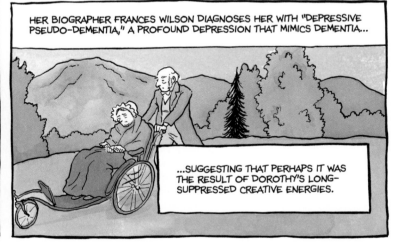

...SUGGESTING THAT PERHAPS IT WAS THE RESULT OF DOROTHY'S LONG-SUPPRESSED CREATIVE ENERGIES.

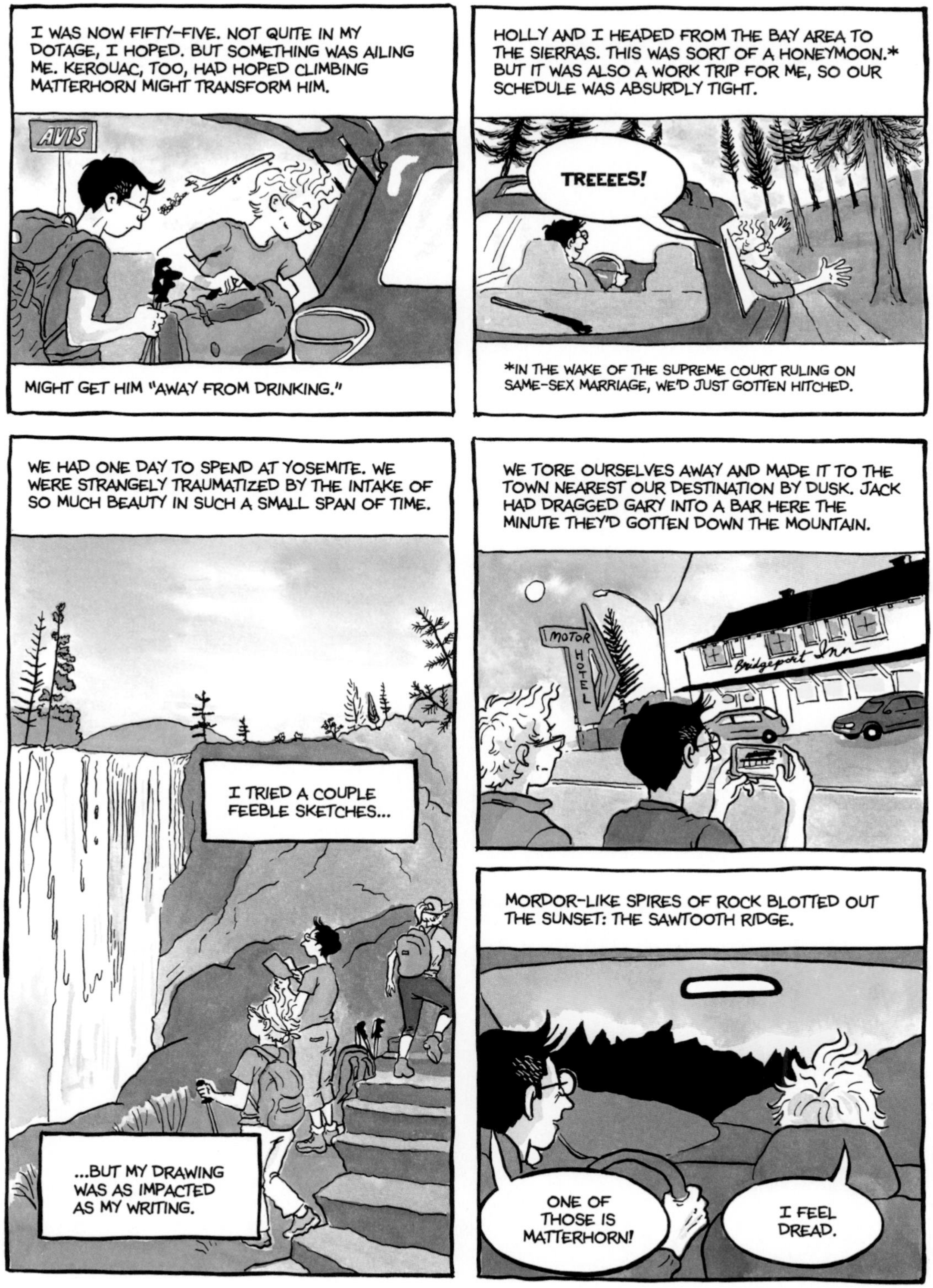
I WAS NOW FIFTY-FIVE. NOT QUITE IN MY DOTAGE, I HOPED. BUT SOMETHING WAS AILING ME. KEROUAC, TOO, HAD HOPED CLIMBING MATTERHORN MIGHT TRANSFORM HIM.
AVIS
MIGHT GET HIM "AWAY FROM DRINKING."
HOLLY AND I HEADED FROM THE BAY AREA TO THE SIERRAS. THIS WAS SORT OF A HONEYMOON.* BUT IT WAS ALSO A WORK TRIP FOR ME, SO OUR SCHEDULE WAS ABSURDLY TIGHT.
TREEEES!
*IN THE WAKE OF THE SUPREME COURT RULING ON SAME-SEX MARRIAGE, WE'D JUST GOTTEN HITCHED.
WE HAD ONE DAY TO SPEND AT YOSEMITE. WE WERE STRANGELY TRAUMATIZED BY THE INTAKE OF SO MUCH BEAUTY IN SUCH A SMALL SPAN OF TIME.
I TRIED A COUPLE FEEBLE SKETCHES...
...BUT MY DRAWING WAS AS IMPACTED AS MY WRITING.
WE TORE OURSELVES AWAY AND MADE IT TO THE TOWN NEAREST OUR DESTINATION BY DUSK. JACK HAD DRAGGED GARY INTO A BAR HERE THE MINUTE THEY'D GOTTEN DOWN THE MOUNTAIN.
MOTOR HOTEL
Bridgeport Inn
MORDOR-LIKE SPIRES OF ROCK BLOTTED OUT THE SUNSET: THE SAWTOOTH RIDGE.
ONE OF THOSE IS MATTERHORN!
I FEEL DREAD.

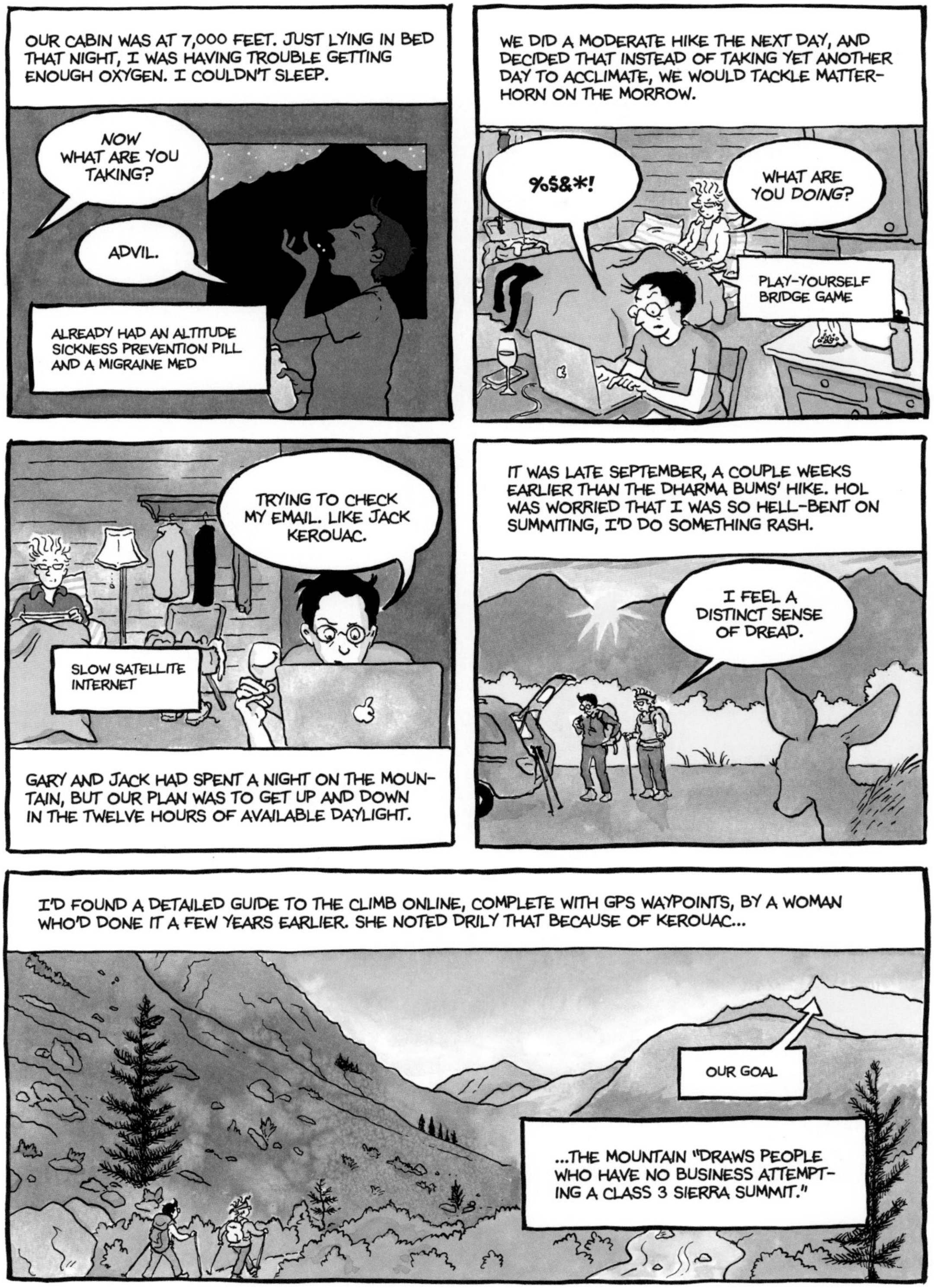
OUR CABIN WAS AT 7,000 FEET. JUST LYING IN BED THAT NIGHT, I WAS HAVING TROUBLE GETTING ENOUGH OXYGEN. I COULDN'T SLEEP.
NOW WHAT ARE YOU TAKING?
ADVIL.
ALREADY HAD AN ALTITUDE SICKNESS PREVENTION PILL AND A MIGRAINE MED
WE DID A MODERATE HIKE THE NEXT DAY, AND DECIDED THAT INSTEAD OF TAKING YET ANOTHER DAY TO ACCLIMATE, WE WOULD TACKLE MATTER-HORN ON THE MORROW.
%$&*!
WHAT ARE YOU *DOING*?
PLAY-YOURSELF BRIDGE GAME
TRYING TO CHECK MY EMAIL. LIKE JACK KEROUAC.
SLOW SATELLITE INTERNET
GARY AND JACK HAD SPENT A NIGHT ON THE MOUN-TAIN, BUT OUR PLAN WAS TO GET UP AND DOWN IN THE TWELVE HOURS OF AVAILABLE DAYLIGHT.
IT WAS LATE SEPTEMBER, A COUPLE WEEKS EARLIER THAN THE DHARMA BUMS' HIKE. HOL WAS WORRIED THAT I WAS SO HELL-BENT ON SUMMITING, I'D DO SOMETHING RASH.
I FEEL A DISTINCT SENSE OF DREAD.
I'D FOUND A DETAILED GUIDE TO THE CLIMB ONLINE, COMPLETE WITH GPS WAYPOINTS, BY A WOMAN WHO'D DONE IT A FEW YEARS EARLIER. SHE NOTED DRILY THAT BECAUSE OF KEROUAC...
OUR GOAL
...THE MOUNTAIN "DRAWS PEOPLE WHO HAVE NO BUSINESS ATTEMPT-ING A CLASS 3 SIERRA SUMMIT."

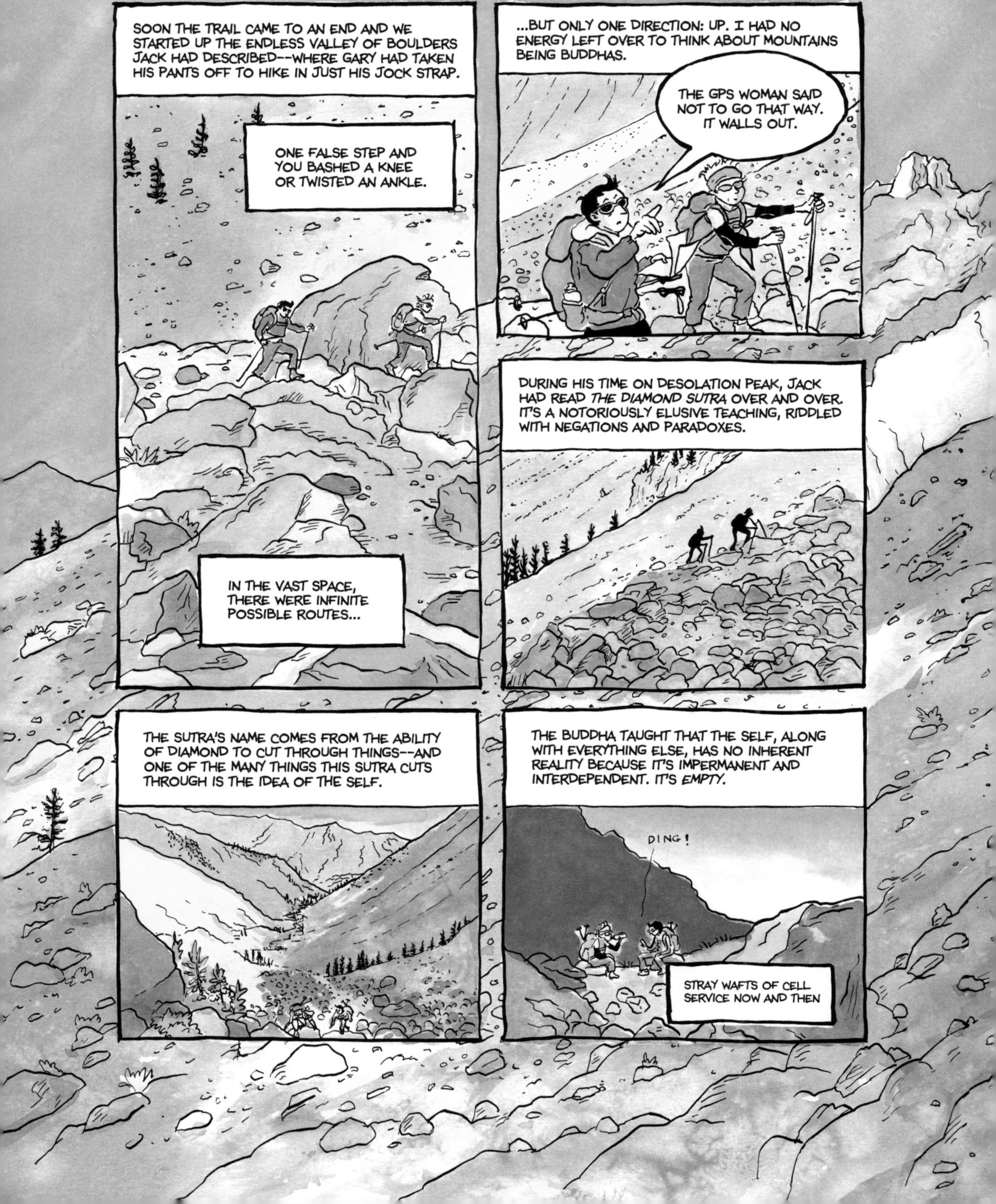

SOON THE TRAIL CAME TO AN END AND WE STARTED UP THE ENDLESS VALLEY OF BOULDERS JACK HAD DESCRIBED--WHERE GARY HAD TAKEN HIS PANTS OFF TO HIKE IN JUST HIS JOCK STRAP.
ONE FALSE STEP AND YOU BASHED A KNEE OR TWISTED AN ANKLE.
IN THE VAST SPACE, THERE WERE INFINITE POSSIBLE ROUTES...
...BUT ONLY ONE DIRECTION: UP. I HAD NO ENERGY LEFT OVER TO THINK ABOUT MOUNTAINS BEING BUDDHAS.
THE GPS WOMAN SAID NOT TO GO THAT WAY. IT WALLS OUT.
DURING HIS TIME ON DESOLATION PEAK, JACK HAD READ *THE DIAMOND SUTRA* OVER AND OVER. IT'S A NOTORIOUSLY ELUSIVE TEACHING, RIDDLED WITH NEGATIONS AND PARADOXES.
THE SUTRA'S NAME COMES FROM THE ABILITY OF DIAMOND TO CUT THROUGH THINGS--AND ONE OF THE MANY THINGS THIS SUTRA CUTS THROUGH IS THE IDEA OF THE SELF.
THE BUDDHA TAUGHT THAT THE SELF, ALONG WITH EVERYTHING ELSE, HAS NO INHERENT REALITY BECAUSE IT'S IMPERMANENT AND INTERDEPENDENT. IT'S *EMPTY*.
DING!
STRAY WAFTS OF CELL SERVICE NOW AND THEN

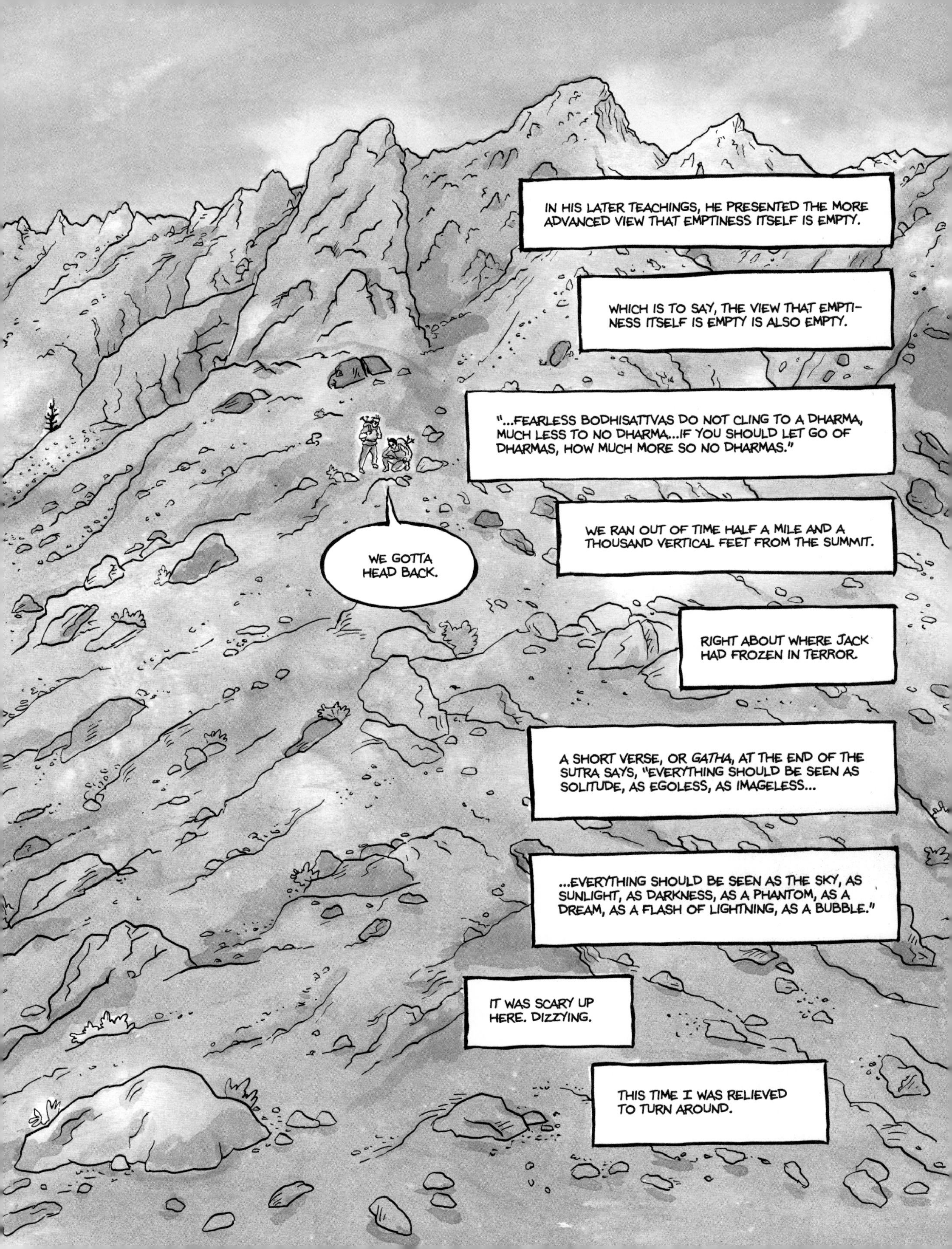
IN HIS LATER TEACHINGS, HE PRESENTED THE MORE ADVANCED VIEW THAT EMPTINESS ITSELF IS EMPTY.
WHICH IS TO SAY, THE VIEW THAT EMPTINESS ITSELF IS EMPTY IS ALSO EMPTY.
"...FEARLESS BODHISATTVAS DO NOT CLING TO A DHARMA, MUCH LESS TO NO DHARMA...IF YOU SHOULD LET GO OF DHARMAS, HOW MUCH MORE SO NO DHARMAS."
WE RAN OUT OF TIME HALF A MILE AND A THOUSAND VERTICAL FEET FROM THE SUMMIT.
WE GOTTA HEAD BACK.
RIGHT ABOUT WHERE JACK HAD FROZEN IN TERROR.
A SHORT VERSE, OR *GATHA*, AT THE END OF THE SUTRA SAYS, "EVERYTHING SHOULD BE SEEN AS SOLITUDE, AS EGOLESS, AS IMAGELESS...
...EVERYTHING SHOULD BE SEEN AS THE SKY, AS SUNLIGHT, AS DARKNESS, AS A PHANTOM, AS A DREAM, AS A FLASH OF LIGHTNING, AS A BUBBLE."
IT WAS SCARY UP HERE. DIZZYING.
THIS TIME I WAS RELIEVED TO TURN AROUND.

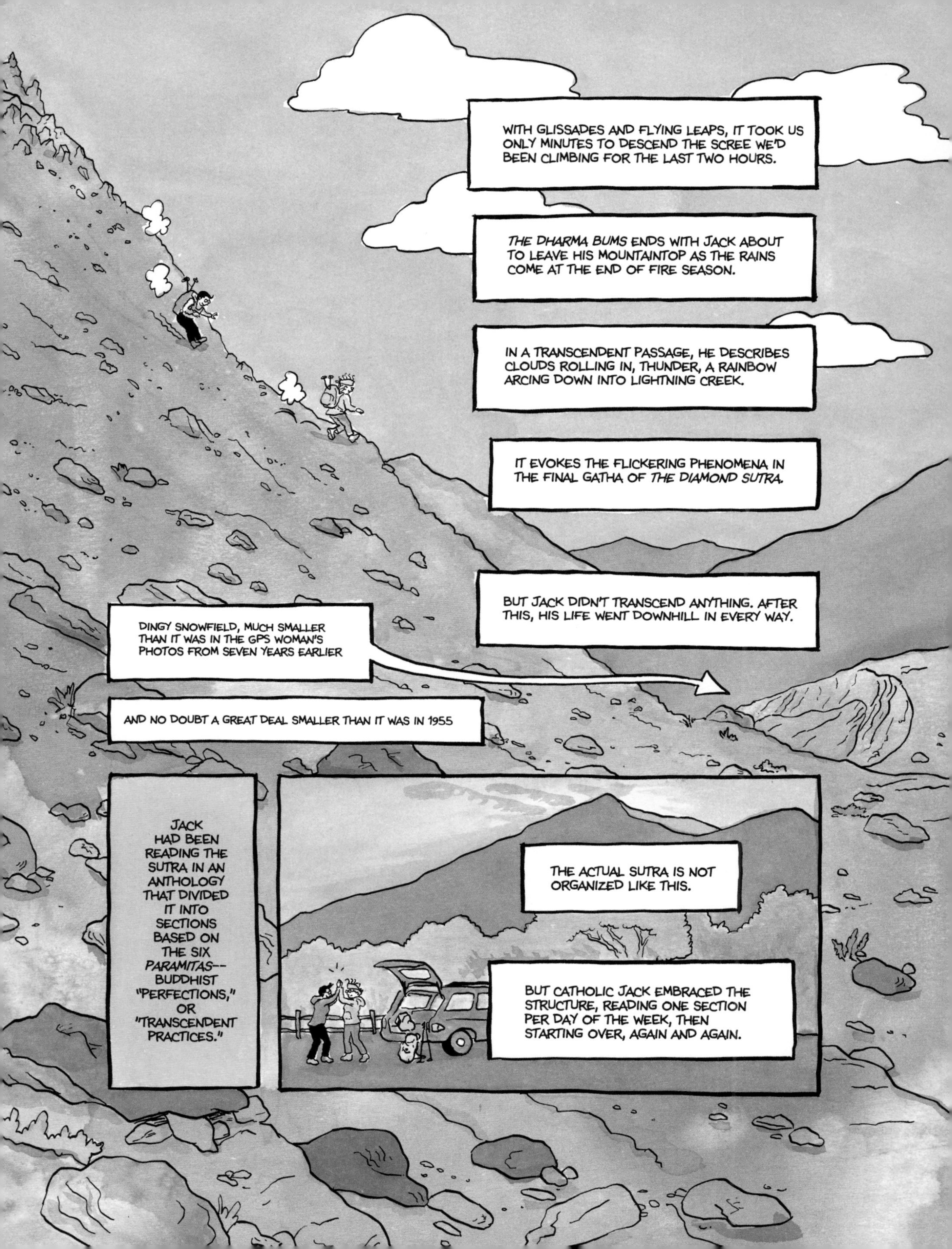
WITH GLISSADES AND FLYING LEAPS, IT TOOK US ONLY MINUTES TO DESCEND THE SCREE WE'D BEEN CLIMBING FOR THE LAST TWO HOURS.
THE DHARMA BUMS ENDS WITH JACK ABOUT TO LEAVE HIS MOUNTAINTOP AS THE RAINS COME AT THE END OF FIRE SEASON.
IN A TRANSCENDENT PASSAGE, HE DESCRIBES CLOUDS ROLLING IN, THUNDER, A RAINBOW ARCING DOWN INTO LIGHTNING CREEK.
IT EVOKES THE FLICKERING PHENOMENA IN THE FINAL GATHA OF *THE DIAMOND SUTRA.*
BUT JACK DIDN'T TRANSCEND ANYTHING. AFTER THIS, HIS LIFE WENT DOWNHILL IN EVERY WAY.
DINGY SNOWFIELD, MUCH SMALLER THAN IT WAS IN THE GPS WOMAN'S PHOTOS FROM SEVEN YEARS EARLIER
AND NO DOUBT A GREAT DEAL SMALLER THAN IT WAS IN 1955
JACK HAD BEEN READING THE SUTRA IN AN ANTHOLOGY THAT DIVIDED IT INTO SECTIONS BASED ON THE SIX *PARAMITAS*-- BUDDHIST "PERFECTIONS," OR "TRANSCENDENT PRACTICES."
THE ACTUAL SUTRA IS NOT ORGANIZED LIKE THIS.
BUT CATHOLIC JACK EMBRACED THE STRUCTURE, READING ONE SECTION PER DAY OF THE WEEK, THEN STARTING OVER, AGAIN AND AGAIN.

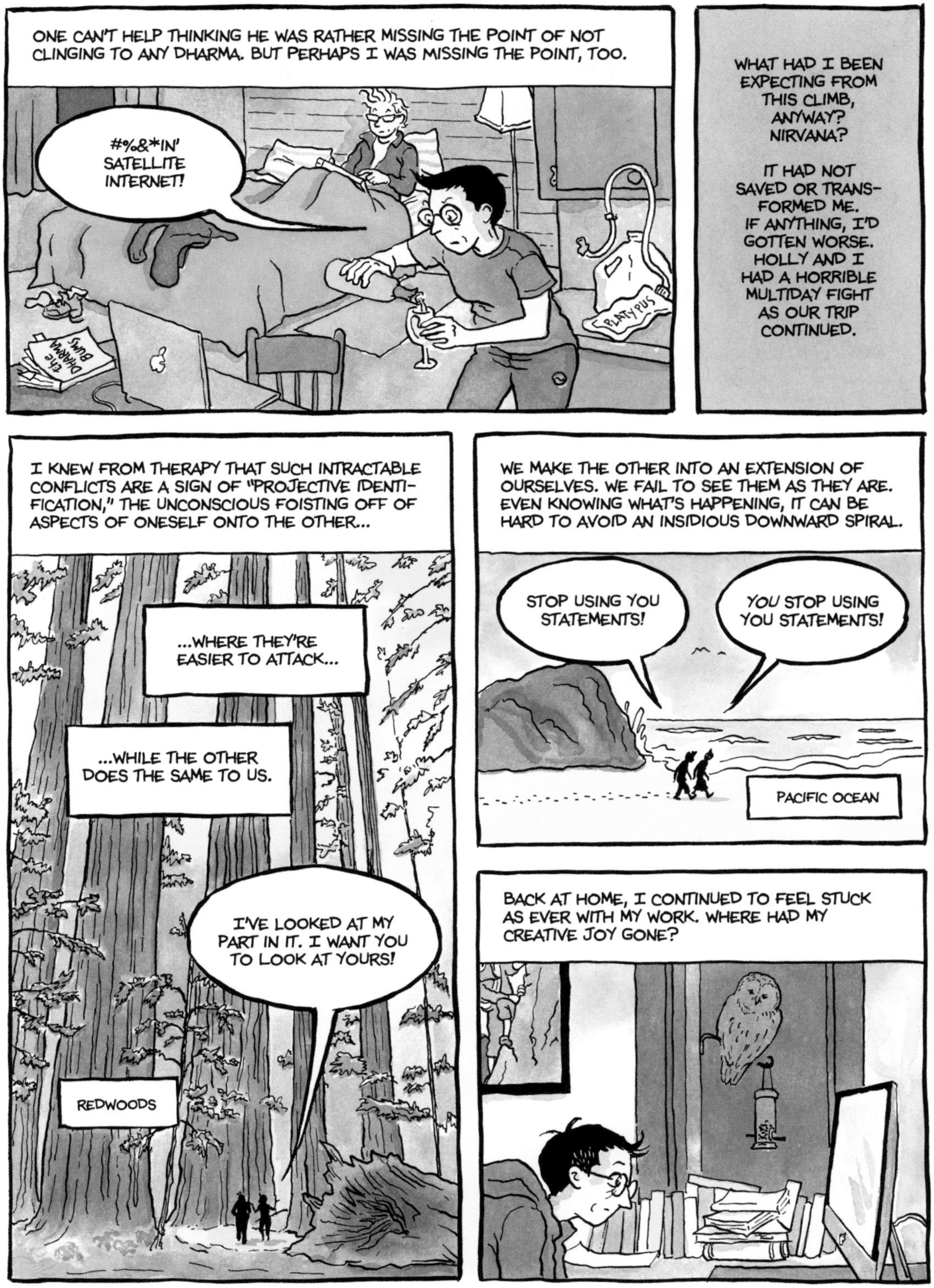

ONE CAN'T HELP THINKING HE WAS RATHER MISSING THE POINT OF NOT CLINGING TO ANY DHARMA. BUT PERHAPS I WAS MISSING THE POINT, TOO.
#%&*IN' SATELLITE INTERNET!
the DHARMA BUMS
PLATYPUS
WHAT HAD I BEEN EXPECTING FROM THIS CLIMB, ANYWAY? NIRVANA?
IT HAD NOT SAVED OR TRANSFORMED ME. IF ANYTHING, I'D GOTTEN WORSE. HOLLY AND I HAD A HORRIBLE MULTIDAY FIGHT AS OUR TRIP CONTINUED.
I KNEW FROM THERAPY THAT SUCH INTRACTABLE CONFLICTS ARE A SIGN OF "PROJECTIVE IDENTIFICATION," THE UNCONSCIOUS FOISTING OFF OF ASPECTS OF ONESELF ONTO THE OTHER...
...WHERE THEY'RE EASIER TO ATTACK...
...WHILE THE OTHER DOES THE SAME TO US.
I'VE LOOKED AT MY PART IN IT. I WANT YOU TO LOOK AT YOURS!
REDWOODS
WE MAKE THE OTHER INTO AN EXTENSION OF OURSELVES. WE FAIL TO SEE THEM AS THEY ARE. EVEN KNOWING WHAT'S HAPPENING, IT CAN BE HARD TO AVOID AN INSIDIOUS DOWNWARD SPIRAL.
STOP USING YOU STATEMENTS!
YOU STOP USING YOU STATEMENTS!
PACIFIC OCEAN
BACK AT HOME, I CONTINUED TO FEEL STUCK AS EVER WITH MY WORK. WHERE HAD MY CREATIVE JOY GONE?

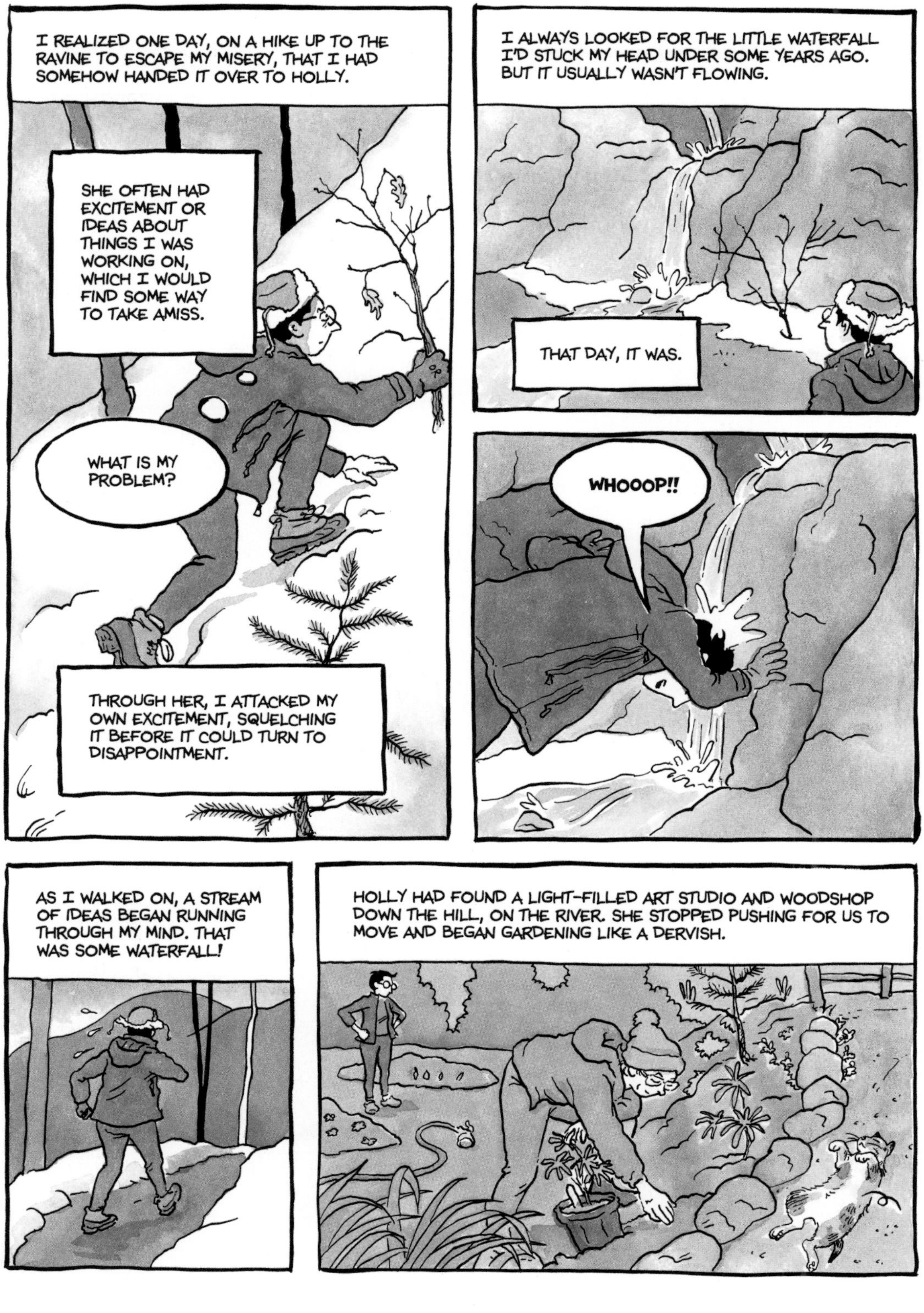
I REALIZED ONE DAY, ON A HIKE UP TO THE RAVINE TO ESCAPE MY MISERY, THAT I HAD SOMEHOW HANDED IT OVER TO HOLLY.
SHE OFTEN HAD EXCITEMENT OR IDEAS ABOUT THINGS I WAS WORKING ON, WHICH I WOULD FIND SOME WAY TO TAKE AMISS.
WHAT IS MY PROBLEM?
THROUGH HER, I ATTACKED MY OWN EXCITEMENT, SQUELCHING IT BEFORE IT COULD TURN TO DISAPPOINTMENT.
I ALWAYS LOOKED FOR THE LITTLE WATERFALL I'D STUCK MY HEAD UNDER SOME YEARS AGO. BUT IT USUALLY WASN'T FLOWING.
THAT DAY, IT WAS.
WHOOOP!!
AS I WALKED ON, A STREAM OF IDEAS BEGAN RUNNING THROUGH MY MIND. THAT WAS SOME WATERFALL!
HOLLY HAD FOUND A LIGHT-FILLED ART STUDIO AND WOODSHOP DOWN THE HILL, ON THE RIVER. SHE STOPPED PUSHING FOR US TO MOVE AND BEGAN GARDENING LIKE A DERVISH.

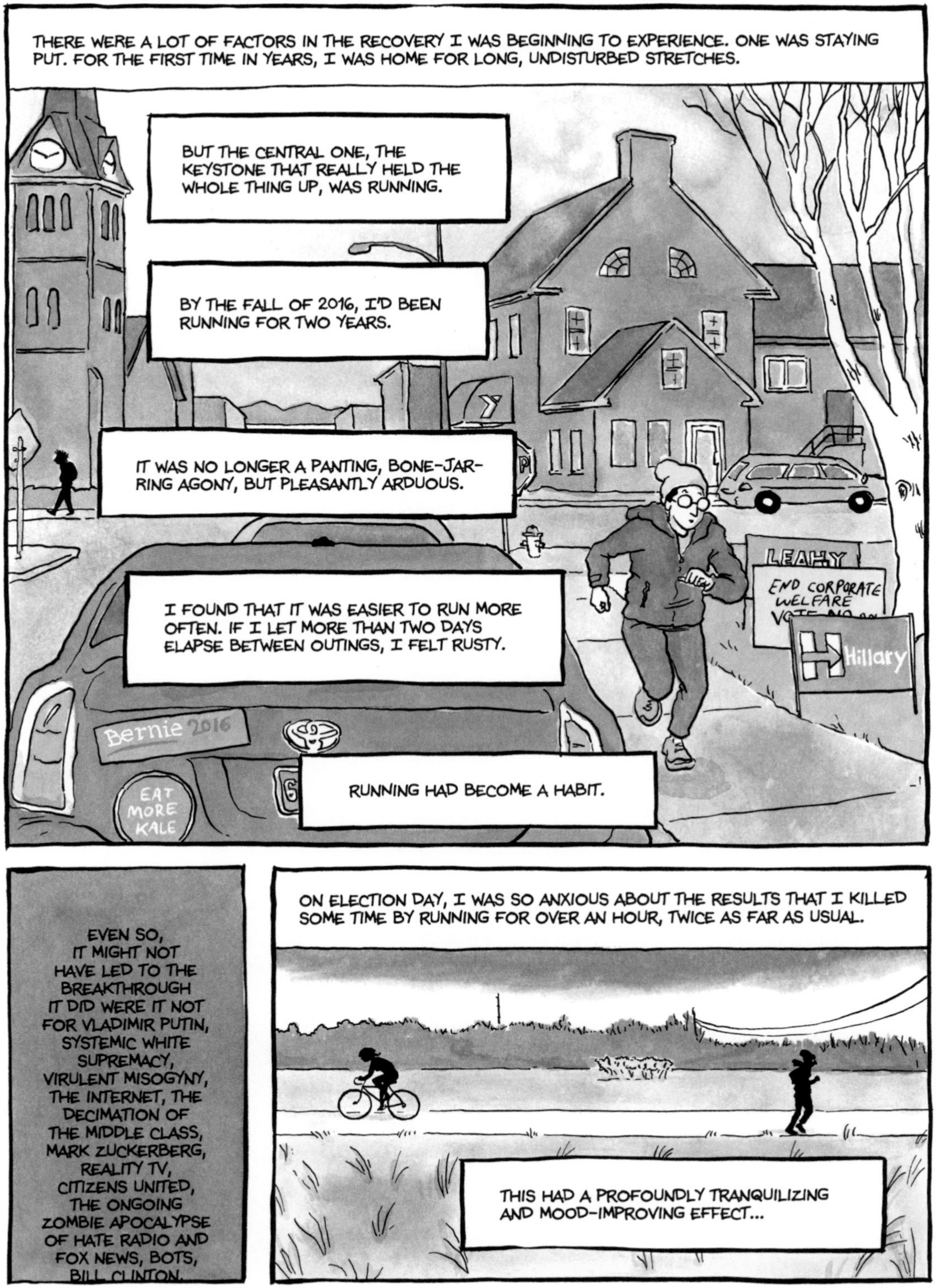
THERE WERE A LOT OF FACTORS IN THE RECOVERY I WAS BEGINNING TO EXPERIENCE. ONE WAS STAYING PUT. FOR THE FIRST TIME IN YEARS, I WAS HOME FOR LONG, UNDISTURBED STRETCHES.
BUT THE CENTRAL ONE, THE KEYSTONE THAT REALLY HELD THE WHOLE THING UP, WAS RUNNING.
BY THE FALL OF 2016, I'D BEEN RUNNING FOR TWO YEARS.
IT WAS NO LONGER A PANTING, BONE-JARRING AGONY, BUT PLEASANTLY ARDUOUS.
LEAHY
END CORPORATE WELFARE
Hillary
I FOUND THAT IT WAS EASIER TO RUN MORE OFTEN. IF I LET MORE THAN TWO DAYS ELAPSE BETWEEN OUTINGS, I FELT RUSTY.
Bernie 2016
EAT MORE KALE
RUNNING HAD BECOME A HABIT.
EVEN SO, IT MIGHT NOT HAVE LED TO THE BREAKTHROUGH IT DID WERE IT NOT FOR VLADIMIR PUTIN, SYSTEMIC WHITE SUPREMACY, VIRULENT MISOGYNY, THE INTERNET, THE DECIMATION OF THE MIDDLE CLASS, MARK ZUCKERBERG, REALITY TV, CITIZENS UNITED, THE ONGOING ZOMBIE APOCALYPSE OF HATE RADIO AND FOX NEWS, BOTS, BILL CLINTON.
ON ELECTION DAY, I WAS SO ANXIOUS ABOUT THE RESULTS THAT I KILLED SOME TIME BY RUNNING FOR OVER AN HOUR, TWICE AS FAR AS USUAL.
THIS HAD A PROFOUNDLY TRANQUILIZING AND MOOD-IMPROVING EFFECT...

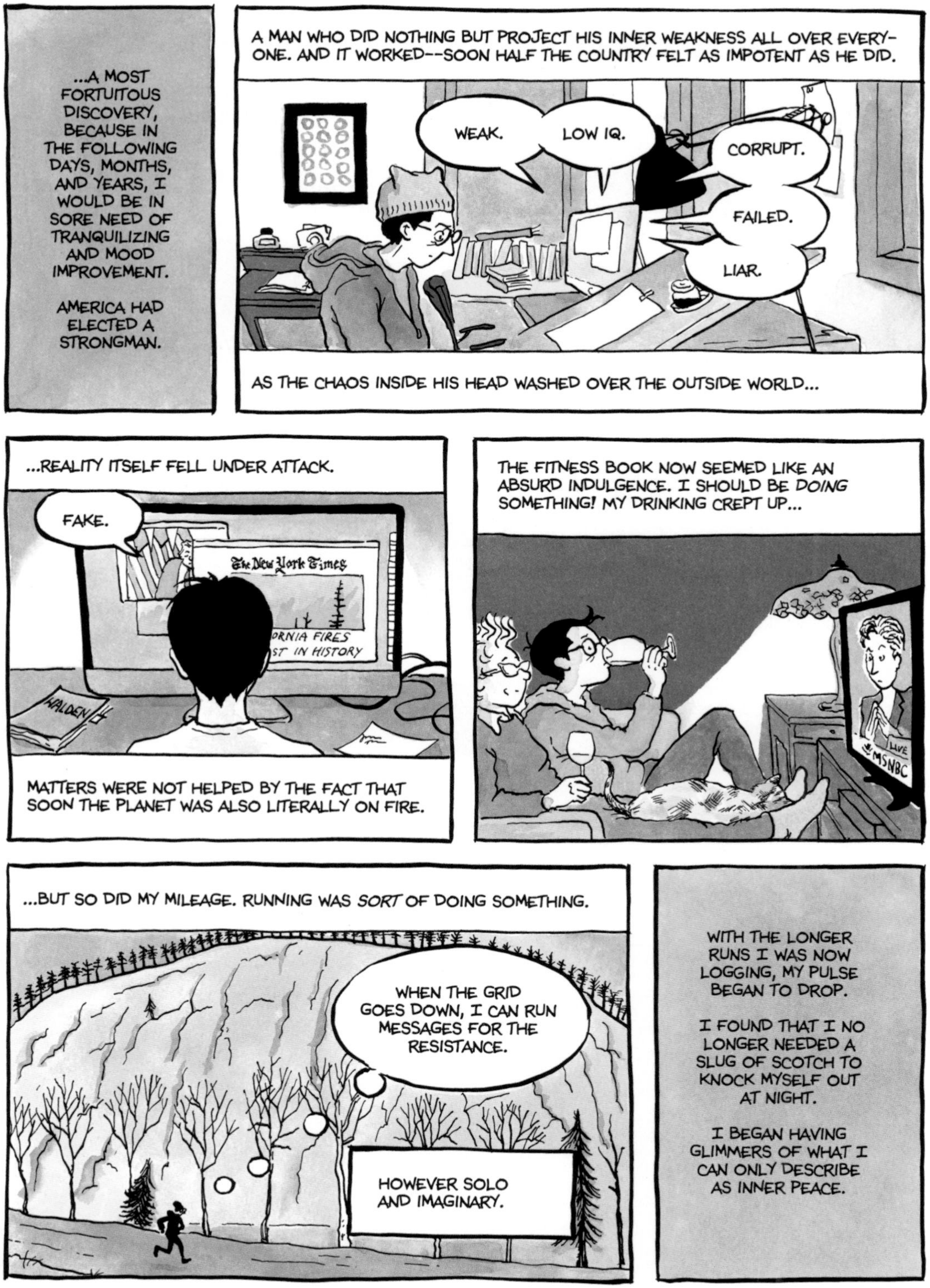
...A MOST FORTUITOUS DISCOVERY, BECAUSE IN THE FOLLOWING DAYS, MONTHS, AND YEARS, I WOULD BE IN SORE NEED OF TRANQUILIZING AND MOOD IMPROVEMENT.
AMERICA HAD ELECTED A STRONGMAN.
A MAN WHO DID NOTHING BUT PROJECT HIS INNER WEAKNESS ALL OVER EVERYONE. AND IT WORKED--SOON HALF THE COUNTRY FELT AS IMPOTENT AS HE DID.
WEAK.
LOW IQ.
CORRUPT.
FAILED.
LIAR.
AS THE CHAOS INSIDE HIS HEAD WASHED OVER THE OUTSIDE WORLD...
...REALITY ITSELF FELL UNDER ATTACK.
FAKE.
The New York Times
WALDEN
MATTERS WERE NOT HELPED BY THE FACT THAT SOON THE PLANET WAS ALSO LITERALLY ON FIRE.
THE FITNESS BOOK NOW SEEMED LIKE AN ABSURD INDULGENCE. I SHOULD BE *DOING* SOMETHING! MY DRINKING CREPT UP...
LIVE
MSNBC
...BUT SO DID MY MILEAGE. RUNNING WAS *SORT* OF DOING SOMETHING.
WHEN THE GRID GOES DOWN, I CAN RUN MESSAGES FOR THE RESISTANCE.
HOWEVER SOLO AND IMAGINARY.
WITH THE LONGER RUNS I WAS NOW LOGGING, MY PULSE BEGAN TO DROP.
I FOUND THAT I NO LONGER NEEDED A SLUG OF SCOTCH TO KNOCK MYSELF OUT AT NIGHT.
I BEGAN HAVING GLIMMERS OF WHAT I CAN ONLY DESCRIBE AS INNER PEACE.

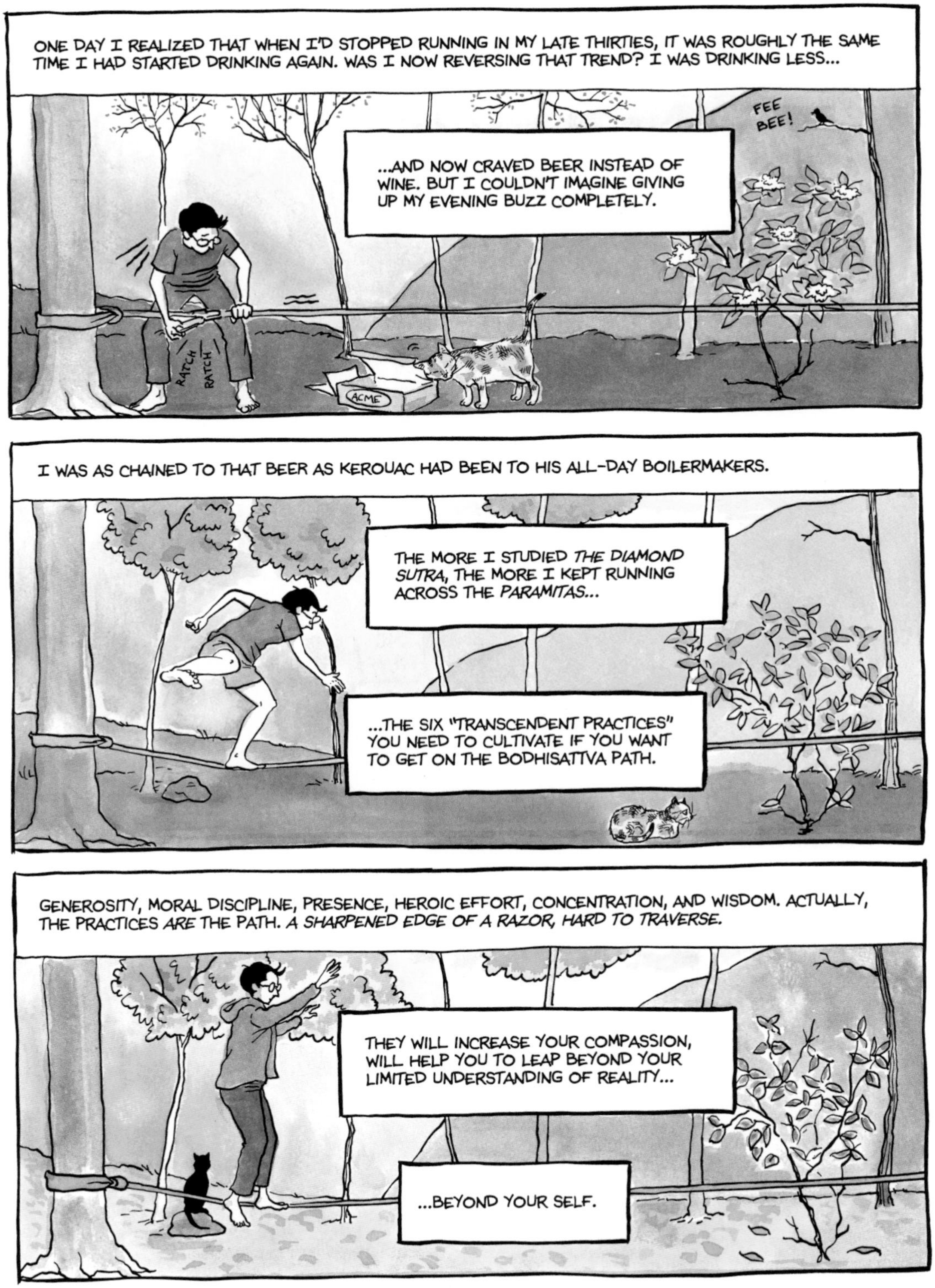
ONE DAY I REALIZED THAT WHEN I'D STOPPED RUNNING IN MY LATE THIRTIES, IT WAS ROUGHLY THE SAME TIME I HAD STARTED DRINKING AGAIN. WAS I NOW REVERSING THAT TREND? I WAS DRINKING LESS...
...AND NOW CRAVED BEER INSTEAD OF WINE. BUT I COULDN'T IMAGINE GIVING UP MY EVENING BUZZ COMPLETELY.
FEE BEE!
RATCH
RATCH
ACME
I WAS AS CHAINED TO THAT BEER AS KEROUAC HAD BEEN TO HIS ALL-DAY BOILERMAKERS.
THE MORE I STUDIED *THE DIAMOND SUTRA*, THE MORE I KEPT RUNNING ACROSS THE *PARAMITAS*...
...THE SIX "TRANSCENDENT PRACTICES" YOU NEED TO CULTIVATE IF YOU WANT TO GET ON THE BODHISATTVA PATH.
GENEROSITY, MORAL DISCIPLINE, PRESENCE, HEROIC EFFORT, CONCENTRATION, AND WISDOM. ACTUALLY, THE PRACTICES *ARE* THE PATH. *A SHARPENED EDGE OF A RAZOR, HARD TO TRAVERSE.*
THEY WILL INCREASE YOUR COMPASSION, WILL HELP YOU TO LEAP BEYOND YOUR LIMITED UNDERSTANDING OF REALITY...
...BEYOND YOUR SELF.

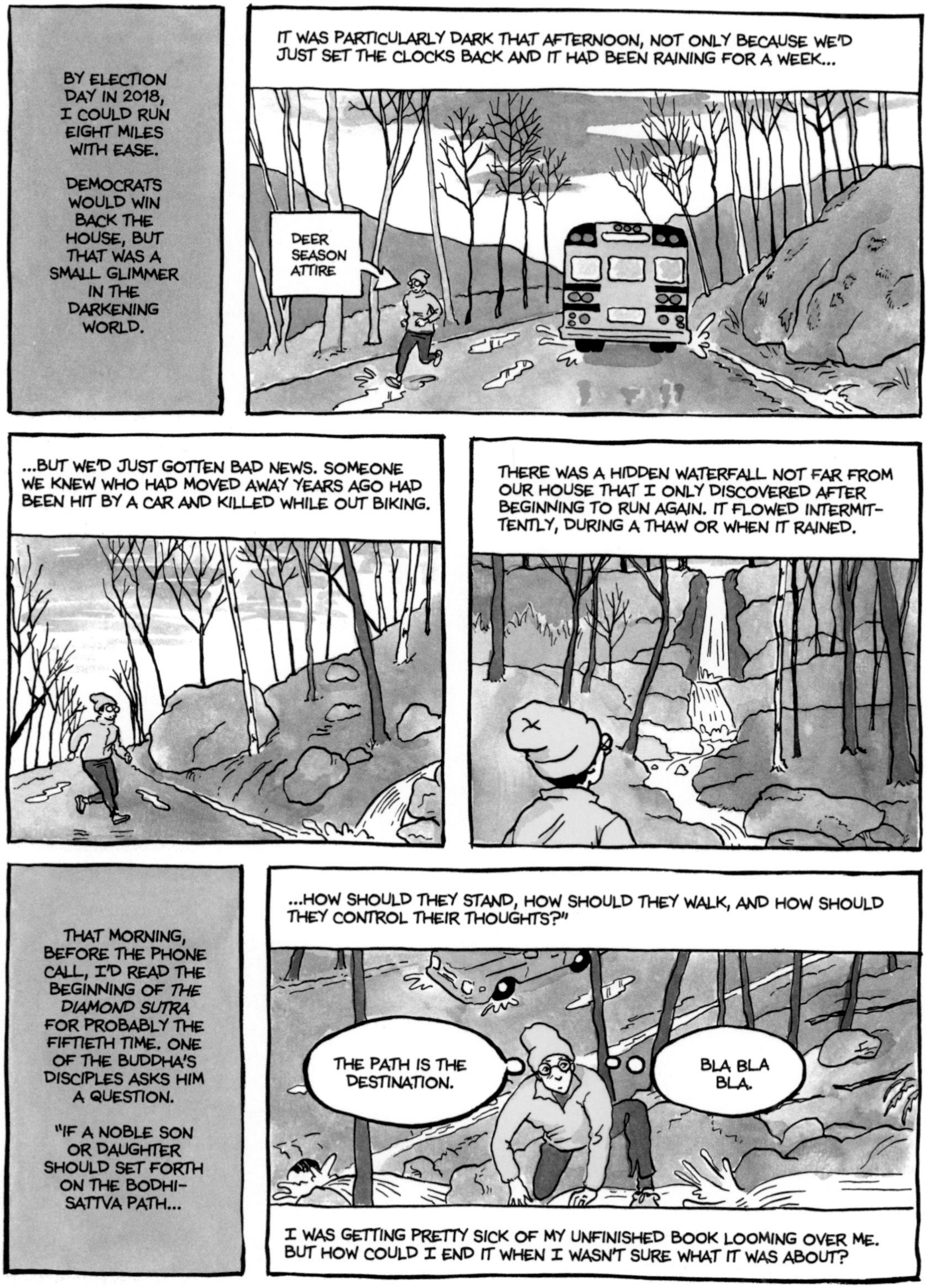
BY ELECTION DAY IN 2018, I COULD RUN EIGHT MILES WITH EASE.
DEMOCRATS WOULD WIN BACK THE HOUSE, BUT THAT WAS A SMALL GLIMMER IN THE DARKENING WORLD.
IT WAS PARTICULARLY DARK THAT AFTERNOON, NOT ONLY BECAUSE WE'D JUST SET THE CLOCKS BACK AND IT HAD BEEN RAINING FOR A WEEK...
DEER SEASON ATTIRE
...BUT WE'D JUST GOTTEN BAD NEWS. SOMEONE WE KNEW WHO HAD MOVED AWAY YEARS AGO HAD BEEN HIT BY A CAR AND KILLED WHILE OUT BIKING.
THERE WAS A HIDDEN WATERFALL NOT FAR FROM OUR HOUSE THAT I ONLY DISCOVERED AFTER BEGINNING TO RUN AGAIN. IT FLOWED INTERMIT-TENTLY, DURING A THAW OR WHEN IT RAINED.
THAT MORNING, BEFORE THE PHONE CALL, I'D READ THE BEGINNING OF *THE DIAMOND SUTRA* FOR PROBABLY THE FIFTIETH TIME. ONE OF THE BUDDHA'S DISCIPLES ASKS HIM A QUESTION.
"IF A NOBLE SON OR DAUGHTER SHOULD SET FORTH ON THE BODHI-SATTVA PATH...
...HOW SHOULD THEY STAND, HOW SHOULD THEY WALK, AND HOW SHOULD THEY CONTROL THEIR THOUGHTS?"
THE PATH IS THE DESTINATION.
BLA BLA BLA.
I WAS GETTING PRETTY SICK OF MY UNFINISHED BOOK LOOMING OVER ME. BUT HOW COULD I END IT WHEN I WASN'T SURE WHAT IT WAS ABOUT?

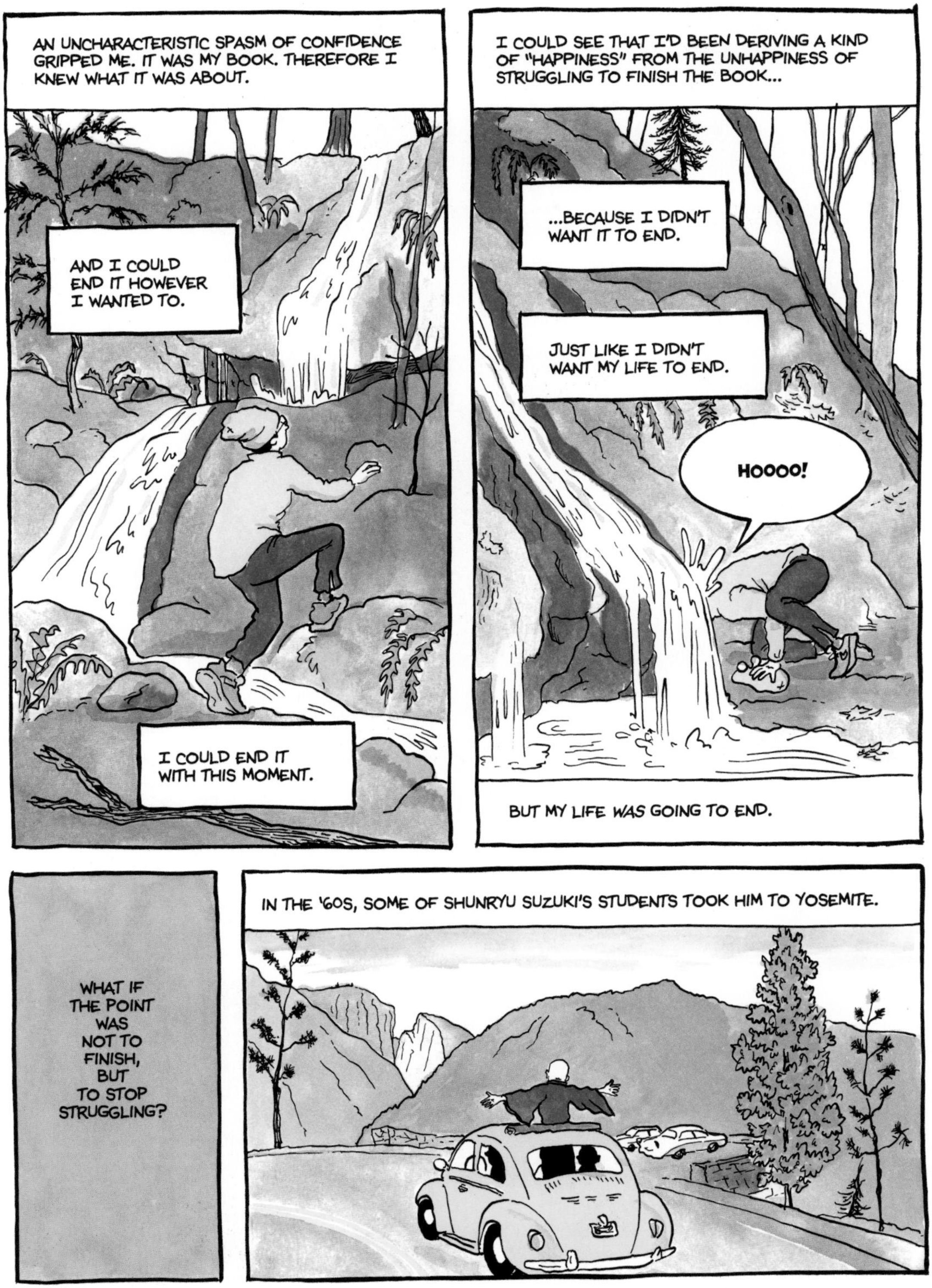

AN UNCHARACTERISTIC SPASM OF CONFIDENCE GRIPPED ME. IT WAS MY BOOK. THEREFORE I KNEW WHAT IT WAS ABOUT.
AND I COULD END IT HOWEVER I WANTED TO.
I COULD END IT WITH THIS MOMENT.
I COULD SEE THAT I'D BEEN DERIVING A KIND OF "HAPPINESS" FROM THE UNHAPPINESS OF STRUGGLING TO FINISH THE BOOK...
...BECAUSE I DIDN'T WANT IT TO END.
JUST LIKE I DIDN'T WANT MY LIFE TO END.
HOOOO!
BUT MY LIFE *WAS* GOING TO END.
WHAT IF THE POINT WAS NOT TO FINISH, BUT TO STOP STRUGGLING?
IN THE '60S, SOME OF SHUNRYU SUZUKI'S STUDENTS TOOK HIM TO YOSEMITE.

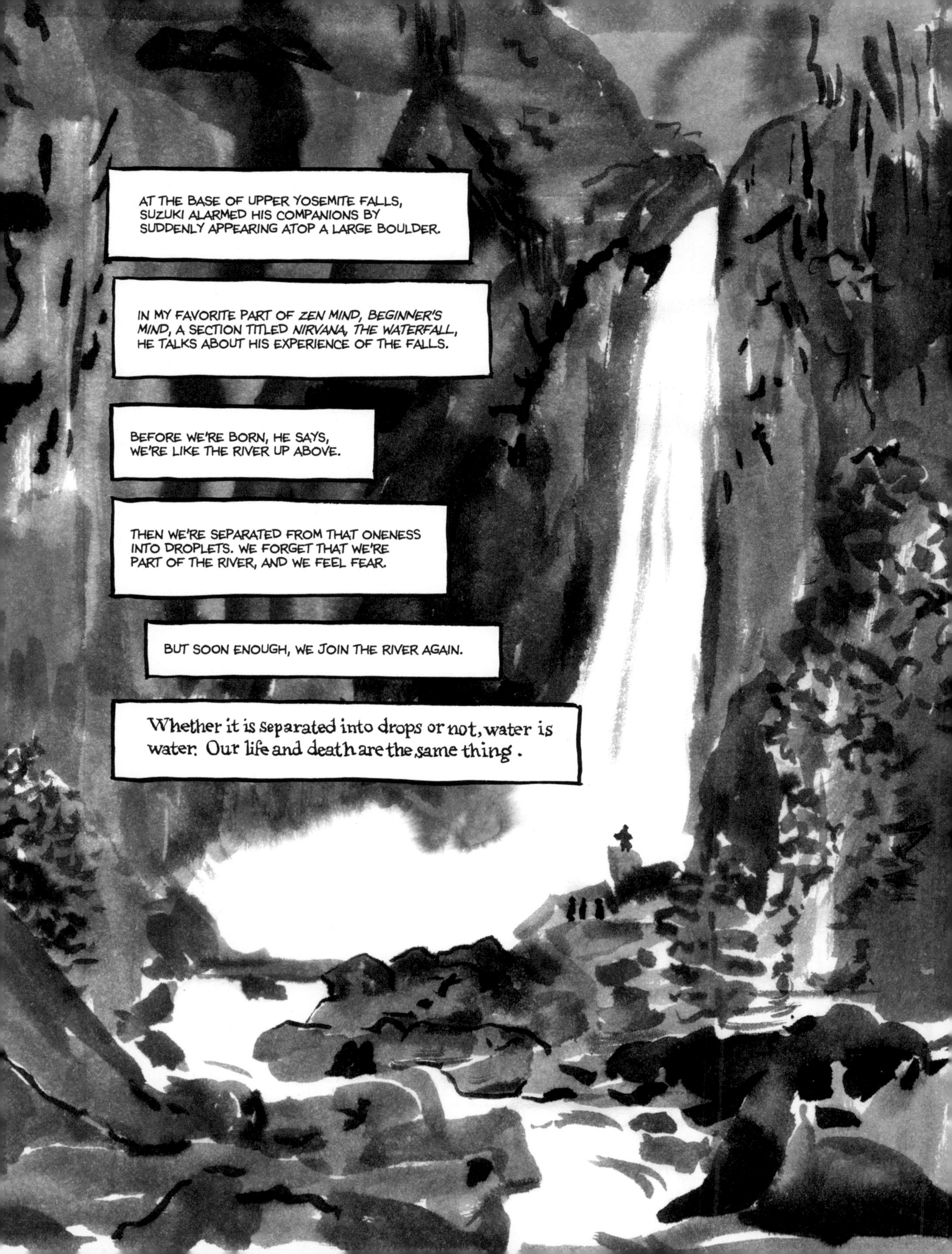
AT THE BASE OF UPPER YOSEMITE FALLS, SUZUKI ALARMED HIS COMPANIONS BY SUDDENLY APPEARING ATOP A LARGE BOULDER.
IN MY FAVORITE PART OF *ZEN MIND, BEGINNER'S MIND*, A SECTION TITLED *NIRVANA, THE WATERFALL*, HE TALKS ABOUT HIS EXPERIENCE OF THE FALLS.
BEFORE WE'RE BORN, HE SAYS, WE'RE LIKE THE RIVER UP ABOVE.
THEN WE'RE SEPARATED FROM THAT ONENESS INTO DROPLETS. WE FORGET THAT WE'RE PART OF THE RIVER, AND WE FEEL FEAR.
BUT SOON ENOUGH, WE JOIN THE RIVER AGAIN.
Whether it is separated into drops or not, water is water. Our life and death are the same thing.

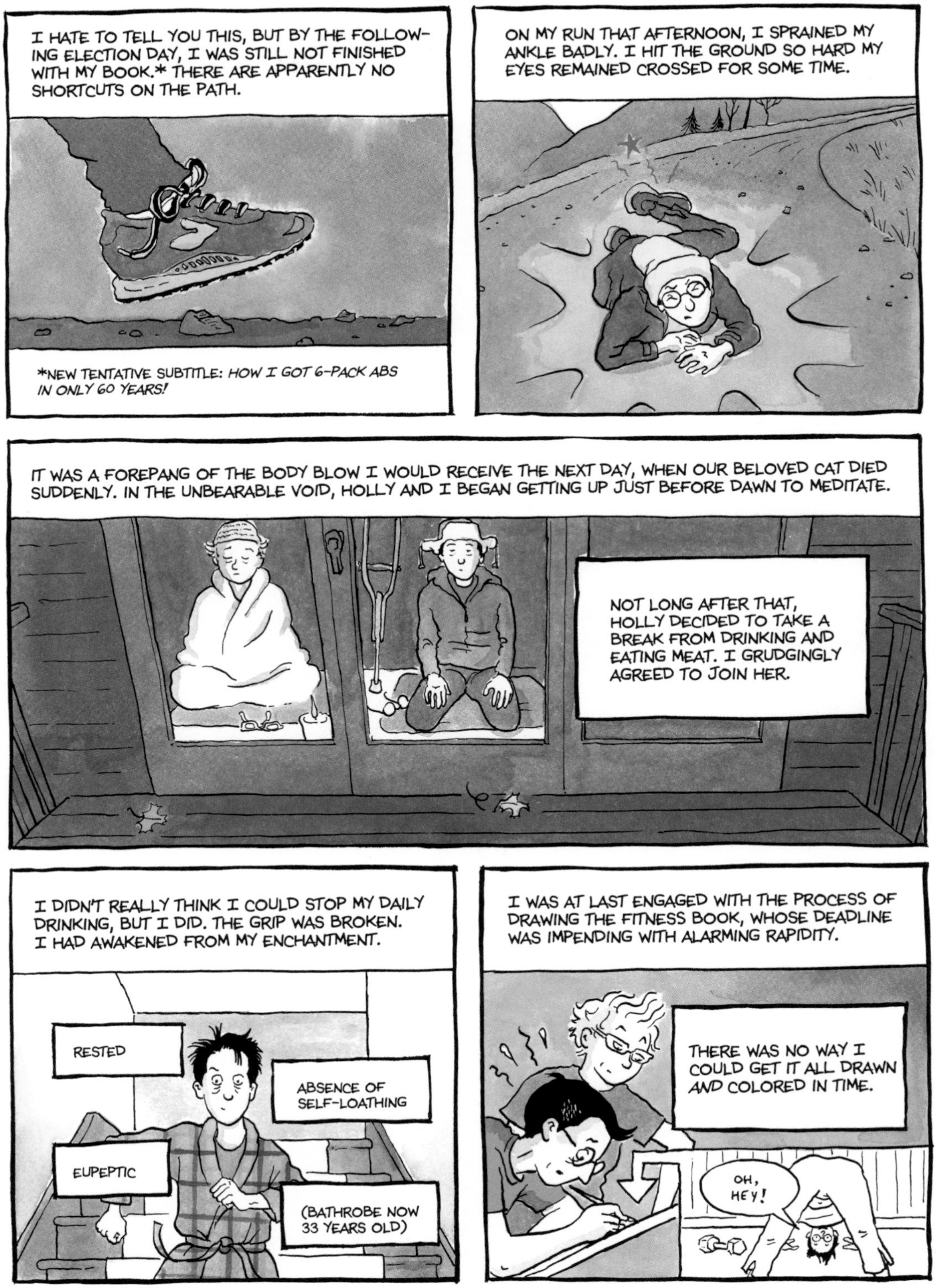
I HATE TO TELL YOU THIS, BUT BY THE FOLLOWING ELECTION DAY, I WAS STILL NOT FINISHED WITH MY BOOK.* THERE ARE APPARENTLY NO SHORTCUTS ON THE PATH.
*NEW TENTATIVE SUBTITLE: *HOW I GOT 6-PACK ABS IN ONLY 60 YEARS!*
ON MY RUN THAT AFTERNOON, I SPRAINED MY ANKLE BADLY. I HIT THE GROUND SO HARD MY EYES REMAINED CROSSED FOR SOME TIME.
IT WAS A FOREPANG OF THE BODY BLOW I WOULD RECEIVE THE NEXT DAY, WHEN OUR BELOVED CAT DIED SUDDENLY. IN THE UNBEARABLE VOID, HOLLY AND I BEGAN GETTING UP JUST BEFORE DAWN TO MEDITATE.
NOT LONG AFTER THAT, HOLLY DECIDED TO TAKE A BREAK FROM DRINKING AND EATING MEAT. I GRUDGINGLY AGREED TO JOIN HER.
I DIDN'T REALLY THINK I COULD STOP MY DAILY DRINKING, BUT I DID. THE GRIP WAS BROKEN. I HAD AWAKENED FROM MY ENCHANTMENT.
RESTED
ABSENCE OF SELF-LOATHING
EUPEPTIC
(BATHROBE NOW 33 YEARS OLD)
I WAS AT LAST ENGAGED WITH THE PROCESS OF DRAWING THE FITNESS BOOK, WHOSE DEADLINE WAS IMPENDING WITH ALARMING RAPIDITY.
THERE WAS NO WAY I COULD GET IT ALL DRAWN *AND* COLORED IN TIME.
OH, HEY!

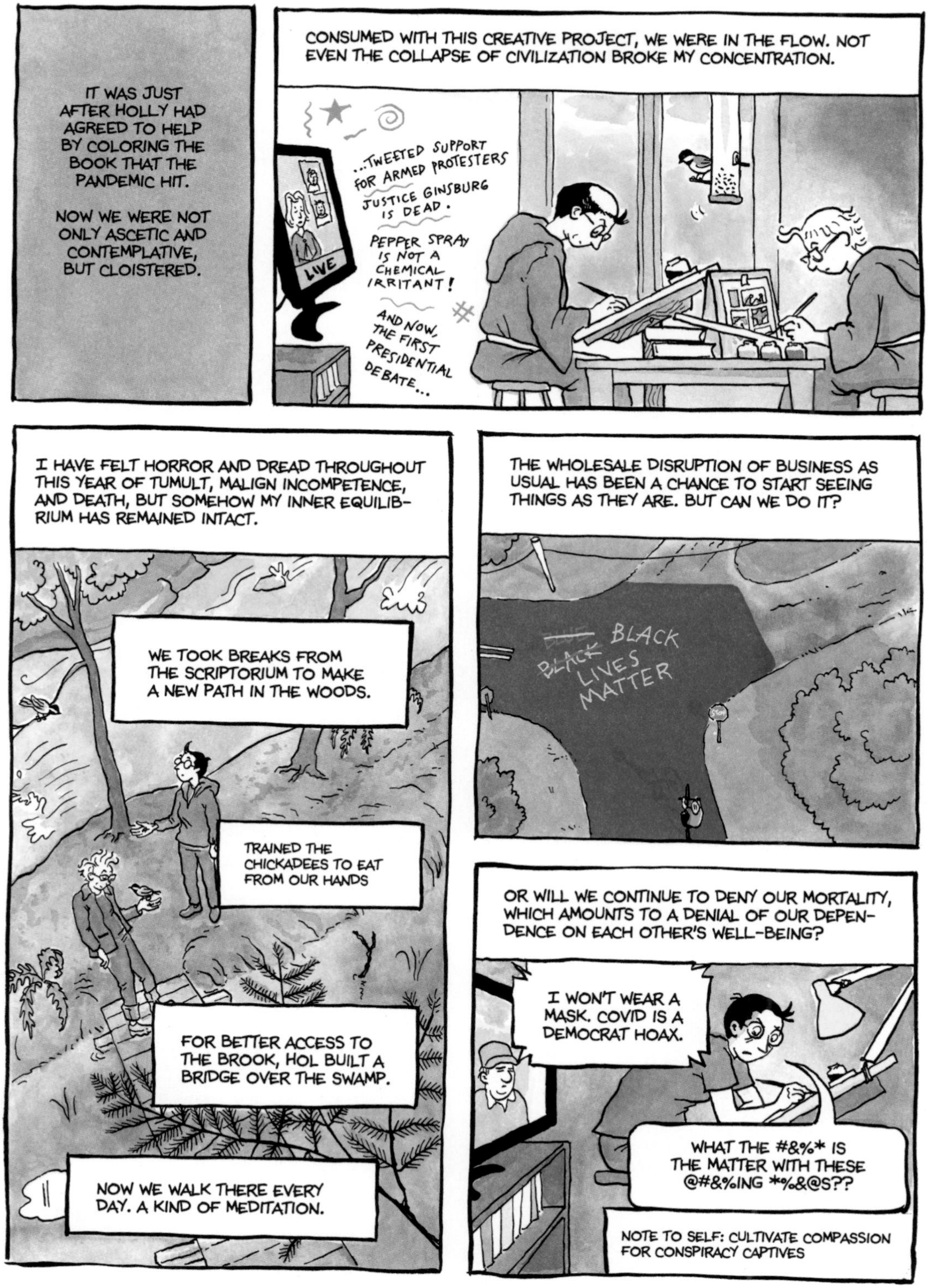

IT WAS JUST AFTER HOLLY HAD AGREED TO HELP BY COLORING THE BOOK THAT THE PANDEMIC HIT.
NOW WE WERE NOT ONLY ASCETIC AND CONTEMPLATIVE, BUT CLOISTERED.
CONSUMED WITH THIS CREATIVE PROJECT, WE WERE IN THE FLOW. NOT EVEN THE COLLAPSE OF CIVILIZATION BROKE MY CONCENTRATION.
LIVE
...TWEETED SUPPORT FOR ARMED PROTESTERS
JUSTICE GINSBURG IS DEAD.
PEPPER SPRAY IS NOT A CHEMICAL IRRITANT!
AND NOW, THE FIRST PRESIDENTIAL DEBATE...
I HAVE FELT HORROR AND DREAD THROUGHOUT THIS YEAR OF TUMULT, MALIGN INCOMPETENCE, AND DEATH, BUT SOMEHOW MY INNER EQUILIBRIUM HAS REMAINED INTACT.
WE TOOK BREAKS FROM THE SCRIPTORIUM TO MAKE A NEW PATH IN THE WOODS.
TRAINED THE CHICKADEES TO EAT FROM OUR HANDS
FOR BETTER ACCESS TO THE BROOK, HOL BUILT A BRIDGE OVER THE SWAMP.
NOW WE WALK THERE EVERY DAY. A KIND OF MEDITATION.
THE WHOLESALE DISRUPTION OF BUSINESS AS USUAL HAS BEEN A CHANCE TO START SEEING THINGS AS THEY ARE. BUT CAN WE DO IT?
BLACK
BLACK LIVES MATTER
OR WILL WE CONTINUE TO DENY OUR MORTALITY, WHICH AMOUNTS TO A DENIAL OF OUR DEPENDENCE ON EACH OTHER'S WELL-BEING?
I WON'T WEAR A MASK. COVID IS A DEMOCRAT HOAX.
WHAT THE #&%* IS THE MATTER WITH THESE @#&%ING *%&@S??
NOTE TO SELF: CULTIVATE COMPASSION FOR CONSPIRACY CAPTIVES

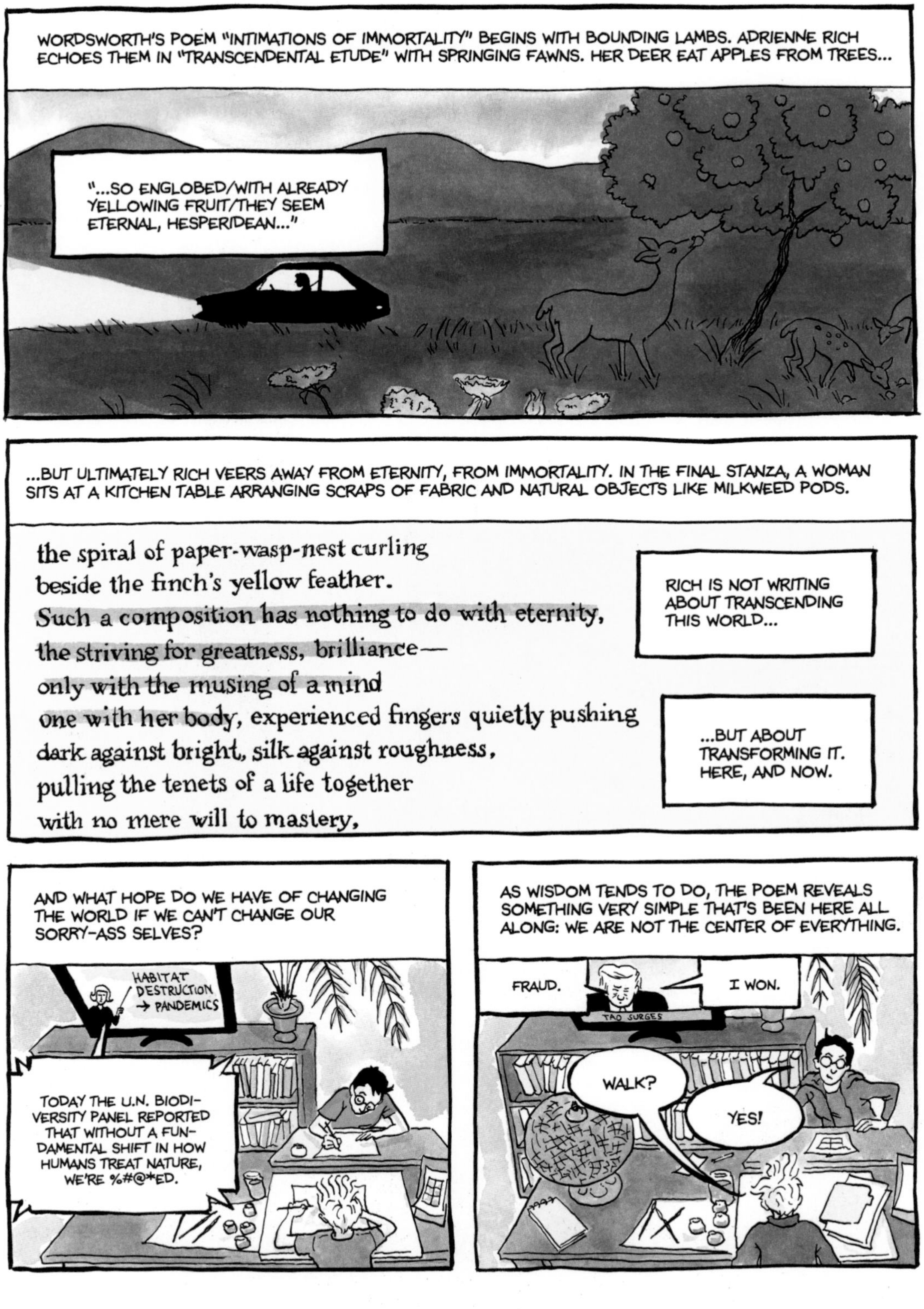
WORDSWORTH'S POEM "INTIMATIONS OF IMMORTALITY" BEGINS WITH BOUNDING LAMBS. ADRIENNE RICH ECHOES THEM IN "TRANSCENDENTAL ETUDE" WITH SPRINGING FAWNS. HER DEER EAT APPLES FROM TREES...
"...SO ENGLOBED/WITH ALREADY YELLOWING FRUIT/THEY SEEM ETERNAL, HESPERIDEAN..."
...BUT ULTIMATELY RICH VEERS AWAY FROM ETERNITY, FROM IMMORTALITY. IN THE FINAL STANZA, A WOMAN SITS AT A KITCHEN TABLE ARRANGING SCRAPS OF FABRIC AND NATURAL OBJECTS LIKE MILKWEED PODS.
the spiral of paper-wasp-nest curling
beside the finch's yellow feather.
Such a composition has nothing to do with eternity,
the striving for greatness, brilliance—
only with the musing of a mind
one with her body, experienced fingers quietly pushing
dark against bright, silk against roughness,
pulling the tenets of a life together
with no mere will to mastery,
RICH IS NOT WRITING ABOUT TRANSCENDING THIS WORLD...
...BUT ABOUT TRANSFORMING IT. HERE, AND NOW.
AND WHAT HOPE DO WE HAVE OF CHANGING THE WORLD IF WE CAN'T CHANGE OUR SORRY-ASS SELVES?
HABITAT DESTRUCTION → PANDEMICS
TODAY THE U.N. BIODIVERSITY PANEL REPORTED THAT WITHOUT A FUNDAMENTAL SHIFT IN HOW HUMANS TREAT NATURE, WE'RE %#@*ED.
AS WISDOM TENDS TO DO, THE POEM REVEALS SOMETHING VERY SIMPLE THAT'S BEEN HERE ALL ALONG: WE ARE NOT THE CENTER OF EVERYTHING.
FRAUD.
I WON.
TAO SURGES
WALK?
YES!

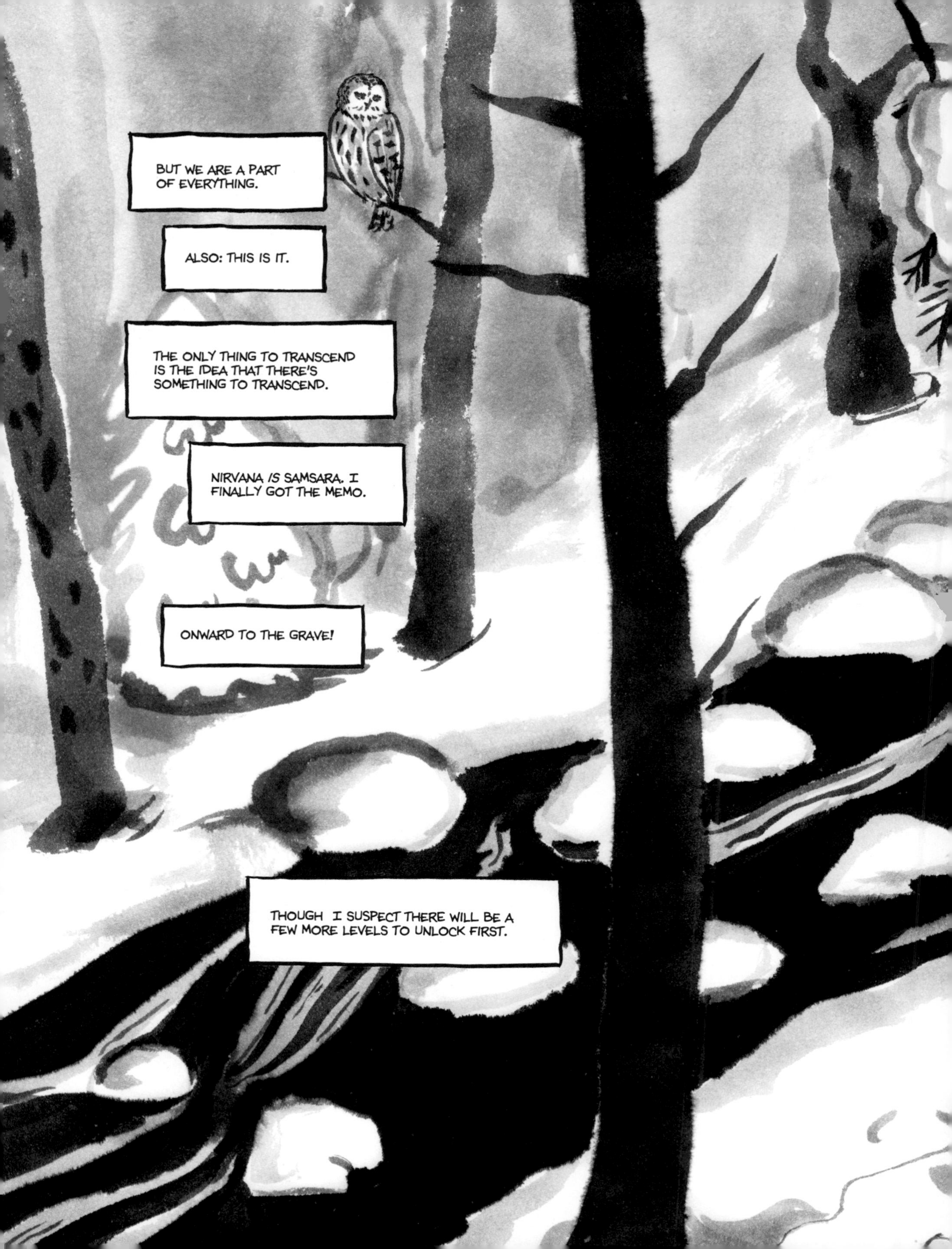
BUT WE ARE A PART OF EVERYTHING.
ALSO: THIS IS IT.
THE ONLY THING TO TRANSCEND IS THE IDEA THAT THERE'S SOMETHING TO TRANSCEND.
NIRVANA *IS* SAMSARA. I FINALLY GOT THE MEMO.
ONWARD TO THE GRAVE!
THOUGH I SUSPECT THERE WILL BE A FEW MORE LEVELS TO UNLOCK FIRST.

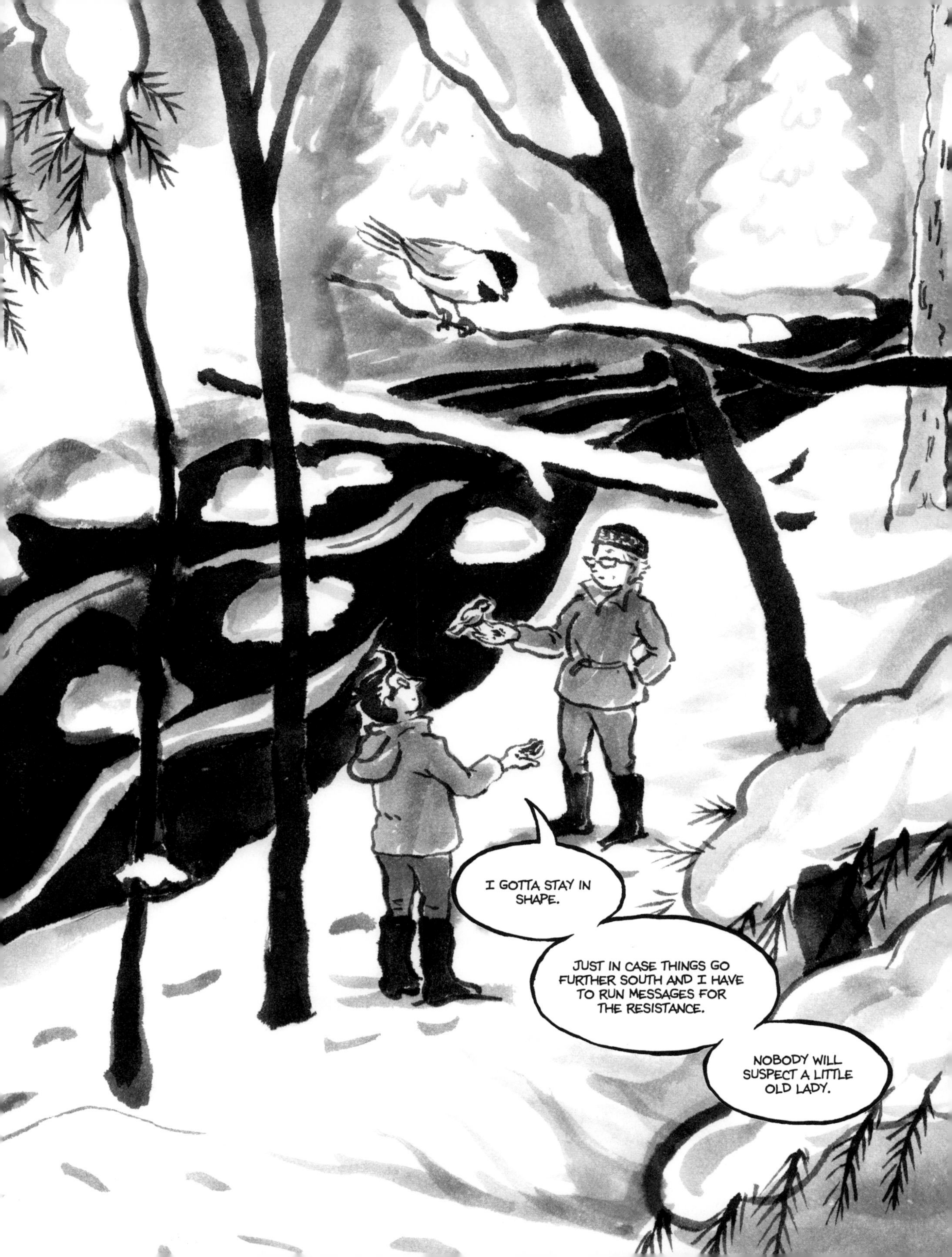
I GOTTA STAY IN SHAPE.
JUST IN CASE THINGS GO FURTHER SOUTH AND I HAVE TO RUN MESSAGES FOR THE RESISTANCE.
NOBODY WILL SUSPECT A LITTLE OLD LADY.

ACKNOWLEDGMENTS

I'M GRATEFUL TO VAL ROHY FOR READING THIS BOOK AS IT EVOLVED, AND FOR HER RESEARCH ASSISTANCE--WITHOUT HER I WOULD NEVER HAVE DISCOVERED THE EDIFYING BOOK *TRANSATLANTIC TRANSCENDENTALISM: COLERIDGE, EMERSON, AND NATURE* BY SAMANTHA C. HARVEY. VAL WAS A GREAT HELP WITH COSTUME DESIGN, TOO, ALONG WITH HER COLLEAGUE ANNAMARIA FORMICHELLA.

THANK YOU TO JANE SHARP FOR TURNING ME ON TO DOROTHY WORDSWORTH'S JOURNALS, NOT TO MENTION THE LAKE DISTRICT ITSELF. I'M ALSO GRATEFUL TO DIANE GAYER FOR PRESSING ON ME HER COPY OF *POETS ON THE PEAKS* BY JOHN SUITER.

MEGAN MARSHALL'S REMARKABLE BIOGRAPHY, *MARGARET FULLER, A NEW AMERICAN LIFE*, SERVED AS A NAVIGATIONAL GUIDE FOR ME, A SORT OF ROPE BRIDGE OVER THE SWAMP OF ALL THE MATERIAL I TRIED TO FIT INTO THIS BOOK. I'M GRATEFUL TO MEGAN AS WELL FOR GIVING ME AN ACTUAL GUIDED TOUR OF CONCORD, MASSACHUSETTS.

MY GRATITUDE TO SOPHIE YANOW FOR HER STAGGERINGLY COMPETENT PRODUCTION ASSISTANCE IN PUTTING THIS BOOK TOGETHER IS REALLY BEYOND MY ABILITY TO EXPRESS IN WORDS. HER PRODIGIOUS CALM IN THE FACE OF MY VARIOUS PANICS WAS ALSO QUITE AWE-INSPIRING. JAMES STURM AND MICHELLE OLLIE OF THE CENTER FOR CARTOON STUDIES EACH VERY GENEROUSLY SHARED IDEAS AND ADVICE EARLY IN MY PROCESS ABOUT HOW TO COLOR THIS THING.

I WOULD BE HOPELESSLY LOST IN THE FOG WITHOUT MY SUPERHUMANLY PATIENT AND INSIGHTFUL EDITOR, DEANNE URMY. I'M DEEPLY GRATEFUL FOR HER STEADY COMPANIONSHIP ON MY CREATIVE TRAVAILS. AND I WOULD HAVE PLUNGED DOWN AN ABYSS LONG AGO WITHOUT SYDELLE KRAMER, MY AGENT AND METAPHORICAL LEAD CLIMBER.

I'M PROFOUNDLY GRATEFUL TO BETH BURLEIGH FULLER AND DAN JANECK FOR THEIR PEERLESS, NAY, BREATHTAKING COPYEDITING.

THANKS TO THE TEACHERS WHO HAVE DEMONSTRATED TO ME THE CONNECTION BETWEEN THE MIND AND THE BODY: SUSAN RIBNER, MY KARATE SENSEI IN THE MID '80S; WILLIAM PROTTENGEIER, MY YOGA INSTRUCTOR IN THE LATE '80S; AND MY SAGACIOUS, AS WELL AS VERY POSSIBLY ACTUALLY ENLIGHTENED ACUPUNCTURIST AND QI GONG INSTRUCTOR, ARTHUR MAKARIS.

THANKS TO THE MACARTHUR FOUNDATION, WHOSE SUPPORT MEANT I COULD ALLOW THIS BOOK TO TAKE AS LONG AS IT NEEDED TO. AND TO THE GUGGENHEIM FOUNDATION--MY PROJECT TURNED OUT RATHER DIFFERENTLY THAN THE ONE I DESCRIBED TO THEM. I'M GRATEFUL TO THE CIVITELLA RANIERI FOUNDATION FOR AN IMMENSELY RESTORATIVE RESIDENCY. I FELT GUILTY FOR ALL THE TIME I SPENT RUNNING AND BIKING IN THE UMBRIAN HILLS, BUT IN THE END I THINK I CAN COUNT IT AS WORK. THANK YOU ALSO TO HEDGEBROOK FOR A BRIEF STAY DURING WHICH I ACCOMPLISHED LITTLE MORE THAN STARING DAZEDLY AT MOUNT RAINIER IN THE DISTANCE. THAT TOO NOW STRIKES ME AS A CONSTRUCTIVE USE OF MY TIME.

THANKS TO SALLY FELLOWS, CATHY HUNTER, AND ALL THE TOWANDANS FOR THE BACKCOUNTRY ADVENTURING. YOU ARE MY INSPIRATION.

EVEN THOUGH I DEDICATED THE WHOLE BOOK TO HOLLY RAE TAYLOR, I MUST THANK HER EXPLICITLY FOR THE HUNDREDS OF HOURS SHE SPENT WORKING ON IT, AND FOR EVERYTHING ELSE SHE DID TO KEEP OUR LIVES AFLOAT WHILE I WAS COMPLETELY ABSORBED. BUT I'M PERHAPS MOST GRATEFUL TO HER FOR THE DRAWING EXERCISES SHE CLEVERLY DEVISED TO JUMP-START MY SLUGGISH CREATIVE ENERGIES. HOL, I LOVE COLLABORATING WITH YOU.

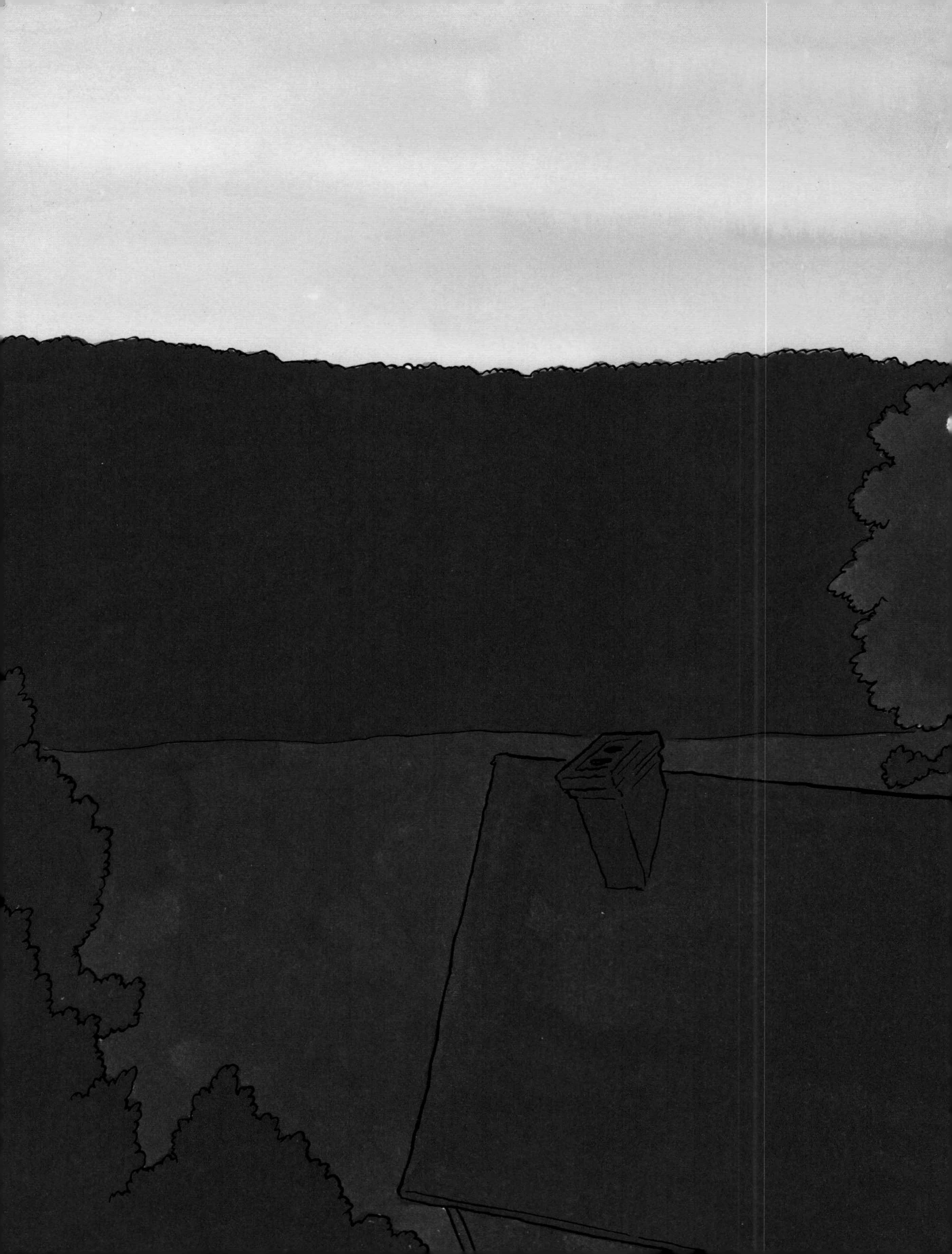